Acute and Critical Care in Adult Nursing

2nd Edition

Acute and Critical Care in Adult Nursing

Desiree Tait, Jane James,
Catherine Williams
and David Barton

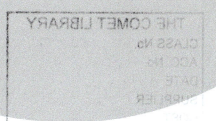
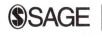 |

Los Angeles | London | New Delhi
Singapore | Washington DC

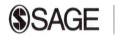

Learning Matters
An imprint of SAGE Publications Ltd
1 Oliver's Yard
55 City Road
London EC1Y 1SP

SAGE Publications Inc.
2455 Teller Road
Thousand Oaks, California 91320

SAGE Publications India Pvt Ltd
B 1/I 1 Mohan Cooperative Industrial Area
Mathura Road
New Delhi 110 044

SAGE Publications Asia-Pacific Pte Ltd
3 Church Street
#10-04 Samsung Hub
Singapore 049483

Editor: Alex Clabburn
Development editor: Richenda Milton-Daws
Production controller: Chris Marke
Project management: Swales and Willis Ltd,
Exeter, Devon
Marketing manager: Tamara Navaratnam
Cover design: Wendy Scott
Typeset by: C&M Digitals (P) Ltd, Chennai, India
Printed in Great Britain by
CPI Group (UK) Ltd, Croydon, CR0 4YY

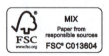

Library of Congress Control Number: 2015950476

British Library Cataloguing in Publication data

A catalogue record for this book is available from
the British Library

ISBN 978-1-4739-1230-4
ISBN 978-1-4739-1231-1 (pbk)

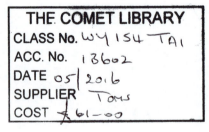

At SAGE we take sustainability seriously. Most of our products are printed in the UK using FSC papers and boards.
When we print overseas we ensure sustainable papers are used as measured by the PREPS grading system.
We undertake an annual audit to monitor our sustainability.

Contents

Contents

Transforming Nursing Practice is a series tailor-made for pre-registration student nurses. Each book in the series is:

○ Affordable
○ Mapped to the NMC Standards and Essential Skills Clusters
○ Full of active learning features
○ Focused on applying theory to practice

Each book addresses a core topic and they have been carefully developed to be simple to use, quick to read and written in clear language.

> "
> An invaluable series of books that explicitly relates to the NMC standards. Each book cover a different topic that students need to explore in order to develop into a qualified nurse... I would recommend this series to all Pre-Registration nursing students whatever their field or year of study
>
> **Linda Robson**
> **Senior Lecturer, Edge Hill University**
>
> The set of books is an excellent resource for students. The series is small, easily portable and valuable. I use the whole set on a regular basis.
>
> **Fiona Davies**
> **Senior Nurse Lecturer, University of Derby**
>
> I recommend the SAGE/Learning Matters series to all my students as they are relevant and concise. Please keep up the good work.
>
> **Thomas Beary**
> **Senior Lecturer in Mental Health Nursing, University of Hertfordshire** "

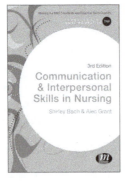

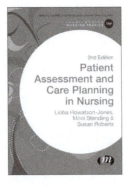

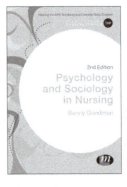

CORE KNOWLEDGE TITLES:

Becoming a Registered Nurse: Making the Transition to Practice
Communication and Interpersonal Skills in Nursing (3rd Ed)
Contexts of Contemporary Nursing (2nd Ed)
Getting into Nursing (2nd Ed)
Health Promotion and Public Health for Nursing Students (2nd Ed)
Introduction to Medicines Management in Nursing
Law and Professional Issues in Nursing (3rd Ed)
Leadership, Management and Team Working in Nursing (2nd Ed)
Learning Skills for Nursing Students
Medicines Management in Children's Nursing
Nursing and Collaborative Practice (2nd Ed)
Nursing and Mental Health Care
Nursing in Partnership with Patients and Carers
Passing Calculations Tests for Nursing Students (3rd Ed)
Palliative and End of Life Care in Nursing
Patient Assessment and Care Planning in Nursing (2nd Ed)
Patient and Carer Participation in Nursing
Patient Safety and Managing Risk in Nursing
Psychology and Sociology in Nursing (2nd Ed)
Successful Practice Learning for Nursing Students (2nd Ed)
Understanding Ethics in Nursing Practice
Using Health Policy in Nursing
What is Nursing? Exploring Theory and Practice (3rd Ed)

PERSONAL AND PROFESSIONAL LEARNING SKILLS TITLES:

Clinical Judgement and Decision Making for Nursing Students (2nd Ed)
Critical Thinking and Writing for Nursing Students (3rd Ed)
Evidence-based Practice in Nursing (2nd Ed)
Information Skills for Nursing Students
Reflective Practice in Nursing (3rd Ed)
Succeeding in Essays, Exams & OSCEs for Nursing Students
Succeeding in Literature Reviews and Research Project Plans for Nursing Students (2nd Ed)
Successful Professional Portfolios for Nursing Students (2nd Ed)
Understanding Research for Nursing Students (3rd Ed)

MENTAL HEALTH NURSING TITLES:

Assessment and Decision Making in Mental Health Nursing
Critical Thinking and Reflection for Mental Health Nursing Students
Engagement and Therapeutic Communication in Mental Health Nursing
Medicines Management in Mental Health Nursing
Mental Health Law in Nursing
Physical Healthcare and Promotion in Mental Health Nursing
Psychosocial Interventions in Mental Health Nursing

ADULT NURSING TITLES:

Acute and Critical Care in Adult Nursing
Caring for Older People in Nursing
Medicines Management in Adult Nursing
Nursing Adults with Long Term Conditions (2nd Ed)
Safeguarding Adults in Nursing Practice
Dementia Care in Nursing

You can find more information on each of these titles and our other learning resources at **www.sagepub.co.uk**. Many of these titles are also available in various e-book formats, please visit our website for more information.

About the authors

Desiree Tait PhD, DNSc, MSc Nursing, DNE, DN, RGN is Senior Lecturer in Adult Nursing at the Faculty of Health and Social Sciences, Bournemouth University. Desi has 35 years' experience in the practice, theory and education of adult acute and critical care nursing and facilitates critical care education at both undergraduate and postgraduate levels. She has a particular interest in the use of blended learning strategies in critical care undergraduate education and is involved in developing and evaluating innovative ways to facilitate student learning by adopting a practice-based approach to education. Her doctoral research looked at nurses' experience of recognising and managing clinical deterioration in patients in hospital, and this continues to be an area of clinical interest.

David Barton PhD, MPhil, BEd, RNT, DipN, RGN was Academic Lead in the Department of Nursing, College of Human and Health Sciences in Swansea University until his recent retirement. David's academic and scholarly interests have focused particularly on advanced clinical nursing, and he has worked to develop nursing networks in Wales and the UK. David was actively involved with the Modernising Careers agenda at a strategic level both in Wales and nationally. He has published widely in healthcare journals and textbooks.

Thomas C. Barton MSc Advanced Clinical Practice in Healthcare, DipN, RGN is an Advanced Nurse Practitioner working for Abertawe Bro Morgannwg University Health Board in Neath Port Talbot Hospital as part of the Advanced Practice Team clinically staffing the inpatient wards. Thomas qualified as an RGN at Swansea University in 2004 and spent his early career in intensive care and cardiothoracic intensive care units before pursuing his development as an Advanced Practitioner. He now works as a ward based clinician focused on the care of older frail people on a junior doctor replacement model. Thomas has specific interests in frailty, advanced life support, pain and is keenly involved in frailty and advanced life support education at local level and is a sessional lecturer/examiner for the Advanced Practice MSc at Swansea University.

David Blesovsky MN, RGN, PGCE(A), DPSN is a Senior Lecturer in Adult Nursing and Admission Tutor in the College of Human and Health Sciences in Swansea University, based in Bronglais Hospital in Aberystwyth. David qualified as an RGN in 1978 from Durham City and specialised in critical care at Newcastle General Hospital where he was Charge Nurse in the ICU and A&E dept. David moved to Aberystwyth in 1985 where he developed the ICU before moving into education. He continues to maintain his involvement with critical care by clinical practice in an ICU. David is involved with adult nursing at a pre- and post-registration level teaching care, critical care and management of people with diabetes. He has a strong interest in health informatics, leading the development of Information for Health from a nursing perspective, and his involvement in the subject – particularly in relation to critical care and enhancing advanced clinical care.

Jane James MSc Nursing, PGCE, RNT, RGN is a Senior Lecturer in Adult Nursing and Admissions Tutor in the College of Human and Health Sciences in Swansea University. Jane's nursing career began in 1980, working in critical care and medical nursing. Her main role is in teaching pre-registration nursing, supporting students throughout the adult programme. She has a particular involvement in clinical skills, with an emphasis on simulation and practical scenarios, and she is module leader for adult acute care nursing. She is also involved in post-registration teaching in critical care and discharge planning, and acts as admissions tutor for the pre-registration adult nursing programme.

Catherine Williams MSc Nursing, BSc (Hons) Nursing, PGCE, RNT, RN is the Undergraduate Programme Director BSc Nursing at the College of Human and Health Sciences and has over 14 years' experience in the practice, theory and education at postgraduate and undergraduate level. Catherine began her nursing career in 1996 and through the following years she has gained a vast array of knowledge and skills in critical care and in burns and reconstructive surgery. Academic and scholarly specialty includes non-medical prescribing, and nursing expertise in burn care, reconstructive surgery and critical care. She has also published in journals and textbooks.

Acknowledgements

The authors and publishers wish to thank the following for permission to reproduce copyright material.

The American College of Chest Physicians for Figure 7.1: The relationships between infection: SIRS, sepsis and severe sepsis, from R C Bone, R A Balk, F B Cerra, R P Dellinger, A M Fein, W A Knaus, R M Schein and W J Sibbald *Definitions for sepsis and organ failure and guidelines for the use of innovative therapies in sepsis.* The ACCP/SCCM Consensus Conference Committee.

Ron Daniels for Figure 7.2: Sepsis and severe sepsis screening, a multidisciplinary assessment, from Ron Daniels, *Surviving Sepsis Campaign* (2011).

The Intensive Care Society for Table 1.1: Defining levels of critical care, from ICS, *Levels of critical care for adult patients* (2009), Intensive Care Society, Churchill House, 35 Red Lion Square, London WC1R 4SG.

National Institute for Health and Clinical Excellence (NICE) for material in Table 1.2; from the NICE NGSO (NICE, 2007).

Foreword

Nurses working in any setting – acute, clinical or community – will need to be prepared to recognise and respond to episodes of acute illness and apply the principles of critical care nursing in emergencies. The authors of this text have a wealth of experience that they bring together to provide second- and third-year student nurses, and post-qualifying nurses who wish to keep current, the essential ingredients to be prepared for such episodes. Acute care is characterised by its rapid, severe onset and is often short-lived. Accurate assessment is vital and nurses need to be confident in their understanding of what is happening and what to do in these circumstances. This text provides expert instruction to undertake rapid clinical assessments and use effective decision-making skills in these situations.

As well as direction on assessment and accurate nursing responses, the authors (Desi Tait, David Barton, Tom Barton, David Blesovsky, Jane James and Catherine Williams) take you through the related pathophysiology of conditions and the all-important rationales underpinning the management of critically ill patients. All too often an acute episode will involve the family and friends of a patient, which is why this text also takes this dimension of care into account in the nursing care plans. The importance of collaborative working is also not overlooked, as an understanding of professional responsibilities, within effective multiprofessional teams, is crucial in these scenarios. Considering these wider features of acute and critical care deepens your knowledge and understanding, which in turn develops your confidence and competence.

The book contains a wealth of information on specific conditions such as respiratory support, chest pain, endocrine disorders, as well as dealing with shock and sepsis, confusion and delirium, and physical trauma. These are dealt with in specific chapters and are explained clearly, with scenarios to enable you to integrate the information in real-life situations. They are helpfully structured into chapters that you can dip into when you need specific information on managing a critically ill person. The final chapter gives you a five-point plan to maintain your knowledge and skills, ensuring you continue in your professional life as a highly competent and skilful nurse. In each chapter the relevant NMC Standards of Proficiency and NMC essential skills are stated, and are a feature of the Transforming Nursing Practice series.

This new edition is a welcome addition to the Transforming Nursing Practice series and I am sure will become essential reading for all nursing students.

Professor Shirley Bach
Series Editor

Introduction

Over the last ten years there has been a strong emphasis in healthcare on the importance of undertaking rapid assessment and management of acutely ill patients who show signs of clinical deterioration (National Patient Safety Agency (NPSA), 2007a). This has led to the development and use of guidelines and policies that promote a structured process for risk assessment, monitoring and fast tracking of clinical information to optimise patient outcome (NICE, 2007). This book aims to show you how you can influence patients' care for the better by learning how to undertake timely risk assessment and have a positive impact on patient outcome in all clinical settings where they are at risk.

People can become critically ill in any clinical or home setting, and prompt management of their condition can reduce the risk of patient morbidity and mortality. The Nursing and Midwifery Council (NMC) has highlighted the recognition of patients' clinical deterioration and the management of unstable and critically ill patients as key skills in the Standards for Pre-registration Nursing Education (NMC, 2010). The purpose of this book continues to be to provide you with the knowledge and professional guidance that you will need to assist you in developing the clinical skills and self-confidence required to care for patients who are unstable, deteriorating or critically ill, regardless of their location.

Each chapter focuses on the development of key clinical assessment and decision-making skills that will support your learning in your second and third years of undergraduate study in nursing and following qualification. In this second edition of the book, we have revisited the existing chapters and updated them according to the latest evidence as well as including chapters on the patient with acute kidney injury and the patient with endocrine disorders. The updated chapters include the use of many new patient scenarios to illustrate the clinical application of the knowledge and skills discussed. Each chapter is person-centred and includes the integration of applied pathophysiology to risk assessment, and management of care. Quick reference guides are used throughout to assist you with the clinical decision-making activities found in the chapters and, where appropriate, you will be asked to reflect on your experiences in practice. Feedback on the activities can be found at the end of each chapter. The core element of each chapter is to assist you in the development of skills in rapid assessment and response to clinical deterioration by using the 'Look: Listen: Feel: Measure/Monitor and Respond' approach in conjunction with ABCDE assessment and management (Resuscitation Council (UK), 2015).

In Chapter 1 you are given an overview of the knowledge and skills required to assess, recognise and respond to acute and critical illness. The chapter introduces you to the levels of dependency for acute and critically ill patients as well as providing quick guides for rapid assessment and response to changes in the patient's condition. The quick reference guides can be applied to all subsequent chapters giving you opportunities to rehearse the process, apply and refine your skills.

In Chapter 2 you are introduced to the breathless patient and are guided through how to undertake a respiratory assessment and the care of patients with type I and type II respiratory failure.

Patient conditions such as pneumonia, chronic obstructive pulmonary disease and asthma are discussed and applied to patient stories.

Chapter 3 builds on the content presented in Chapter 2 and explores the assessment and management of patients who need advanced respiratory support. The chapter focuses on key assessment skills including the interpretation of arterial blood gases and acid-base balance and the assessment and monitoring of patients who require non-invasive and invasive respiratory support.

In Chapter 4 you are introduced to the patient with chest pain and you will be guided through the process of chest pain assessment and management according to national guidelines. Key areas of assessment also include rhythm identification and the significance of ST elevation to the management of patients with cardiac pain.

Chapter 5 focuses on the patient in pain and explores the significance of pain in relation to the patient experience and the impact of pain on the development of critical illness. Pain assessment and management is considered in the context of holistic and collaborative care.

In Chapter 6 you will be guided through the process of assessing, recording and responding to patients in shock. There is also an opportunity for you to practise risk assessment and early recognition of patients in shock and steps to prevent the progression of shock.

Chapter 7 focuses on the risk assessment and management of patients at risk of developing sepsis and the management of patients with severe sepsis (including septic shock). You will be guided through how to use sepsis screening and care bundles in the context of patient scenarios.

In Chapter 8 you are introduced to patients with delirium. The chapter focuses on the risk assessment of patients who have the potential to develop delirium and how to plan ways in which to prevent and/or manage patients in a state of delirium. You have an opportunity to reflect on patients you have nursed and how you may influence practice development in the care of patients with delirium.

Chapter 9 is a new chapter which focuses on the risk assessment and prevention of acute kidney injury in patients in a variety of critical care settings. You will have an opportunity to recognise the difference between acute kidney injury and chronic kidney disease as well as the impact of acute kidney injury on patient morbidity and mortality.

In Chapter 10 you are introduced to the assessment and management of patients who have experienced physiological trauma. The chapter links well with Chapter 6 and includes the care of patients with soft tissue injuries including burns as well as patients with traumatic fractures.

Chapter 11 focuses on explaining the causes and management of the unconscious patient. The focus is on prioritising care and reducing the risks of side effects associated with loss of consciousness. Neurological assessment is discussed together with an evidence base for practice. Opportunities to practice neurological assessment and recognition of clinical deterioration in levels of consciousness are included.

Chapter 12 is new and introduces you to patients with endocrine disorders. The dominant feature of this chapter concerns the risk assessment and management of patients experiencing acute hyperglycaemia and hypoglycaemia. It takes you through the clinical decision-making skills required to maintain patient safety and reduce the risk of morbidity and mortality for people living with both type 1 and type 2 diabetes.

The book concludes by offering a summary of lessons learnt and an action plan for practice. You will be able to consider how you can develop either a career in acute and critical care and/or continue to utilise the lessons learnt in both hospital and community-based care.

Chapter 1
Assessing, recognising and responding to acute and critical illness

Desiree Tait

NMC Standards for Pre-registration Nursing Education

This chapter will address the following competencies:

Domain 3: Nursing practice and decision-making
Generic competencies:
3. All nurses must carry out comprehensive, systematic nursing assessments that take account of relevant physical, social, cultural, psychological, spiritual, genetic and environmental factors, in partnership with service users and others through interaction, observation and measurement.

Field-specific competencies:
7.1 Adult nurses must recognise the early signs of illness in people of all ages. They must make accurate assessments and start appropriate and timely management of those who are acutely ill, at risk of clinical deterioration, or require emergency care.

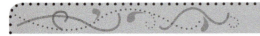

NMC Essential Skills Clusters

This chapter will address the following ESCs:

Cluster: Organisational aspects of care
9. People can trust the newly registered graduate nurse to treat them as partners and work with them to make a holistic and systematic assessment of their needs; to develop a personalised plan that is based on mutual understanding and respect for their individual situation promoting health and well-being, minimising risk of harm and promoting their safety at all times.

By entry to the register:
 xx. Acts autonomously and appropriately when faced with sudden deterioration in people's physical, or psychological condition or emergency situations, abnormal vital signs, collapse, cardiac arrest, self-harm, extremely challenging behaviour, attempted suicide.
 xxi. Measures, documents and interprets vital signs and acts autonomously and appropriately on findings.

Chapter aims

By the end of this chapter, you should be able to:

- identify the terms used to define levels of acute and critical care;
- describe how to undertake a rapid assessment of a changing clinical situation;
- describe how to collate accurate data from a variety of sources and analyse the results;
- demonstrate how to communicate the findings to staff at the appropriate level.

Introduction

Scenario: Susan's story

I am a second year student and this is my first day on the acute medical admissions unit. Up until now my only experience has been working in a nursing home and on a surgical day unit. I arrived just as a new patient was being admitted; her name was Sally Smith, and she was 67 years old. She was being admitted with a six day history of malaise, vomiting, falls and confusion. Her husband was with her and he seemed very anxious. He suggested we call his wife Sally because she seemed to respond better to that name. We transferred Sally onto the bed and I was asked to make sure she kept her oxygen mask on while she was assessed. We documented her vital signs on the observation chart for NEWS (National Early Warning Score) and the patient scored six. This was the first time that I had looked after someone with a score higher than three and I began to feel very anxious about the situation. What does six mean, what was going to happen, what was I going to do? I began to realise that risk assessing a sick patient was complex and involved much more than a numerical score. I looked at the patient as if for the first time. The medical team had been informed that the patient was now in the ward and a nurse from the critical care outreach team had arrived to assess her. The outreach nurse began asking Sally's husband questions about the last week and was able to obtain detailed information about the progression of Sally's illness and how she had come to be admitted. At the same time another set of clinical observations were being completed and fluid balance monitored. All the time the outreach nurse remained calm and continued to observe Sally very closely, while quietly reminding me to help Sally to keep the oxygen mask on. I felt completely out of my depth but was reassured by the calm efficiency of my mentor and the outreach nurse. I had a lot to learn!

Within five minutes we had obtained the following data.

__Situation:__ Sally Smith, age 67 years has been ill for six days, provisionally with a three-day history of decreasing appetite and vomiting, diagnosed by her GP as viral gastritis. By day five the patient was still unable to tolerate food but was able to take sips of water. She was also complaining of loin pain when trying to pass urine. According to her husband Sally had fallen twice when attempting to get to the bathroom and had periods when 'she didn't seem to make sense'. As a consequence Sally received a

(Continued)

continued . . . •

home visit from her GP on day five who diagnosed a urinary tract infection. He asked Sally's husband to send a urine sample from his wife to the pathology department in the local hospital and prescribed a broad spectrum antibiotic. Twenty-four hours later the patient was not improving and she was admitted as an emergency at the GP's request.

Background: *Past medical history of hypertension controlled by lisinopril 20 mg.*

Next of kin: *Husband, no children.*

Assessment on admission

Airway: *Patent.*

Breathing: *R 19/minute; oxygen saturation (SpO₂): 92% (oxygen 40% prescribed in the emergency unit to maintain SpO₂ at 96–98%).*

Circulation: *P 88/minute; sinus rhythm; BP 126/82 mmHg; T: 37.4°C; cool hands and feet; has not passed urine for approximately six hours. Infusion of 0.9% saline commenced in the emergency unit at 125 ml/hr. White cell count 10.4 10⁹/L.*

Disability: *Drowsy and disorientated; glucose: 6.5 mmol/L.*

Exposure: *Skin appears dry to touch and the patient's face looks drawn and hollow; weight 73 kg (11 st 7 lbs) prior to her illness; height 1.6 m (5 ft 4 in); she has a red area over her right hip.*

Recommendation from the outreach nurse

Continue with continuous oxygen therapy.

Assessment and monitoring of the patient's fluid and electrolyte balance and continue with IV hydration.

Continue with hourly monitoring of physiological parameters and risk assess for sepsis.

Check the result of the first sample and send a repeat urine sample.

Review antibiotics.

What Susan's story illustrates is that assessing, risk assessing and managing care can require complex skills and a multidisciplinary approach that combines knowledge and experience of the following.

- The patient.
- Bio-psychosocial systems.
- Observation and interpersonal skills.
- Relevant clinical experience.

- The ability to interpret patterns of illness and behaviour beyond a numerical score.
- The ability to interpret and manage care in rapidly changing situations.

Within this chapter we will explore Sally's assessment and highlight the core skills required for recognising and interpreting, communicating and acting on an episode of clinical deterioration. As a student you have the opportunity to observe, learn and practise these skills under supervision before you embrace them as a registered and accountable practitioner. While this book cannot equip you with all of these skills, it does highlight core skills and landmarks to guide you towards competent practice.

Why is assessing and monitoring care important?

In 1860 Florence Nightingale recognised the significance of clinical observation and monitoring, and argued that it is a nursing responsibility to recognise and consider the cause of any change in a patient's clinical condition in order to save life and promote health. Nightingale wrote (1860, p105):

> *The most important practical lesson that can be given to nurses is to teach them what to observe – how to observe – what symptoms indicate improvement – what the reverse – which are of importance – which are of none – which are the evidence of neglect – and what kind of neglect. All this is . . . an essential part, of the training of every nurse.*

Assessing and monitoring of the patient's condition has been a central role of the nurse for 150 years and yet a growing body of evidence recognises that nurses and other healthcare practitioners have been unable to provide safe care to a consistent standard for acutely ill patients and this has resulted in evidence of unnecessary distress and patient deaths on an international scale. A review of these findings is included in the research summary below.

Research summary: Suboptimal care

Empirical evidence of suboptimal care can be traced back to the 1990s. In the USA Franklin and Matthew (1994) undertook a retrospective study of patient signs and symptoms before cardiac arrest and demonstrated that in 25% of the 150 cases studied there was evidence that the nurse had documented deterioration but failed to inform the medical team. They also found significant failings in the medical management of the patients. In the UK case studies of patients admitted to intensive care from the ward by McQuillan et al. (1998) and McGloin et al. (1999) found evidence of suboptimal care in 50% and 30% respectively of the cases studied. Both studies identified that nursing and medical staff had failed to

(Continued)

(Continued)

recognise and/or report the urgency of the situation and that there was evidence of lack of continuity of care, poor supervision of junior staff and other organisational failings. The NPSA Report (2007b) further reinforced the concerns by publishing that out of 425 reported deaths in acute care, 64 were related to patient deterioration not being recognised or acted upon (15%). All of these research studies are based on retrospective analysis of case studies and cannot be considered to be gold standard evidence, but the nature and implications of the findings have triggered a national and international campaign to improve the recognition of and response to clinical deterioration (Institute for Healthcare Improvement (IHI), 2011a; NICE, 2007; Royal College of Physicians (RCP), 2012).

The assessment, recognition, communication and management of patients with clinical deterioration is a vital part of the nurse's role and supports collaborative practice. According to Coulter Smith et al. (2013), recognising and responding to clinical deterioration requires not only physiological measurement but the combination of rapid, detailed assessment and skilled clinical judgement concerning the history and context of the person's illness. Key factors that influence the quality of care provided when patients deteriorate include the following (Massey et al., 2009; Quirke et al., 2011).

- The knowledge and experience of the healthcare workers and their ability to appreciate the clinical urgency of the situation.
- The medical complexity of the patient balanced with available nursing skill mix and resources.
- Communication, clinical leadership and team working.
- Organisational and strategic changes affecting healthcare.

In the remainder of the chapter we will begin to introduce and explore these factors by focusing on how you can provide a safe but rapid assessment and response to patients with acute and critical illness by using physiological measurement, clinical judgement and effective communication.

Knowing and understanding the acutely ill patient

In order to know and understand the acutely ill patient you need to be able to define what acute care is and then the patient's potential for clinical deterioration. The Department of Health (2000) set out guidance for patient dependency levels, and these have subsequently been updated by the ICS (Intensive Care Society) (2009). The levels of care definitions follow a numerical pattern from 0 to 3 and are listed in Table 1.1. These levels of care have been used to assist in the risk assessment of patients as well as in the identification and justification of decisions made about the skill mix requirements for individual wards and units (NICE, 2007; Smith, 2009). Knowing and understanding your patient can begin before you meet them and, in some cases, begin with the patient's handover, followed by meeting and assessing the patient and ensuring continuity of patient-centred care.

Level of critical care criteria	Patient/clinical examples
Level 0 • Requires hospitalisation: needs can be met through normal ward care.	• Jennifer Harris is admitted for routine minor surgery. Her planned length of stay is two days and she will need post-operative monitoring and intravenous therapy for 24 hours during her stay.

Level 1
 	
• Patients recently discharged from higher levels of care.
• Patients in need of additional monitoring, clinical interventions, support or advice.
• Patients requiring critical care outreach service support.
	• Fred Johnson has been discharged to your care from the high dependency unit, where he received respiratory support and interventions for acute respiratory failure.
	• This includes any patient who requires a minimum of four-hourly observations with one or more of the following.
	
	   o Continuous oxygen therapy for impaired respiratory function.
	   o Fluid resuscitation, at risk of renal failure.
	   o Intravenous or epidural pain management.
	   o Presence of a tracheostomy, central venous catheter, chest drain.
	   o Requiring neurological assessment.
	   o Presence of co-morbidities such as diabetes.

Level 2 • Patients needing pre-operative optimisation in order to stabilise their condition prior to surgery. • Patients needing extended post-operative care. • Patients stepping down from level 3 to level 2 care. • Patients who are receiving single organ support/basic respiratory support/basic cardiovascular support.	• Mr Brown needs stabilisation and invasive monitoring of his cardiac and haemodynamic function prior to receiving a general anaesthetic for planned surgery. He has an arterial and central venous line. • Mary Simpson was admitted to high-dependency care for 24 hours following a surgical carotid endarterectomy to remove plaque from the carotid artery. The surgery carries a risk of stroke and haemorrhage, and Mary requires hourly invasive haemodynamic monitoring and neurological assessment.

(Continued)

Table 1.1   (Continued)

Level of critical care criteria	Patient/clinical examples
• Patients receiving advanced cardiovascular/ renal/ neurological/dermatological support.	• Harry Green required 14 days of invasive ventilation and is now being weaned from full respiratory support to spontaneous breathing. He has a tracheostomy, is confused at times and tires quickly. • Jane Morris has been admitted with sepsis and requires invasive haemodynamic support and oxygen therapy. • Paul Stone was admitted following a road traffic incident. He has sustained bilateral fractured shafts of femur and a fractured pelvis. He requires advanced cardiovascular support following emergency surgery to stabilise the fractures.
Level 3 • Patients receiving advanced respiratory support alone or support for a minimum of two organs.	• Ben Williams was transferred from an acute medical ward after showing signs of clinical deterioration. He is diagnosed with pneumonia, acute respiratory distress syndrome, severe sepsis and acute renal failure. He requires invasive ventilation, invasive haemodynamic support and renal replacement therapy.

Table 1.1: Defining levels of critical care

Source: ICS, 2009.

In Susan's story her patient meets the criteria for level 1 patient dependency for the following reasons.

- She is receiving continuous oxygen therapy for impaired respiratory function.

- She requires fluid resuscitation.

- She is at risk of renal failure and sepsis.

- Initially, she required the support of the outreach nurse.

During handover

The levels of patient dependency also allow you to risk assess, from a distance, the potential for patient deterioration; if the patient's dependency level is noted during handover, then you have already started to prioritise your patients' needs. Other related factors, identified during handover and/or during the patient assessment, may influence the potential for the patient to deteriorate (Elliot et al., 2014). These include the following:

- *Age*: increasing age in the older adult is associated with increased vulnerability to co-morbidities, infection, multiple medications.

- *Hydration*: over- or under-hydration can increase the risk of clinical deterioration.

- *Nutrition*: malnutrition can prolong recovery, wound healing and increase the risk of infection.

- *Pain*: a patient in pain is likely to have impaired mobility and increased risk of venous thrombosis, chest infection and a longer length of stay in hospital.

- *Mobility*: reduced mobility increases the risk of pressure ulcers, sepsis and lethargy.

- *Mood/psychological*: anxiety, fear and low mood can negatively impact on the speed and progress of a patient's recovery.

- *Mental health*: knowledge and understanding of patients' mental health problems can enhance your understanding of their ability to cope with other health problems.

- *Learning difficulties*: knowledge of underlying physiological disorders related to their learning difficulties can be crucial and vital to risk assessment of these patients.

- *Co-morbidities and medication*: the presence of combined bio-psychosocial problems such as diabetes, heart disease and the patient's requirement for a hip replacement will increase the risk associated with surgery. Drugs such as prednisolone are steroids that, when prescribed, can lead to a suppressed immune response, hypertension and raised blood glucose.

- The patient has been previously admitted to intensive care during this hospital stay.

Recognising the significance of these factors in patients will alert you to the potential for deterioration.

Meeting and assessing the patient

This should always begin with a rapid assessment of your patient's safety (illustrated in Table 1.2). If you are concerned, complete the rapid assessment and report your concerns without delay (NICE, 2007; NPSA, 2007a). The difference between a routine assessment and a rapid assessment of a patient's condition is the ability to anticipate, recognise and respond in a timely manner to any aspect of concern you have for the patient's condition. The National Institute for Health and Care Excellence (NICE, 2007) recommends that in these circumstances you should initiate and perform the admissions, recognition and response bundles and monitor the patient's condition illustrated in Table 1.2.

Central to the use of these bundles is the integration of the physiological track and trigger score, and the use of emergency outreach teams for the provision of patient and staff support. The National Early Warning Score (NEWS) has been developed in order to standardise risk assessment across the UK (RCP, 2012). The RCP proposes that standardising the numerical score and tracking the changes in the patient's condition provides objective evidence of deterioration, justifies calling the rapid response team for support and optimises standards for education and training of all healthcare staff. However, a systematic review of the effectiveness of physiological track and trigger tools by Gao et al. (2007) concluded that the validity, reliability and sensitivity of the tools in use were poor when used as a single indicator for evidence of deterioration.

However, Smith et al. (2013) found that NEWS has a greater ability to discriminate patients at risk of deterioration than 33 other early warning scoring systems. A study by Ludikhuize et al. (2012) highlights another area of concern, finding that in a retrospective study of 204 patients in an acute hospital the collection of vital signs and track and trigger scores were incomplete in the majority of cases. This suggests that future studies need to focus on measuring the effectiveness of NEWS implementation and the use of clinical judgement in recognising and responding to clinical deterioration.

Bundle of care	Bundle purpose	Interventions
Admission bundle: multidisciplinary	To achieve a baseline of patient data within two hours of admission, collected and communicated to the medical team.	1. Minimum data to collect on admission to your practice area: T, P, R, BP, level of consciousness (LOC), oxygen saturation (SpO_2). 2. Document a clear monitoring plan including the type and frequency of observations to be undertaken. 3. Ensure that all members of the multidisciplinary team know and agree the monitoring plan.
Recognition bundle	Early identification and risk assessment of the deteriorating patient.	1. Monitor physiological signs at least 12 hourly for all patients. 2. Record track and trigger score. 3. Perform risk assessment according to the assessment and trigger score. 4. Consider the possibility of sepsis/severe sepsis. 5. Communicate the information to the medical team.
Response bundle	Optimal and timely treatment of the at-risk patient.	1. If there is clinical concern. 2. If the trigger score is in the low-risk range, increase the frequency of the observations. 3. If the trigger score is in the medium-risk range, contact the patient's medical team urgently and/or the critical care outreach team. 4. If the trigger score is in the high-risk ranges (excluding cardiac arrest), contact the critical care outreach team urgently. 5. In all cases communicate and document communication using the SBAR (situation, background, assessment, recommendation) tool.

Table 1.2: Rapid response to acute illness: admission, recognition and response bundles
Source: NICE, 2007; NHS Wales, 2010.

Clinically effective detection and management of clinical deterioration therefore begins with nurses being alerted to or recognising signs of clinical deterioration and using a systematic, comprehensive and holistic approach to managing care.

When meeting and assessing the patient, it is important not to make assumptions about your patient's bio-psychosocial and spiritual needs until you have verified this with the patient and the healthcare team. Has your patient made a choice about resuscitation? Does your patient have a living will? The provision of patient-centred care should take into account patients' individual needs and wishes where possible. You should be encouraging patients to make informed decisions about their care, and this includes advanced care planning for decisions about cardiopulmonary resuscitation when it is appropriate to do so, for example, in the following patient case study (British Medical Association (BMA), Resuscitation Council (UK) and RCN, 2014). ✓

Case study: Tom Jones

Tom is 74 years old and has a 20-year history of chronic respiratory disease. For the last ten years he has been admitted to level 2 and/or 3 care for management of acute exacerbations of his chronic respiratory problem during the winter months. Last year he was in hospital for a period of 12 weeks, four weeks of which were in intensive care. Tom has made it clear to his family and the nursing team that he doesn't want to go through 'that torture' again. He has expressly wished that he does not want to be **'intubated** *and put on a* **ventilator'***. A collaborative team meeting with Tom and his family resulted in clear documented guidelines for active treatment of his chest infection with a ceiling of treatment noted: 'He will receive active and full support for his condition excluding invasive respiratory support of any kind and cardiopulmonary resuscitation.' The documentation was agreed and signed, with review dates and criteria agreed with the patient and family.*

Knowledge of your patient will enable you to make informed decisions about your patient's progress. Where possible, plan for continuity of care using a collaborative team approach to organising patient-centred care with clear lines of responsibility. ✓

Why do patients deteriorate?

A person is at risk of clinical deterioration in any situation where damage to the body's cells, organs and systems is left unchecked. Causes of cellular injury can be categorised into three groups. These include:

- damage as a result of a deficiency in oxygen and nutrients as illustrated in patients with hypoxia (Chapters 2 and 3);
- patients with ketoacidosis or problems with blood glucose levels (Chapters 8 and 12);
- patients in shock (Chapters 6 and 7); damage through intoxication including drugs, alcohol and infection (Chapter 7); damage through trauma or injury (Chapter 10; Woodrow, 2012). ✓

Evidence-based rapid assessment and interpretation of the patient's condition

The purpose of undertaking a rapid assessment and interpretation of a patient's condition is to:

- anticipate potential risks;
- prevent deterioration;
- ensure timely interventions to provide optimal outcome.

The Airway – Breathing – Circulation – Disability – Exposure 'ABCDE' approach to assessment advocated by the Resuscitation Council (UK) (2015) provides a simple but systematic and priority-driven approach that focuses initially on assessing patient safety and then provides a focus for more in-depth assessment once the patient's safety has been established. When the ABCDE approach is combined with clinical assessment processes – including look, listen, feel, measure, monitor, collate evidence and finally respond – you will have the basis of preliminary but detailed assessment data that can be used to communicate and collaborate with the medical team in order to achieve an effective response.

This chapter and subsequent chapters introduces you to the ABCDE algorithm and encourages you to apply this in the context of patient assessment, clinical interpretation and management of care. In the remainder of this chapter you will be taken through the rapid assessment process by using the core skills: Look: Listen: Feel: Measure, monitor and collate evidence: and Respond.

Each element of the process is summarised in table format and provides a working guide that you can apply to scenarios in this book and in clinical practice. In the following tables each assessment activity is prioritised and listed using A-B-C-D-E; there are columns that illustrate normal and abnormal signs and tips for drawing conclusions and taking action.

It is important to note that while, for the purpose of this book, these core skills have been listed in separate tables, in practice you will be using these skills concurrently and consistently in order to manage patient care.

Assessing your patient: Look/Listen/Feel

Look: As you approach the patient, your initial observation of them begins and your priority is to look and assess for any evidence of patient distress. Nurses often say that they only have to look at a patient to know there is something wrong: what they are actually doing is using their skills of visual perception, combined with knowledge and clinical experience, to interpret a picture of the patient before them (Tait, 2009; Thompson and Dowding, 2002).

Listen: Once you have approached the patient, the second sense to use is listening. This includes listening for signs of a patient's physiological distress such as noisy and laboured breathing and/or signs of psychological distress such as crying. Assessment skills related to listening include the active process of gathering verbal data from the patient and/or relatives, receiving handover from clinical staff and the process of linking relevant data to form clinical judgements.

Feel: The use of touch in professional caring can be described as being involved with functional nursing activities related to physical aspects of care as well as therapeutic nursing activities related to communication and psychological care. When undertaking a rapid assessment of a patient, your priority is to focus on factors affecting circulation. This includes assessing for evidence of cardiac activity and changes to the patient's circulation.

Airway			
Assessment data	**Normal signs**	**Abnormal signs**	**Drawing conclusions/taking action**
Are they breathing?	Quiet regular respiratory pattern: 10–20/min.	Absent breathing: no rise and fall of the chest or abdomen. No response to verbal stimulation.	Absent breathing (apnoea). If the patient does not respond and is not breathing normally after you have opened the airway and checked for airway obstruction then follow the guidelines for basic life support (Resuscitation Council (UK), 2015).
Is there an airway obstruction?	Regular rise and fall of the chest.	Laboured breathing. Choking behaviour. Irregular pattern of breathing with paradoxical chest movements (see-saw respirations). Unequal chest expansion (may be a sign of a pneumothorax or haemothorax).	Untreated airway obstruction leads to a lowered level of oxygen in the arterial circulation (hypoxia) and increases the risk of hypoxic damage to the brain, kidneys and heart. This situation can lead to cardiac arrest and death. Open the patient's airway, suction the airway and consider the use of an oropharyngeal airway. Anticipate the need for tracheal intubation in a medical emergency. Commence high concentration oxygen using a mask with an oxygen reservoir. Aim for oxygen saturations of 97–100% (Resuscitation Council (UK), 2015).

Table 1.3: Quick guide to rapid assessment and response to clinical deterioration: Look/Listen/Feel: Airway

The process of collating additional information begins with your rapid assessment of the patient and becomes a vital part of the data collection process that informs your decision making and that of the healthcare team. This includes collating a record of the patient's recent history, past medical and social history as well as spiritual needs and agreed existing treatment plans. Table 1.8 gives you some pointers for what you should be asking and analysing.

Breathing			
Assessment data	Normal signs	Abnormal signs	Drawing conclusions/taking action
Is the breathing noisy?	Quiet relaxed respirations.	Respiratory stridor indicates narrowing or partial obstruction to the upper airways. Respiratory wheeze is consistent with narrowing of the bronchi due to bronchospasm. Rattle indicates sputum or liquid in the apices of the lung.	For airway obstruction see Table 1.3. Assess the patient history for a diagnosis of asthma or chronic obstructive pulmonary disease (COPD). If the patient has COPD provide oxygen therapy to achieve oxygen saturations (SpO_2) of 90%.
Does the patient have a cough?	No cough.	Cough present. Dry cough. Chesty cough. Productive cough with sputum. Sputum green/yellow/black/pink/thick, tenacious, copious amounts (fills a tissue in one cough). Rapid shallow breathing (may be related to diabetic ketoacidosis, sepsis, exhaustion).	If the cough is dry and wheezy this may indicate an acute asthma attack. If the patient is producing yellow/green sputum this may indicate an infection. Obtain a sputum sample for microbial culture. If the sputum is black and there is a recent history of exposure to fire this may indicate inhalation of smoke/inhalation burns. Frothy pink sputum may indicate pulmonary oedema.
Is there evidence of abdominal breathing or use of accessory muscles to breath?	Quiet relaxed respirations.	Use of accessory muscles indicates there is increased work of breathing. The use of abdominal breathing without chest expansion may indicate an injury to the cervical spine.	Does the patient have a history of chronic respiratory disease? Does the patient have a pneumothorax or fluid obstructing the lung space in the thorax? Risk assess for and assume spinal injury until this cause has been ruled out or confirmed.

Table 1.4: Quick guide to rapid assessment and response to clinical deterioration: Look/Listen/Feel: Breathing

Circulation			
Assessment data	**Normal signs**	**Abnormal signs**	**Drawing conclusions/taking action**
What can you interpret from looking and feeling the skin?	Skin is pink or brown with pink mucosa. Skin is warm to touch and well perfused.	Skin is pale. Lips and mucosa pale blue or purple. Skin shows signs of central cyanosis. Cold hands and feet with a blue tinge to the skin on fingers and toes. Skin shows signs of peripheral cyanosis. Skin is warm, flushed and red. One or more limbs pale and cold with absent pulses.	Pale skin may indicate early signs of shock. Central cyanosis is an indication of hypoxia. Peripheral cyanosis may indicate poor peripheral perfusion/ peripheral shutdown and in the presence of other clinical factors indicates shock. A flushed skin indicates peripheral vasodilation, present in anaphylaxis. A patient with severe sepsis may present with warm flushed skin. Localised peripheral changes may indicate localised trauma and loss of circulation.
Pulse?	Pulse is present and regular. Pulses present in the peripheral pulse points.	Carotid pulse is absent. Pulse is weak and thready. Pulse is full and bounding. Pulse is irregular. Pulse is absent or altered in one or more of the following: pedal, radial, femoral.	If the patient has no carotid pulse and cardiac output is absent follow the Resuscitation Council (UK) (2015) algorithm on basic life support or in-hospital life support. A weak thready pulse indicates reduced cardiac output. A full and bounding pulse may indicate sepsis. A rapid irregular pulse indicates an increased risk of embolus development and/or a failing cardiac output. Localised peripheral changes may indicate localised trauma and loss of circulation.

Table 1.5: Quick guide to rapid assessment and response to clinical deterioration: Look/Listen/Feel: Circulation

Disability			
Assessment data	**Normal signs**	**Abnormal signs**	**Drawing conclusions/taking action**
Is the patient alert and responding?	The patient is alert and responding to questions in a logical manner when assessed using the AVPU algorithm (Alert/responds to Voice/responds to Pain/no response Unconscious).	The patient responds to voice, pain or is unconscious.	Consider possible causes including: • hypoxia • ketoacidosis (smell the breath for the presence of ketones – pear drops) • head injury • drugs • stroke. Place patient in the recovery position unless a spinal injury is suspected.

Table 1.6: Quick guide to rapid assessment and response to clinical deterioration: Look/Listen/Feel: Disability

Exposure/Examination			
Assessment data	**Normal signs**	**Abnormal signs**	**Drawing conclusions/ taking action**
Is there evidence of trauma/injury?	No signs of physical damage to the person, comfortable in any position. Calm facial expression.	Unresponsive patient with facial grimacing, frowning. Signs of bruising, physical trauma, foreign object in the person, abnormal movement of the chest, immobility.	Attempt to open the airway where safe and possible for the patient. If you suspect the person may have a cervical spine injury, open the airway using a jaw thrust rather than a head tilt (Resuscitation Council (UK), 2015).
Is there evidence of factors that may be related to the patient's condition?	A safe environment.	Causes of injury or trauma include: empty medication packets, empty bottle of alcohol, sharp objects, etc.	Look for causes of injury or trauma.

| Is there evidence of fluid loss, blood loss? | No signs of loss of body fluids. | Evidence of vomiting and/or diarrhoea. Blood loss. Loss of fluid through burns. | Risk assess for hypovolaemic shock (see Chapters 6 and 10). |

Table 1.7: Quick guide to rapid assessment and response to clinical deterioration: Look/Listen/Feel: Exposure

Assessment data	Normal signs	Abnormal signs	Drawing conclusions/taking action
Have you listened to the patient's or relative's story of events?	Patient is able to give you a clear account of their problem and history.	Patient is unable to respond, unconscious, confused and unable to give appropriate answers. A relative or others are able to give an account of the events.	Always listen and be alert to information regardless of the source: it may be important!
Do you know the patient?	The patient has a named nurse.	The patient is registered 'do not resuscitate' and this has been dated and signed with an agreed time frame. Patient has been admitted in the last 24 hours and has no prescribed limiting directives. Patient is not known by the staff.	If the patient is not for resuscitation this does not mean that active treatment has been withheld. Therefore always check to obtain a collaborative agreement of the patient's care plan. If the patient is a recent admission and no information is available then assume that all active treatment continues. If the patient does not have a recent history of continuous care by the nursing staff then ensure that a baseline of assessment details is recorded for comparison.

Table 1.8: Quick guide to additional information gathering when undertaking a rapid assessment and response to clinical deterioration

Assessment data	Normal signs	Abnormal signs	Drawing conclusions/ taking action
Respiration (R)	R: 12–20/min	R: <12, >20	Assess the patient in context: are you concerned about your patient?
Oxygen saturation (SpO_2)	SpO_2: 97–100%	SpO_2: <96%	Is there evidence to support this from your 'Look: Listen: Feel' assessment?
Arterial blood gas analysis (ABG)	ABG: • pH: 7.35–7.45; • PaO_2: 11.5–13.5 kPa; • $PaCO_2$: 4.5–6.0 kPa; • HCO_3: 24–27 mmol/L.	ABG • Respiratory acidosis: pH: <7.35; $PaCO_2$: >6.0 kPa. • Respiratory alkalosis: pH: >7.45; $PaCO_2$: <4.9 kPa. • Metabolic acidosis: pH: <7.35; HCO_3: <22 mmol/L. • Metabolic alkalosis: pH: >7.45; HCO_3: >26 mmol/L.	If so, what information is there and can you see a pattern or trend in deterioration? Has the NEWS score changed? Is there evidence of sepsis? (see Chapter 7) Is there a recent history of head trauma?
Pulse (P)	P: 51–90/min	P: <50, >90/min	
Blood pressure (BP)	BP: 110/70–140/90 mmHg	BP: <110/70 mmHg, >140/90 mmHg	
Electrocardiogram (ECG)	Sinus rhythm.	Evidence of any abnormal-looking complexes and irregularities in rate.	
Urine output	≥ 0.5 ml/kg body weight/hr (≥ 1000 ml/24hrs).	Urine output: • oliguria (acute renal failure): <0.5 ml/kg body weight/hr; • polyuria (diabetes, diabetes insipidus). Negative urine balance despite rigorous fluid replacement.	

Fluid balance	Fluid balance should be equal (=) based on a minimum input of 2 L/24hrs.	Fluid balance < or > = based on a minimum input of 2 L/24hrs.
Central venous pressure (CVP)	Mid-axilla: 2–6 mmHg (5–10 cm water).	Mid-axilla: • hypovolaemia. CVP: <2–6 mm Hg; • hypervolaemia/ cardiac failure. CVP: >2–6 mmHg.
Level of consciousness (LOC)	APVU score: A GCS score: 15	APVU score indicating PVU. GCS: <15
Pain assessment	Pain managed effectively.	Elevated pain score.
Blood results Glucose Urea and creatinine Electrolytes Microbiology	Glucose: 4–8 mmol/L Urea: 3.5–6.5 mmol/L Creatinine: 60–120 micromol/L Na: 135–145 mmol/L K: 3.5–4.5 mmol/L Mg: 1.25–2.5 mmol/L Cl: 95–108 mmol/L WCC: 4–12 10^9/L	Glucose: <4 or >7.7 mmol/L Urea: <or >3.5–6.5 mmol/L Creatinine: >60–20 micromol/L Na: < or >135–145 mmol/L K: < or >3.5–4.5 mmol/L Mg: < or >1.25–2.5 mmol/L Cl: < or >95–108 mmol/L WCC: <4 or >12 10^9/L

Table 1.9: Quick guide to rapid assessment and response to clinical deterioration using objective clinical measurement

Measure and collate evidence of clinical change

The core assessment skills of 'Look: Listen: Feel' can be completed within a few minutes of meeting the patient. The process of measuring and collating evidence for clinical change involves bringing together the objective data that can be collected on a patient through the assessment of vital signs, blood glucose, fluid and electrolyte balance, and other relevant investigations. This process also begins when you meet the patient and runs concurrently with the look, listen and feel assessment. According to Adam et al. (2010) there is strong evidence to suggest that changes in respiratory rate are associated with clinical deterioration, along with a decline in patient oxygen saturation levels, changes in pulse and blood pressure, and level of consciousness. It is at this stage that evidence of your concerns becomes apparent and, if necessary, triggers the next step. See Table 1.9.

The outreach nurse in Susan's story was able to demonstrate expertise and clinical reasoning in the context of the clinical situation. This resulted in him being able to quickly obtain a clinical grasp of the situation, anticipate and prevent potential problems. This is what Benner et al. (2011, p2) describe as *habits of thought and action* (problem identification, clinical problem solving, anticipating and preventing potential problems) that rely on a dynamic process of knowledge acquisition, experience, pattern recognition and critical reflection. The development of these skills occurs over time and is always dependent on the history, knowledge and experience of the nurse (Higgs et al., 2008). In the activity below you have a chance to practise rapid assessment and management of a patient.

Activity 1.1   *Risk assessment and decision making*

Isabel Campbell is 85 years old and lives a full and active life. She lives alone but has adult children living nearby. Isabel routinely takes an ACE inhibitor to control hypertension and aspirin as a preventer for stroke and heart disease. This evening Isabel has been experiencing some abdominal discomfort and nausea but she put it down to eating rich food and went to bed. Two hours later she awoke and vomited a large amount of brown liquid over the bed. She felt very faint and dizzy so called her daughter who arranged for an ambulance. She has now been admitted to the medical assessment unit.

1. What knowledge and skills would you use to assess Isabel on admission?

   On assessment the following data were collected regarding her condition.

   - R 28/min.
   - SpO_2 94%.
   - Skin pale and drawn.
   - P 98/min.
   - BP 105/93 mmHg.

- Has not passed urine since teatime at home.
- Alert.
- T 37.3°C.

2. What concerns would you have and what will you do about your concerns?

There are sample answers to this question at the end of the chapter.

Communicating and collaborating with patients, relatives and staff to achieve appropriate and timely interventions

Risk assessment is a continuous process. If, however, you are concerned about your patient and you wish to seek advice or help, the next stage of the process is to communicate your concerns to the relevant person or team using the recognition and response bundles (NICE, 2007) referred to in Table 1.2.

- If you have a clinical concern about the patient and the data indicates the patient to be at low risk, then increase the frequency of the observations (minimum 4–6 hourly) and monitor the patient.

- If you have a clinical concern about the patient and the data indicates the patient to be at medium risk, then contact the patient's medical team urgently. If necessary contact the critical care outreach team in order to get an urgent assessment by a clinician with core competencies to assess the acutely ill patient.

- If you have a clinical concern about the patient and the data indicates the patient to be at high risk, then contact the critical care outreach team urgently and consider transfer to critical care.

When communicating with the medical team or critical care outreach team it is vital that the date, time and nature of your concern are identified and documented. It is this process of documentation that provides a timeline and audit trail for the review of practice.

SBAR is a structured communication tool that has been recommended by the Institute for Healthcare Improvement (IHI, 2011a) and NICE (2007) as a framework for improving inter-professional communication and patient safety. SBAR is an abbreviation for 'Situation: Background: Assessment: Recommendation', and as a tool it meets the quality requirements for safe and effective clinical documentation of care.

- Situation: identify yourself, your location and the patient. Describe the problem, your concern and reason for calling.

- Background: provide the patient's reason for admission, diagnosis and relevant history.

- Assessment: provide both your subjective concerns and objective data. Offer a provisional diagnosis of the problem or clarify your concern.
- Recommendations: explain what you need, when and where.

According to Dayton and Henriksen (2007) SBAR works because it provides a shared and logical structure for communicating core details of a patient's situation either verbally or through written communication. The tool can be used to communicate urgent and non-urgent clinical information.

In the example in Table 1.10, we have returned to our student nurse Susan and her patient Sally, who we met at the beginning of the chapter. There has been a change in Sally's condition and using the SBAR approach we will recap and see what has changed.

Date and time of initial call: *05/11/14 at 18.00 hrs* Date and time of response: *05/11/14 at 18.05 hrs*	Patient's name: *Sally Smith aged 67 years* Nurse's name: *Susan Brown* Name of person called: *Specialist registrar (Brian James)*	
Situation: reason for the call	*I am concerned about Sally Smith; she was admitted today at 16.00 hrs after being diagnosed with dehydration and possible urinary tract infection. Her condition has deteriorated despite receiving fluid resuscitation, oxygen 40% and her first dose of trimethoprim 200 mg. She now meets the criteria for sepsis.*	
Background	*Known to have hypertension controlled by lisinopril 20 mg but has been unable to take her medication for six days.*	
Assessment	*Previous assessment data: 17.00 hrs* **Airway:** *patent* **Breathing:** *R: 19/min;* *SpO₂: 95%* **Circulation:** *P: 88/min;* *sinus rhythm;* *BP 126/82 mmHg;* *T: 37.4°C; cool hands and feet.* *Has not passed urine for approximately six hours.* *Infusion of 0.9% saline commenced in the emergency unit running at 125 ml/hour.*	*New assessment data: 18.00 hrs* **Airway:** *patent* **Breathing:** *R 26/min;* *SpO₂: 89%* **Circulation:** *P: 97/min;* *sinus tachycardia* *BP 102/45 mmHg;* *T: 37.7°C; cool hands and feet.* *Urine output 50 ml of cloudy urine (positive to blood and protein).* *White cell count 11.2 10⁹/L*

	White cell count 10.4 10$_9$/L *Glucose: 6.5 mmol/l*	*Glucose: 7.9 mmol/l*
	Disability: *drowsy and disorientated*	**Disability:** *responding to voice.*
	NEWS = 5	*NEWS = 11*
Recommendations and response	What you are requesting? Urgent ward visit: *Yes.* Telephone advice: – Prescription: – Other: *Sally Smith requires an urgent review and risk assessment for sepsis.* *I have contacted the outreach nurse who reviewed her two hours ago and he will meet you on the ward.* *Sally's husband is aware of the change in her condition and is with her.* *Is there anything else you would like me to get ready for you?* Action taken and registrar's response: *Thank you. Can you increase the oxygen therapy immediately according to the sepsis guidelines (see Chapter 7) and I will come and reassess the patient. Please have ready the equipment for taking blood cultures, etc. and I will be on the ward in five minutes.* Signatures: *Signed by both the staff nurse and the registrar following Sally's assessment and management.*	

Table 1.10: Communicating concern using the SBAR approach

In our patient Sally's case there were a number of reasons why her condition may have deteriorated. These include:

- dehydration and the resultant hypovolaemia (see Chapter 6);
- urinary tract infection that has progressed to sepsis with a risk of acute kidney injury (see Chapters 7 and 9);
- a risk of acute heart failure (Chapter 4).

At this stage of her care the priorities include supporting Sally physiologically and psychologically by:

- supporting her airway, breathing and circulation in order to reduce the risk of further deterioration;
- providing information and reassurance to her and her husband.

Providing standardised and optimal care during all stages of the patient's journey

A registered nurse has a professional responsibility to ensure safe and clinically effective care in order to support an agreed patient outcome and to accurately document any changes in the patient's condition or variance from the care pathway. The adoption of a care pathway and a care bundle approach by NICE (2011) has given all healthcare providers an opportunity to standardise practice while continuing to provide patient-focused care. The emphasis is now on you as a nurse to recognise and adopt the most clinically appropriate pathway of care, but at the same time to recognise, record and respond to any variances in the care package. In this context those variances have to be justified and evidence based. The seven points below are a useful guide to what should be provided to ensure the quality of nursing documentation (Jeffries et al., 2010).

Good nursing documentation:

- is patient centred and includes extracts from the patient's description of their illness experience;
- reflects the objective clinical judgement of the nurse so that every statement has an objective descriptor, for example:
  - subjective comment: the patient seemed a bit tipsy;
  - objective comment: the patient was walking with an unsteady gait, his speech was slurred and his breath smelt of alcohol;
- contains the actual work of nurses including bio-psychosocial interventions;
- is presented in a logical sequence;
- is written as events occur so that it remains up to date;
- records all variances in care, in a clear and concise way without repetition;
- fulfils legal and professional requirements according to *The Code* (NMC, 2015).

In a busy and acute clinical setting nurses and healthcare professionals can be easily distracted. The safety of patients, however, should be paramount and the prevention of patient deterioration is a multidisciplinary goal that can only be achieved through assessment, communication and collaboration between the patient and all professional groups.

Managing and organising care using the appropriate skill mix

The ability to know and understand your patients is dependent on you and your team having a balanced skill mix, evidence of continuity of care, effective communication channels and effective teamwork so that you are able to assess and respond to the patient's immediate needs in an emergency (Scott, 2003; Duffield et al., 2010).

There is a wide range of skill mix in acute care across hospitals and even in the same hospital because of changes in nurse education strategies and the loss of nursing apprentices (Scott, 2003; Duffield et al., 2010). In acute care the number of healthcare assistants has increased at a faster rate than that of registered nurses, leading to a dilution of professionally registered nurses in the skill mix (Scott, 2003). Furthermore, staffing levels often vary because of staff sickness, unexpected patient turnover and the use of bank or agency nurses.

Within this climate of change in models of healthcare provision, there is evidence to support the use of a collaborative team approach to care (Royal College of Nursing, 2003; Zwarenstein et al., 2009). A team may consist of all the providers of care for a group of patients, including nurses, healthcare assistants, medical staff and other health professionals. Nonetheless, the focus should remain on patient-centred care where continuity of care is provided by the team, with each team member ensuring effective communication. Task-based team nursing, where management of care is based on a series of tasks rather than focusing on patient need, should be avoided as this has been found to reduce the quality of care (Fairbrother et al., 2010).

Activity 1.2   *Reflection*

Think back to your experiences in the clinical setting.

- Can you identify a situation where you have been unable to understand how the nurse was able to know or anticipate clinical changes in a deteriorating patient?
- If you can, write down the story and look back on the incident after reading this chapter.
- Using the chapters as a guide, try to write down an action plan of how you might manage a similar situation in the future.

Hint: These reflective questions will help you to practise the skills of rapid assessment and management of a patient.

There is no outline answer at the end of the chapter as this activity is based on your own reflections.

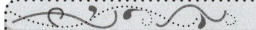

Chapter summary

Within this chapter we have introduced you to the skills and processes involved in the rapid assessment of and response to deteriorating patients. The core skills focus on risk assessment, prevention and timely intervention of care. The tables included have been designed to provide you with an aide-memoire that you can apply to the patient examples in the remainder of the book.

Activities: brief outline answers

Activity 1.1: Risk assessment and decision making (pages 22–3)

1. The knowledge and skills you would use relate to clinical assessment and in particular rapid assessment skills. These include using 'ABCDE' as a guide: look at the patient; listen to the patient, family, handover from other staff, listen for physiological signs of distress; feel the patient's skin and note any abnormal signs; measure the patient's physiological signs. Interpret the clinical signs and assess the findings against the normal range.

2. Increased respiratory rate with a lower than normal SpO_2 suggests respiratory distress and requires immediate action: call for help from a senior member of staff and administer oxygen guided by the local protocol (Chapter 2). Isabel also has signs of haemodynamic insufficiency indicated by rapid respirations, rapid pulse and low BP. She is considered to be at medium risk of deterioration and requires at least hourly observations of vital signs and fluid resuscitation. She is also at risk of further fluid loss and requires urgent management of a possible peptic ulcer (see Chapter 6).

Further reading

Royal College of Nursing (RCN) (2004) *Nursing Assessment of Older People: RCN Tool Kit.* London: RCN.

This resource provides general guidance and tools for assessing older people and offers useful background detail on collaborative assessment processes.

Rushforth, H (2009) *Assessment Made Incredibly Easy.* London: Wolters Kluwer/Lippincott Williams and Wilkins.

This book provides information on detailed systematic assessment of all clinical situations and is a useful revision guide to assessment skills.

Useful websites

www.resus.org.uk/pages/dnar.htm

This resource provides information and guidance by the Resuscitation Council on ethical decisions related to resuscitation.

www.resus.org.uk/pages/alsABCDE.htm

This resource provides a summary of the ABCDE assessment using a multidisciplinary approach.

www.londonccn.nhs.uk/_store/documents/national-early-warning-score-standardising-assessment-acute-illness-severity-nhs.pdf

National Early Warning Score (2012).

www.londonccn.nhs.uk/_store/documents/news-observation-chart-with-explanatory-text.pdf

NEWS observation chart (with explanatory notes).

www.londonccn.nhs.uk/_store/documents/outline-clinical-response-to-news-triggers-with-explanatory-text.pdf

NEWS clinical response outline (with explanatory notes).

www.londonccn.nhs.uk/_store/documents/news-thresholds-and-triggers-with-explanatory-text.pdf

NEWS thresholds and triggers (with explanatory notes).

The NEWS resources provide you with the national guidance on assessing and risk assessing patients for clinical deterioration and is now part of standard practice.

Chapter 2
The breathless patient

Jane James

continued . . .

develop a personalised plan that is based on mutual understanding and respect for their individual situation promoting health and well-being, minimising risk of harm and promoting their safety at all times.

By entry to the register

xx. Acts autonomously and appropriately when faced with sudden deterioration in people's physical or psychological condition or emergency situations, abnormal vital signs, collapse, cardiac arrest, self-harm, extremely challenging behaviour, attempted suicide.

xxi. Measures documents and interprets vital signs and acts autonomously and appropriately on findings.

Chapter aims

By the end of this chapter, you should be able to:

- identify causes of breathlessness;
- describe the clinical features of breathlessness in relation to cardiac failure, type I and II respiratory failures, pneumonia, chronic obstructive pulmonary disease (COPD) and asthma, and the clinical implications for the patient;
- demonstrate awareness of how to undertake respiratory assessment;
- diagnose and differentiate between possible causes of patient deterioration and identify most appropriate interventions;
- reflect on clinical examples illustrated in the chapter and relate to your own clinical practice.

Introduction

Breathlessness relates to perceived difficulty in breathing and is a sensation experienced by people in many circumstances of health and illness. In some circumstances, such as exercise, it is normal to feel breathless, but there is an expectation that breathing will return to normal during rest. In other abnormal circumstances, breathlessness will persist until adequate corrections are made to the condition causing the breathlessness.

This chapter gives an overview of some of the possible causes of breathlessness that are included in Table 2.1 and examines in detail the care of patients suffering with breathlessness related to:

- cardiac failure;
- pneumonia;
- COPD;
- asthma.

Underlying physiology, social psychology and ethical implications of all four types of patients will be discussed in the context of risk assessment and collaborative management and care.

Cardiac	Lung	Neuromuscular	Other
Cardiac failure	Lung infections such as pneumonia	Pain	Exercise
Angina pectoris	Pneumothorax	Rib fractures	Anaemia
Myocardial infarction (heart attack)	Pulmonary embolism	Myasthenia gravis	Systemic infection
		Muscular dystrophy	Distended abdomen
Abnormal heart rhythms	Pleural effusion	Kyphoscoliosis	Allergy/anaphylaxis
Cardiac tamponade	Chronic obstructive pulmonary disease		Metabolic causes such as acidosis
	Asthma		Stress, anxiety, fear
	Emphysema		Brain injury
	Carcinoma of the lung tissue or bronchus		
	Fibrotic lung disease		

Table 2.1: Some conditions that cause breathlessness

The chapter begins with the case study of a patient with cardiac failure, followed by an explanation of breathlessness. This leads to an overview of the knowledge and skills required to recognise, assess, prioritise and manage care for patients with breathlessness. You will see how the degree of breathlessness represents the severity of the circumstances and thus dictates the level and speed of response required.

This chapter introduces the need for respiratory support and the concept of arterial blood gas analysis, but these are discussed in detail in Chapters 3 and 10.

Case study: Cardiac failure

Susan had been allocated a small caseload of patients to visit while on her final community placement. One of her patients was 76-year-old Charlie Morris, who had been having a chronic leg wound redressed twice weekly. When Susan arrived at his house on her second visit, she found Mr Morris sitting in a chair dressed in his pyjamas. He said he was having trouble getting going and was very tired because he had not slept very well. His wife added that he had woken several times during the night short of breath, had sat on the edge of the bed and asked her to open the window. He seemed better once morning

(Continued)

continued . . . •••

came. Mr Morris said that this happened to him sometimes, but not usually this bad. He normally rested and felt better after a while.

When Susan went to look at Mr Morris's wound, she found the leg of his pyjamas was very tight. In helping her to access his wound, he struggled to remove his pyjamas, becoming more breathless and needing time afterwards to get his breath back. Susan also found the wound bandage was constricting Mr Morris's leg, which appeared swollen; his toes were cold and pale. She wondered if she had applied the bandage too tightly on her previous visit and contacted her mentor, Bridget, to ask for advice.

Bridget called by and assessed Mr Morris. First she checked his respirations, pulse and blood pressure, then asked questions about his regular medication and his fluid intake and output, felt both Mr Morris's ankles and listened carefully to what Mrs Morris told her. Susan was confused by the fact that Bridget did not seem concerned about Mr Morris's leg wound, but instead requested the GP to visit, saying that she thought he might have an exacerbation of his heart failure.

Susan's experience highlights the fact that patients with chronic conditions often have more than one problem. Susan thought that she was visiting Mr Morris for a straightforward dressing change, but his other health problems were more serious at that time.

The fact that Mr Morris was feeling tired and lethargic was not simply due to a poor night's sleep. The reason why his sleep was disturbed was significant in that he was waking up from sleep feeling breathless, and this happened several times. It was also worth noting that his breathlessness worsened on physical exertion and speaking.

When Bridget heard Mrs Morris's story and saw that Mr Morris was still breathless at rest and had swollen legs, she recognised some important indicators and knew from her experience that it could be a worsening of Mr Morris's heart failure. Susan had only seen Mr Morris once previously and had been concentrating on being professional and doing the dressing correctly. She was glad that she had contacted her mentor, even though her reason was misdirected.

Susan visited Mr Morris to do a dressing but found that he was tired and breathless. His main problem was not his wound but related to his heart. What can we learn from this?

The important messages in Susan's story are these.

- Take every opportunity in all clinical settings to assess your patients holistically and systematically (see Chapter 1); assimilate your findings and keep an open mind.

- Listen carefully to your patient's complaints or concerns about things such as breathlessness that affect their daily activities, as these are often significant.

- If you are concerned about your patient, seek advice and support according to local risk assessment protocol (see Chapter 1).

- The seat of the problem may not necessarily be what you think, and breathlessness alone or combined with other symptoms needs further exploration.

Breathlessness

Breathing is vital for life and is part of the mechanism depended upon to supply oxygen to the tissues. All cells in the human body require a continuous supply of oxygen otherwise they die. As oxygen is used, carbon dioxide is produced as a waste product. While it is important for the body to take in oxygen, it is also important to remove the carbon dioxide at the same rate that oxygen is supplied. Essentially, this is respiration, and it contributes to maintaining homeostasis – a state of balance and stability within the cells to keep them working. If the cells receive insufficient amounts of oxygen, they become hypoxic. This state is known as tissue hypoxia. It can lead to anaerobic metabolism, which causes increased acid production resulting in cell death (Kumar and Clark, 2012). Likewise, if the carbon dioxide is not removed efficiently, it builds up in the blood (CO_2 retention) creating hypercarbia and has the effect of increasing blood acid levels.

Acidity and alkalinity, body temperature and fluid levels are also involved in homeostasis, and respiration plays an important part in controlling and responding to changes in these factors to achieve the narrow range of normality required (Grossman and Porth, 2013). Adaptations in response from various other body systems also play a part. These include metabolic processes and the circulatory, neuromuscular and renal systems. While respiration itself comprises four processes (Table 2.2), in the first instance, we notice our patients' bodies attempting to achieve homeostasis by changes in their breathing.

Process	Dependent upon	Measured by	Clinical examples
Pulmonary ventilation: the movement of air in and out of the lungs.	Respiratory centres in the brain. Chemoreceptors in aorta, carotid body and medulla oblongata.	Respiratory observations: rate; depth; sound; effort; volumes.	1. Diane suffered a head injury affecting her brain stem.
	Nerves: phrenic, intercostal. Muscles: diaphragm, intercostal, accessory.		2. Jean has **Guillain Barré syndrome** affecting the nerves supplying her intercostal muscles and reducing the size of her breaths.
	Pressure changes within thoracic cavity. Patent airways.		3. Phil was trapped in a fire and breathed in hot smoke causing pharyngeal oedema.

(Continued)

Table 2.2   (Continued)

Process	Dependent upon	Measured by	Clinical examples
	Elasticity of lungs.		4. John has fibrosed lungs due to chronic disease, causing his lungs to be stiff and unable to stretch.
	Lung capacity.		5. Peter sustained broken ribs when a tree fell on him, causing pneumothorax and precluding him from taking deep breaths.
External respiration: the exchange of oxygen and carbon dioxide between the alveoli in the lungs and the pulmonary capillaries.	Tidal volume > physiological dead space. Fresh supply of oxygen to alveoli. Gas pressure changes (oxygen and carbon dioxide). Diffusion. Presence of blood supply (pulmonary capillaries). Proximity of pulmonary blood flow to alveoli.	Inspired/ expired gas analysis.	1. Mary took an overdose of her sleeping tablets and has very shallow breaths. 2. Chris is climbing Mount Everest and developed pulmonary oedema due to lower air pressure at altitude. 3. Brian has COPD with emphysema and atelectasis. 4. Ross was recovering from hip surgery when he suffered a pulmonary embolism. 5. Siobhan has pneumonia and secretions have consolidated the bases of both lungs.
Transport of gases: the carriage of oxygen from the lungs to the tissues and carbon dioxide from the tissues to the lungs in the blood.	Circulation of blood. Patency of vessels. Uninterrupted flow.	Oxygen saturations. Arterial blood gas analysis (ABG).	1. Charlie has heart failure and reduced cardiac output. 2. Trudy is anaemic after months of heavy periods. 3. Margaret had a thrombosis that lodged in her popliteal artery causing her foot to become ischaemic.
Internal respiration: the delivery of oxygen to the body cells and the collection of carbon dioxide from the cells	Gas pressure changes. Blood supply to cells. Correct environment within the cell.	ABGs – level of metabolic acidosis. Lactate levels.	1. Bob's gas fire was faulty and he suffered carbon monoxide poisoning. 2. Andy fell into the river and suffered hypothermia.

Table 2.2: Processes of respiration

When different factors of homeostasis are disturbed and the body tries to adjust to put things back to normal (compensation), it does this initially by altering the rate and pattern of breathing.

So anyone who is breathless (dyspnoeic) is in the process of trying to normalise their body's internal environment by drawing on compensatory or corrective mechanisms. Their degree of breathlessness often indicates the severity of imbalance within their cells, and could be caused by problems with any one of the four processes involved in respiration as shown in the clinical examples in Table 2.2. These processes can be affected by other body systems as demonstrated by Mr Morris's heart failure in the previous case study. As his heart failed to pump effectively, there was inadequate circulation to maintain his blood pressure and internal respiration, resulting in poor tissue oxygenation. Mr Morris's frequent episodes of breathlessness during the night resulted from his body trying to compensate.

Mr Morris also had swelling (**oedema**) of his lower legs, and this was a key indicator to Bridget that Mr Morris was retaining fluid. She knew that Mr Morris's heart was probably working harder and that his lungs might well be congested due to the increased fluid in his body, thus affecting his external respiration. When she found that he was hypotensive as well as dyspnoeic and tachycardic, she was satisfied with her assessment.

Because breathlessness can result from the body's compensation in relation to the respiratory, circulatory, neuromuscular, renal and metabolic systems, you will find breathless patients of all ages and in all clinical settings. Breathing rates change quickly in response to demands from body systems, so breathlessness is an early indicator of acute illness and should not be ignored (NICE, 2007; NPSA, 2007a). In order to prevent further deterioration you need to be alert to breathless patients and undertake an initial rapid assessment using the ABCDE approach (Resuscitation Council (UK), 2011), as outlined in Chapter 1, including a detailed assessment of breathing. This needs to be combined with the clinical assessment process of 'Look: Listen: Feel: Measure', which will then enable you to respond appropriately to your patients' needs in a timely manner (Smith, 2009).

Breathing assessment

As part of the ABCDE approach to organising rapid assessment, it is important to ensure that your patient's airway is patent before going on to assess breathing. On assessing your patients, you will be aware of several aspects of breathing, and noting these can be very useful in identifying risks and changes in your patients' conditions.

Activity 2.1   *Critical thinking*

Consider the patients in Table 2.2 and note down how many different aspects of breathing you can think of. Remember to use the 'Look: Listen: Feel: Measure: Respond' approach discussed in Chapter 1.

A table of what you could identify is given at the end of the chapter.

Bridget rapidly assessed Mr Morris when she arrived to see him. She could see that he was alert, as he replied to her when she greeted him. This suggested that his brain was receiving adequate oxygenation to maintain consciousness and verified that his airway was clear. She could see that he was breathing and that it seemed to be fast, so continued to assess his breathing in detail using the 'Look: Listen: Feel: Measure: Respond' approach to determine where the problems lay. She could see that he was pale and his chest was rising equally on both sides. He was breathing fast and deep. He did not look distressed, but he was using his accessory muscles (pulling his shoulders up and pushing his abdomen out). Breathing looked hard work for him and his nostrils were flaring slightly on inspiration. This informed Bridget that he was trying to get more air into his lungs and that he might be short of oxygen.

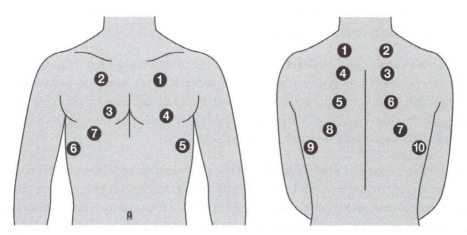

Figure 2.1: Position and sequence for stethoscope placement when listening to breathing sounds as shown by numbered dots

Bridget went on to listen, and she could hear the air moving in and out of Mr Morris's nose. It was audible as she knelt next to him, but was not noisy. She then listened with a stethoscope to the front and back of his chest. She moved her stethoscope systematically over the chest, listening at specific points identified in Figure 2.1.

On listening with the stethoscope, Bridget could hear the air moving in and out of Mr Morris's lungs as he breathed normally. She also asked him to take some deeper breaths in order to improve the quality of the breath sounds she could hear. There were crackles all over his chest at the end of inspiration and a faint wheeze on expiration. This suggested to her that he had fluid accumulating in the tissues of his lungs (pulmonary oedema), which would obstruct external respiration.

When Bridget put her hands flat on Mr Morris's chest, she felt his chest expanding equally on the left and the right and she could feel the movement of fluid as Mr Morris breathed in and out. His skin felt cool and clammy, suggesting that his peripheral circulation was poor.

Bridget counted Mr Morris's breaths (in and out) for one minute to measure his respiratory rate at 32 breaths per minute (bpm). She also noted that he could speak four or five words between breaths. She had been very mindful to ask open questions in order to measure this, but subsequently asked only closed questions to avoid additional undue breathlessness. Her hand-held oxygen saturation monitor told her that his oxygen saturations (SpO_2) were 94%, indicating that he was just achieving the target range of 94–98% recommended by O'Driscoll et al. (2008).

Activity 2.2   *Evidence-based practice and research*

Visit the 3M™ Littman® Stethoscopes website education page below and follow the link 'About Stethoscopes' to find information about the components of a stethoscope and how to use it.

http://www.littmann.com/wps/portal/3M/en_US/3M-Littmann/stethoscope/littmann-learning-institute/about-stethoscopes/stethoscope-use

After gaining consent, practise the 'Look: Listen: Feel: Measure' approach to perform a respiratory assessment on a well person and on your patients with breathlessness.

Practise using your stethoscope to listen to the areas of the chest identified on Figure 2.1. Make notes and compare your findings.

There is a link on the website to 'Heart and Lung Sounds'. Follow this link to hear some different breathing sounds to compare with your findings.

As this answer is based on your own observations, there is no outline answer at the end of the chapter.

Following assessment of Mr Morris's breathing, Bridget confirmed signs of circulation by noting the colour and temperature of Mr Morris's skin and by quickly checking his pulse for rhythm and volume as she took his hand. Checking his blood pressure would give more detailed information so Bridget completed her assessment of his circulation by feeling and measuring his pulse rate and blood pressure. Bridget noted Mr Morris's answers to her brief questions, quickly assessing his level of consciousness in relation to disability, and in relation to exposure as she looked at all other areas of his body, feeling where necessary. She could see that his lower legs were swollen.

Bridget also considered other information she had gained on questioning Mr and Mrs Morris and her previous knowledge of his medical history. She recognised that his main problem was breathlessness, but tachycardia, hypotension and leg oedema supported her respiratory assessment to conclude that Mr Morris had worsening heart failure. She now needed to get him the required treatment and care.

Why is oxygen important?

Scenario: Pneumonia

Imagine you are working in the Accident and Emergency Department (A&E) when Siobhan French, a 38-year-old physical education teacher, is brought in with breathing difficulties, pain in her chest and confusion.

(Continued)

continued . . . •

*The paramedics report that she has had influenza-like symptoms for the past four days and seems to be getting worse. They give details of their assessment and interventions: due to her **tachypnoea**, respiratory distress and oxygen saturations of 90%, they have given high-flow oxygen via a non-rebreathing mask (Figure 2.2), and inserted an intravenous cannula into her left hand.*

You see that Siobhan is sitting up and talking, but she appears weak and unable to support herself. You have difficulty getting her to concentrate on what you are telling her and asking her to do. Your mentor asks you to do her observations while she goes to get the doctor, and you find that Siobhan's respiratory rate is 38 bpm. She is still wearing the non-rebreathing oxygen mask that the paramedics gave her and this is delivering oxygen to her at around 70%. Siobhan's oxygen saturations are now 92%. Her pulse rate is 122 bpm and her blood pressure is 105/48 mmHg (normal adult blood pressure 100–140 mmHg systolic, 60–90 mmHg diastolic). She has a temperature of 38.6°C.

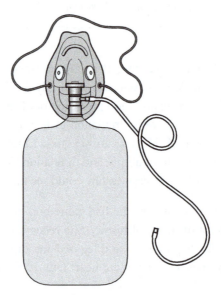

Figure 2.2: A non-rebreathing mask with reservoir bag. The reservoir fills with oxygen and the mask delivers up to 70% oxygen. These masks are used for patients who are in severe respiratory distress

Activity 2.3   *Decision making*

Look carefully at Table 1.1 (on pages 9–10), and identify which level of critical care Siobhan French falls into and give your reasons for your decision. Then, using Table 1.2 (page 12), apply the admission, recognition and response bundles of care to Siobhan.

An outline of how these apply to Siobhan is given at the end of the chapter.

Your main concern for Siobhan is that her SpO_2 levels are too low and have improved only marginally from 90% to 92% since receiving high-flow oxygen at about 70% via the non-rebreathing mask. These levels are worrying because the target saturations for an adult are 94–98%, and in health these are normally achieved without added oxygen (O'Driscoll et al., 2008). It is worth considering the accuracy of the reading, but you note that she is still dyspnoeic, tachypnoeic, tachycardic and confused. These are signs of low blood oxygen levels (hypoxaemia). From your rapid assessment and the track and trigger score, you can calculate that she is at high risk of deterioration.

Siobhan is already receiving high-flow oxygen and you must consider other ways of improving her oxygenation because she has not responded sufficiently; she needs more oxygen delivered to her body cells and you cannot increase the oxygen further by face mask. Despite her blood pressure being borderline low, it is important for her to sit as upright as possible in order to max-imise her pulmonary ventilation (Table 2.2). Gravity helps to increase lung compliance (elasticity) and lung volume by allowing her accessory muscles to work more easily, thus enabling larger breaths for less effort (Fleming and Todd, 1998). Breath size is important as not all inspired air reaches the alveoli. No gas exchange takes place in the nasal passages, trachea, bronchi and bronchioles, known as anatomical dead space, and these constitute approximately 150 ml of inhaled air. It is more effective for Siobhan to increase her breath size, known as tidal volume (the volume of air inhaled and exhaled at each breath), than her respiratory rate (the number of breaths taken within a set amount of time, typically 60 seconds); she is already breathing very fast and is getting tired. She needs to get more oxygen into her blood to cope with the demands of her body cells. The medical team needs to perform further investigations to give an indication of how this might be achieved. These should include a chest X-ray to give a picture of lung infla-tion and blood tests for full blood count (FBC), urea and electrolytes (U&E), liver function tests (LFT), arterial blood gas analysis (ABG) and blood cultures. Together these will give indications of blood oxygen carrying capacity (haemoglobin from FBC), renal function (U&E levels), hydra-tion (U&E levels plus haematocrit from FBC), presence of and response to infection (blood cultures and white cell count from FBC) and Siobhan's ability to exchange inspired oxygen for carbon dioxide (ABG). Arterial blood gas analysis will also indicate the acidity of Siobhan's arterial blood and whether she has progressed to anaerobic metabolism due to reduced oxygenation.

Scenario

Things happen very quickly from this point. Your mentor returns with the doctor and blood is taken to be tested for FBC, U&E, LFT, ABG and blood cultures to rule out causes such as poisoning or renal failure, and to confirm suspected infection as a cause of Siobhan's respiratory distress and altered con-sciousness. Intravenous fluids are commenced and a portable chest X-ray performed as well as a 12-lead electrocardiograph. The anaesthetist who is on call reviews Siobhan and decides that she should be quickly transferred to the high dependency unit with a diagnosis of type I respiratory failure secondary to community-acquired pneumonia. She needs respiratory support to improve her oxygenation and close monitoring of her ABGs, breathing and consciousness. Temperature, heart rate and rhythm, blood pressure, oxygen saturations and fluid balance will also be monitored and recorded, as well as any pain.

How did Siobhan become so ill so quickly when she is so young and usually very fit? Siobhan has been suffering with influenza-like symptoms, most probably from a virulent infection of her upper airways. Bacteria have been aspirated into her lungs during breathing, where they have caused inflammation of the bronchioles and alveoli. The air spaces have filled with exudate (escaping fluid containing cell debris and pus), which in turn filled with white blood cells and fibrin to create a solid mass known as consolidation (Wheeldon, 2013). This blocks inhaled oxygen from contact with the alveolar surface, thus restricting external respiration.

Siobhan reports localised, sharp chest pain known as pleuritic pain, which results from inflammation spreading to the pleura. The pain restricts her ability to take deep breaths and combined with the inefficient external respiration, she has quickly become hypoxaemic and breathless. Despite her young age and usual health, Siobhan's defence mechanisms are failing to cope with the virulence of the infection. Without intervention to control the infection, clear secretions and correct her poor oxygenation, Siobhan is at serious risk of death from pneumonia and respiratory failure. Lim et al. (2009) recommend the CURB65 score to ascertain risk from community-acquired pneumonia. One point is awarded for each symptom.

- C – confusion of new onset.
- U – urea level >7 mmol/litre.
- R – respiratory rate >30 bpm.
- B – blood pressure: systolic <90 mmHg or diastolic <60 mmHg.
- 65 years of age or more.

A score of 2 or more indicates moderate to high risk of death and the need for treatment in hospital with a minimum of 12-hourly medical review, whilst intensive care assessment should be considered for patients scoring 3 or more (NICE, 2014a; Lim et al., 2009).

From the nursing assessment we can see that Siobhan scores a minimum of 3, and following blood results indicating her urea level, she may score 4, confirming the need for level 2 care.

pH	7.37	(7.35–7.45)
$PaCO_2$	5.2	(4.5–6.0 kPa)
PaO_2	7.8	(11.5–13.5 kPa)
HCO_3	21	(24–27 mmol/L)
Base excess	–1.4	(–2–+2)
SpO_2	91%	(97%)

Table 2.3: Siobhan's ABG result with normal values shown in brackets

The clinical examination and chest X-ray confirm Siobhan's diagnosis of pneumonia, and the blood test results indicate how her body is responding and coping with the infection. The ABG analysis gives important information about her blood acidity or alkalinity (pH), levels of oxygen (PaO_2), carbon dioxide ($PaCO_2$) and bicarbonate levels (involved in CO_2 carriage), which are detailed in Table 2.3. The information is relevant to diagnosing the extent of her respiratory failure and shows the degree of deviation from normal. It also gives an accurate arterial oxygen saturation reading. This indicates her respiratory status and metabolic environment (how her cells are working) and gauges the body's ability to maintain homeostasis. Factors other than respiration and gas exchange contribute to this and will be discussed in more detail in Chapter 7.

Types of respiratory failure

Type I respiratory failure is characterised by:

- PaO$_2$ less than 8 kilopascals (kPa);
- low or normal PaCO$_2$.

It is also known as hypoxaemic respiratory failure and can progress to type II respiratory failure if not treated.

Type II respiratory failure is characterised by:

- PaO$_2$ less than 8 kPa;
- PaCO$_2$ more than 5.5 kPa (hypercarbia);
- respiratory acidosis.

Type II respiratory failure is also known as ventilatory respiratory failure.

Type I respiratory failure

Case study

Siobhan's ABG results show that the pH is normal, but tending towards low, her PaCO$_2$ is normal and her PaO$_2$ is low, confirming type I respiratory failure.

Her bicarbonate level is also low.

Siobhan has type I respiratory failure indicated by hypoxaemia. This must be treated to prevent progression to type II respiratory failure and the risk of tissue hypoxia, whereby insufficient oxygen is available for cell metabolism. Without adequate levels of oxygen for aerobic cell metabolism, anaerobic metabolism begins, thus producing lactic acid. Anaerobic metabolism is less efficient, and if prolonged, cells begin to swell and cell death can occur (Kumar and Clark, 2012).

Siobhan is already trying to compensate by breathing faster and trying to increase her pulmonary ventilation. She is receiving as much oxygen as can be given to her via oxygen mask and her SpO$_2$ readings of 92% and her confusion tell us that her body is failing to compensate. NICE (2014a) recommend that she needs dual antibiotic treatment of the infection. Because she is so unwell, the antibiotics will need to be given intravenously and she needs additional interventions such as humidification and nebulisers to loosen the viscous secretions that are blocking external respiration (O'Driscoll et al., 2008). If her cough is too weak to expectorate the thick sputum, Siobhan may need chest physiotherapy, and consideration should be given to controlling her pain to facilitate this. If her condition does not improve and she becomes more tired, she may need respiratory support by non-invasive **ventilation** (NIV), which will help her to take bigger breaths with less effort. This system uses a very tight fitting face mask so that extra air and oxygen can be pushed into the lungs via a series of pipes. The larger breaths help to improve gaseous exchange at the alveoli, whilst Siobhan's demand for oxygen should be reduced due to not needing to work so hard. Similarly, if Siobhan's ability to sustain spontaneous breathing is further reduced, she may need invasive positive pressure ventilation (IPPV) in the intensive care unit. In this instance Siobhan will need to have an endotracheal tube inserted to have her breathing totally controlled by a ventilator (see Chapter 3). Both invasive and non-invasive respiratory support carry risks, so for this reason, it is important to continually monitor Siobhan using the 'Look: Listen: Feel: Measure: Respond' approach. Her respiratory rate, SpO_2 against inspired oxygen, pulse, blood pressure, mental state and temperature should be closely observed and recorded (Lim et al., 2009). Any changes should be reported immediately to prompt a timely response.

You must ensure that measurements recorded are accurate to facilitate administration of the most appropriate treatment and care for Siobhan. Accurate monitoring of SpO_2 requires good peripheral perfusion, which can be assessed by measuring capillary refill. This is the time taken in seconds for colour to return after compressing a fingernail bed (you could practise this on your own fingernail). Capillary refill should be used as part of holistic assessment, although its value is sometimes questioned. In altered pathophysiology states, such as peripheral vascular disease, results can mislead interpretation (Creed and Spiers, 2010). Reliability of oxygen saturations can be affected by poor peripheral perfusion, anaemia, hypothermia, false or painted nails, bright environmental lights or incorrect probe positioning (Creed et al., 2010).

Because Siobhan is acutely ill, her peripheral perfusion may be compromised, affecting the accuracy of her SpO_2 reading. The reading is most significant when considered against the inspired oxygen percentage. A low reading recorded on breathing room air is less worrying than a low reading on high-flow oxygen. As Siobhan is receiving high-flow oxygen, it is important to check her ABGs again to evaluate the effectiveness of any treatment and care. Results should be considered alongside other findings from clinical assessment.

Activity 2.4   *Evidence-based practice and research*

In clinical practice where an oxygen saturations monitor with finger probe is available, ask your mentor if you and a fellow student can experiment to test the accuracy of oxygen saturations measurement on a healthy person (each other). If you ask your teacher you may also be able to do this in your university clinical skills laboratory. Apply the following variances.

- Apply a blood pressure cuff.
- Hold the arm up in the air for a few minutes.

- Apply nail polish.
- Shine a bright light close to the probe.

Note the variations in results of these actions and consider how these things apply to your patients.

As this answer is based on your own observations, there is no outline answer at the end of the chapter.

Type II respiratory failure

Case study: Chronic obstructive pulmonary disease

Pav, a student nurse, was asked to look after 64-year-old Brian Carter who was known to have COPD and previous type II respiratory failure. He was well known on the ward, having been an inpatient on several previous occasions. Three days ago he was admitted with an infected exacerbation of COPD. Following medical review, Brian was prescribed care including intravenous antibiotics, nebulisers, steroid therapy and oxygen at 24% via a venturi device (Figure 2.3) to keep his oxygen saturations above 92%.

Pav went to do Brian's observations and found that he looked quite uncomfortable. On further ABCDE assessment he found Brian's respiratory rate was 36 bpm and his oxygen saturations were reading 88% on his ear probe. His pulse rate was 127 bpm and his blood pressure was 98/52 mmHg. Pav noticed that Brian's fingers were slightly blue and his nose and lips were also rather dusky coloured. Pav tried to comfort Brian and asked how he was feeling, but his answers were difficult to hear because he seemed so short of breath and sounded wheezy. Brian looked as if he was working hard to breathe, pulling his chest up by his shoulders and breathing through pursed lips while his oxygen mask hung around his neck. He looked frightened and his hand was shaking as he reached out for a glass of water.

From Pav's assessment based upon 'Look: Listen: Feel: Measure: Respond', we can deduce that Brian is in respiratory distress. This is a serious situation with risk of further deterioration if appropriate action is not taken. Brian is struggling to get air into his lungs and his oxygen saturation levels are too low, suggesting hypoxaemia and respiratory failure; without ABG analysis to indicate Brian's $PaCO_2$ levels we do not know whether Brian is in type I or type II respiratory failure. Brian is, however, showing signs that he is in type II respiratory failure. We know this because Pav noticed the tachycardia under circulation assessment and under exposure should find dilation of Brian's peripheral veins and hand tremor, which are due to the effects of hypercarbia on the vascular system and central nervous system (Green et al., 2003). Pav now needs to organise his findings to enable him to prioritise his response in order to reduce the risk of Brian deteriorating further.

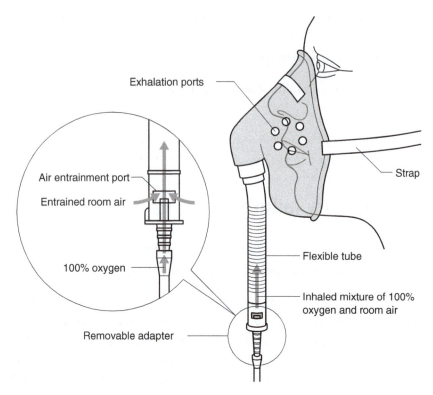

Figure 2.3: Venturi device used to administer controlled oxygen. The inhaled mixture of oxygen and room air comprises varied percentages of oxygen, depending upon the size of the air entrainment port

As a student nurse it is important that he gets help to deal with this situation, but Pav should not leave Brian alone. He can summon his mentor by use of the bedside emergency call bell. The aim is to make breathing easier for Brian, thus improving his oxygenation and reducing his carbon dioxide levels. Considering the different phases of respiration, Pav is able to help with pulmonary ventilation and the supply of oxygen, but is unable to control other respiratory processes.

Case study

Pav explained to Brian what he was going to do and summoned his mentor. He sat Brian more upright by using the profiling action of the bed. He helped Brian to take some sips of water and made sure that the oxygen was flowing through the mask correctly, then replaced it over Brian's nose and mouth. He checked the accuracy of the oxygen saturations probe by repositioning it and continued to observe Brian's breathing effort, rate and depth. When his mentor arrived, Pav asked if he should increase the oxygen in view of Brian's breathlessness and low oxygen saturation readings, but he was advised not to. Instead he was asked to give two litres of oxygen via nasal cannulae while giving Brian an air-driven nebuliser. The mentor asked Pav to stay with Brian to reassure him and to make sure that he breathed in all the nebulised liquid. Pav's mentor also adjusted the bed so that it formed a chair shape. She asked Pav to call her when the nebuliser started to splutter.

> After some time and two further nebulisers, Brian's breathing slowed down and he looked more comfortable. The physiotherapist helped him to have a good cough. He expectorated large amounts of thick green-yellow sputum.

Why did Pav's mentor insist on these interventions for Brian? Sitting Brian upright would immediately make a difference to his pulmonary ventilation (see Table 2.2) by enabling larger breaths for less effort. Lowering his legs and making the bed into a chair shape reduces intra-abdominal pressure, thus allowing more space for chest expansion. As with Siobhan, it is more effective for Brian to increase his breath size than his respiratory rate, thus promoting better intake of oxygen and allowing exhalation of carbon dioxide. Brian may have felt anxious and acutely aware of the effort required to breathe, so it was important that Pav stayed to help and reassure him. The simple act of helping Brian take sips of water relieved the stress of discomfort from a dry mouth, caused by mouth breathing and the use of oxygen.

Once Pav had improved Brian's pulmonary ventilation, quickly checking and replacing Brian's oxygen mask over his nose and mouth would ensure that Brian was receiving the prescribed level of oxygen. Pav could not know how long Brian had been without the extra oxygen, and so it was sensible to check and reposition the oxygen saturations probe to ensure a good pulse was sensed, thus ensuring accuracy of the reading. Pav could then also check that the displayed pulse rate corresponded to Brian's palpated pulse rate.

Even though Brian's oxygen saturations were low at 88%, Pav's mentor was correct to advise him not to increase the oxygen, but to give two litres/min via nasal cannulae while also giving an air-driven nebuliser via a face mask. Inpatients with COPD and the risk of hypercarbic respiratory failure should aim for oxygen saturations of 88–92% using only 24% oxygen via a venturi mask until ABG analysis is available (O'Driscoll et al., 2008). Brian's COPD was longstanding, and whereas hydrogen ions resulting from synthesis of carbon dioxide would normally be a major stimulus for breathing, people such as Brian, with long-term increased carbon dioxide levels, cease to respond to this stimulus. Instead, they depend on stimulation provided by a sensed reduction in oxygen levels (Grossman & Porth, 2013). This means that had Pav increased Brian's oxygen to achieve normal oxygen saturation levels and Brian's chemoreceptors sensed adequate oxygen levels, the stimulus to breathe would be lost, causing Brian to have a respiratory arrest.

Brian's hypoxaemia required continued low-level oxygen therapy to correct it, but it was equally important to reduce his carbon dioxide level. Nebulising prescribed drugs, such as salbutamol and ipratropium bromide to treat bronchoconstriction and reduce air trapping, help to reduce the feeling of breathlessness and aid smoother air flow through the airways (Merritt, 2009). NICE (2010c) recommends increasing the frequency of nebulisers in exacerbations of COPD and to drive them with air in patients at risk of hypercarbic respiratory failure. Pav's mentor gave him accurate instructions and observed guidelines that the nebuliser is ineffective once it starts to splutter (Kelly and Lynes, 2011).

Brian's inability to exhale sufficient carbon dioxide (CO_2 retention) was probably caused by sputum retention, although poor posture and air trapping could also contribute. Physiotherapy can help with clearing sputum by helping to shake it loose, precipitating coughing. Brian was able to do as the physiotherapist asked, cough and expectorate sputum, but had he been unable to do so, insertion of a naso-pharyngeal airway, through which secretions can be removed by suctioning, should be considered. Because Brian was already receiving antibiotic therapy for his exacerbation of COPD, it would be necessary to review their effectiveness in relation to available sputum culture results, which would indicate the antibiotic sensitivity.

Pav was quick to respond to Brian's respiratory distress by immediate ABCDE assessment using the 'Look: Listen: Feel: Measure: Respond' approach. He responded by asking for help, sitting Brian up, ensuring correct oxygen delivery and continually monitoring Brian while he received nebuliser therapy. Pav's interventions under his mentor's guidance were instrumental in preventing deterioration that could have led to the need for NIV (Chapter 3) or respiratory arrest.

Monitoring to prevent breathlessness

Scenario: Asthma

You are working alongside the hospital respiratory nurse specialist and you are asked to gather initial information from patients as they arrive for asthma clinic appointments. You meet 24-year-old Liz Gardiner, who appears anxious, wheezy and a little out of breath. She tells you she has been rushing and that she will be fine in a few minutes.

Activity 2.5	*Critical thinking*

Make a list of the possible causes of Liz's symptoms and try to prioritise them in order of significance from very important to not important. Give reasons for your answer.

A list of symptoms and significance is given at the end of the chapter.

It is important that you observe Liz as she waits to see the respiratory nurse. She may be well enough to walk into the department and be convincing in her story, but she has an appointment time lasting only a few minutes and then she will leave again. You have very little time to determine whether or not Liz has health needs that require immediate attention by way of investigation, intervention or education. Anything that is not attended to now may have to wait six months, and during that time Liz may be at risk of severe respiratory problems leading to hypoxia and associated with uncontrolled asthma, infection or allergy. Any of these may require hospital admission, which would put her more at risk.

Liz already has a diagnosis of asthma: a chronic inflammatory lung disorder that causes obstruction of airflow. The fact that she attends hospital appointments suggests that she has had problems in the past with control of her asthma or acute, life-threatening episodes

(BTS and SIGN, 2014). Liz's breathlessness and wheeze on arrival are significant and warrant further exploration. After allowing her to rest for a few minutes, you should note her degree of recovery and inform the respiratory nurse. She will want to know what triggers Liz's wheeze and **dyspnoea**, the frequency that Liz has been experiencing symptoms such as breathlessness, wheeze, chest tightness or a cough, how she deals with them and how long they last (BTS and SIGN, 2014).

The respiratory nurse should review Liz's use of any asthma medication, such as inhalers for prevention or treatment of symptoms. She should check that Liz uses the correct techniques when using her inhalers, to ensure that medication is effectively administered. Inhaler technique has important clinical consequences and while 98% of people think they use their inhalers correctly, only 8% of people actually do (BTS and SIGN, 2014). Liz may well need some additional advice to improve her technique. Any psychosocial factors that could contribute to exacerbating Liz's asthma should be considered, and it would be useful for Liz to use a peak flow meter to monitor and keep a diary of her peak expiratory flow rate (PEFR). Peak flow measurements give an indication of airway resistance by measuring the force of expiration in litres per minute (Wheeldon, 2013). Normal values of PEFR vary depending upon age, sex and height of the individual, and recordings of 70% of expected value or less indicate airway obstruction (BTS and SIGN, 2014). Peak flow trends are more useful than single values recorded, as they highlight deviations from normal for individual patients. These can serve to warn of potential instability in response to infection or other asthma triggers, thus allowing the patient to take appropriate preventative action. More information on peak flows can be obtained from the peak flow website listed at the end of the chapter.

Identifying the lowest level of treatment to maintain control for Liz's asthma and preventing life-threatening episodes depends upon her understanding her condition, being involved in monitoring and her honesty and concordance with prescribed therapy and health promotion advice, such as inhaler technique. For this reason, the relationship that you develop with Liz on your first encounter could have implications for her lifelong respiratory health.

Activity 2.6 — *Practical health promotion skills*

Visit the Asthma UK website on the link below to see demonstrations of how techniques vary for different kinds of inhalers.

http://www.asthma.org.uk/knowledge-bank-treatment-and-medicines-using-your-inhalers

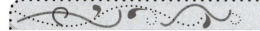

Chapter summary

Within this chapter we have used examples of patient situations to demonstrate why patients become breathless, how we can specifically assess breathing and the most appropriate interventions for some common clinical situations. We have considered patients in a variety of healthcare settings to demonstrate how acute situations can arise and how your response can have a significant impact upon patient outcomes.

Activities: brief outline answers

Activity 2.1: Critical thinking (page 35)

Assessment method	Making note of	Significance
Look	Rate of breaths – how many per minute. Rhythm. Depth. Symmetry. Smoothness. Effort used.	Breathing should be effortless 10–20 breaths per minute. Bradypnoea (>10 bpm) could be a sign of central nervous system depression. Tachypnoea (<20 bpm) could indicate hypoxia but is normal after exercise. Both sides of chest should rise equally and evenly.
	Facial expression – pursed lips, nasal flaring, grimace with pain. Skin colour Use of accessory muscles. Ratio I:E (inspiration time: expiration time). General distress.	Asymmetrical inflation could signify injury, pneumonectomy or pneumothorax. Mucous membranes should be pink and moist; pale mucous membranes could indicate low oxygen saturations or low haemoglobin content. Skin – should be pink and warm. Breathing should not be painful – pain could indicate infection of lungs, airways or inflammation of pleura. Distress, use of accessory muscles and facial expressions are evidence of hypoxia and need for patient to take bigger breaths.
Listen (with and without stethoscope)	Is breathing noisy or quiet? Where does the sound come from: throat, upper or lower airways? What type of sound? At what stage of the breath does the sound occur – inspiration or expiration? Beginning or end? Equality/symmetry. Front and back. Sound of each breath in and out. Airflow noise.	Is normally quiet in clear airways and is quieter on expiration than inspiration. Different noises can indicate bronchospasm (intermittent closing of the airways), blockage, sputum retention, pulmonary oedema. Visit the following website to listen to different breathing sounds. **http://www.littmann.com/wps/portal/3M/en_ US/3M-Littmann/stethoscope/littmann-learning- institute/about-stethoscopes/stethoscope-use** When using a stethoscope you will hear better quality sounds than without. Inability to complete sentences in one breath indicate hypoxia.

	Quality of breath sounds. Ability to speak – how many words?	
Feel	Breath/air movement on hand. Chest expansion – rise and fall. Sensations on chest movement. Skin temperature. Movement.	Feeling for air movement can augment other methods of assessment to confirm what you see or hear, especially if breathing is shallow or you are in a noisy environment. Different sensations can indicate sputum retention (rattles), surgical emphysema (like crepe paper) or pulmonary oedema (boggy). Skin should be warm and dry to touch – cold clammy skin can indicate hypoxia.
Measure	Number of breaths per minute. Size of breaths in millilitres. Force of breaths millilitres per second. Oxygen saturations. Acid base balance results from ABG analysis. Number of words spoken between breaths.	Respiratory rate (RR), number of complete breaths (in and out) per minute, also known as respiration rate, respiratory frequency (R_f), ventilation rate (VR), ventilation frequency (V_f), breathing frequency (B_f) or pulmonary ventilation rate. These abbreviations may be seen on respiratory support equipment. The size in millilitres of a normal exhaled breath (without force) is known as (expiratory) tidal volume. This can only be effectively measured through a tracheostomy or endotracheal tube. Peak flow measures force of breaths and is useful to establish effects of therapy. Oxygen saturations in conjunction with therapy response: 98–100% in normal. 94–98% aim in acute. 88–92% in risk of HRF. Levels of oxygen in peripheral circulation and carbon dioxide in blood = type of respiratory failure. Gives an indication of degree of improvement or deterioration in breathing efficiency.

Table 2.4: Answer to Activity 2.1: different aspects of breathing that can be assessed

Activity 2.3: Decision making (page 38)

Siobhan French has more than one vital sign that falls outside normal ranges – her respiratory rate, pulse rate and temperature are high while her SpO_2 is low and her blood pressure is borderline low. She is currently receiving high-flow oxygen via a non-rebreathing mask and her saturations are still low. This suggests that she will need further support and continued oxygen therapy and continual monitoring.

It is clear that the level 1 indicators apply to Siobhan, but as she is receiving single organ support (respiratory support) she really requires level 2 care and will need to be nursed in the high dependency unit.

Admission bundle   So far you have collected data relating to respirations, oxygen saturations, pulse, blood pressure and temperature, but you need to determine Siobhan's level of consciousness. Because your findings indicate that Siobhan is at high risk of deterioration, you will plan to monitor all of the above parameters continuously, and you will want your medical and nursing colleagues to be aware of these facts.

Recognition bundle   You will be constantly monitoring Siobhan and will have calculated her risk score in relation to your local track and trigger score. This will be high due to the fact that she has abnormalities in all categories. She has several indicators that should trigger consideration of sepsis (see Chapter 7), and you will want to tell the medical team about this.

Response bundle   Siobhan is at high risk of deterioration, so the critical care outreach team need to be contacted urgently. You will need to document and communicate your findings and concerns to them using the SBAR tool.

Activity 2.5: Critical thinking (page 46)

The possible reasons why Liz is anxious, wheezy and out of breath are given in order of importance.

1. She may have a chest infection: secretions and inflammation within the airways as a result of chest infection will narrow her airways and make Liz more prone to bronchospasm, which creates the wheeze. If the wheeze is audible without a stethoscope, it is significant. Wheeze indicates constriction of the airways, thus airflow is restricted and Liz will find it harder to breathe in the oxygen she needs, particularly if she is rushing and using more energy. This is the priority problem as it needs to be treated with antibiotics and Liz will need to temporarily increase the use of her inhalers, making sure that she takes both the preventer and reliever. She will also need to monitor her peak flows to make sure that her asthma symptoms are being adequately controlled. If Liz does not get early treatment for a chest infection, she could have severe respiratory difficulties, leading to hospitalisation and intensive care (BTS and SIGN, 2014).
2. Liz's asthma may not be as well controlled as she says it is. If she is getting anxious prior to her appointment and this is triggering wheeziness and shortness of breath, it is important to ascertain what Liz understands about her asthma symptoms and the medication she takes, how often she takes it, what time of day she takes it and her technique. She may need to increase her medication, she may need to be taught better inhaler techniques or she may not be taking her medication as prescribed. Liz may need some information to help her decision making. She may also need information about peak flow monitoring so that she can see clearly when her asthma is not well controlled. It would be useful to find out what triggers Liz's symptoms and to reiterate when Liz needs to seek help from her doctor or respiratory nurse. Giving Liz good health promotion advice can help to prevent her asthma getting severely out of control and necessitating hospital admission.
3. Liz may have been subjected to an allergen that triggers her asthma symptoms while on her journey. Much of the educational and health promotion information detailed in Answer 2 still applies as it is important that Liz responds quickly when her asthma is triggered.
4. She may just have been rushing and may have had a stressful journey. However, she is clearly showing symptoms of asthma, which should ideally be better controlled. Good health promotion advice is needed as in Answer 2.

Further reading

Higginson, R and Jones, B (2009) Respiratory assessment in critically ill patients: airway and breathing. *British Journal of Nursing,* 18(8): 456–61.

This article gives a good overview of respiratory assessment and the skills needed by ward nurses as well as critical care nurses. There is clear advice about use of oxygen masks.

O'Driscoll, B R, Howard, L S and Davison, A G (2008) *Guidelines for Emergency Oxygen Use in Adult Patients: Executive Summary.* London: British Thoracic Society.

These are the guidelines for oxygen use that should be applied nationally. This is information that all nurses need to know.

Robinson, T and Scullion, J E (2009) *Oxford Handbook of Respiratory Nursing.* Oxford: Oxford University Press.

This book is a pocket-sized resource giving practical advice and current best practice for a range of respiratory conditions.

Useful websites

www.lunguk.org

The British Lung Foundation website has information about most lung conditions, including pneumonia and COPD.

http://www.littmann.com/wps/portal/3M/en_US/3M-Littmann/stethoscope/littmann-learning-institute/about-stethoscopes/stethoscope-use/

The 3M™ Littman® Stethoscopes website offers informative advice about the use and care of stethoscopes as well as having audio clips of heart and lung sounds.

www.peakflow.com/top_nav/normal_values/PEFNorms.html

The Mini-Wright Peak Flow Meter site offers clear information about peak flow monitoring and devices used. There is patient information as well as professional information and links to other useful organisations.

www.asthma.org.uk/index.html

The Asthma UK website gives a lot of information about asthma including inhalers and nebulisers. There is useful information for both professionals and patients.

Chapter 3
The patient who needs respiratory support

Desiree Tait

NMC Standards for Pre-registration Nursing Education

This chapter will address the following competencies:

Domain 3: Nursing practice and decision-making

Generic competencies:

3. All nurses must carry out comprehensive, systematic nursing assessments that take account of relevant physical, social, cultural, psychological, spiritual, genetic and environmental factors, in partnership with service users and others through interaction, observation and measurement.

4. All nurses must ascertain and respond to the physical, social and psychological needs of people, groups and communities. They must then plan, deliver and evaluate safe, competent, person-centred care in partnership with them, paying special attention to changing health needs during different life stages, including progressive illness and death, loss and bereavement.

Field-specific competencies:

3.1. Adult nurses must safely use a range of diagnostic skills, employing appropriate technology, to assess the needs of service users.

4.1. Adult nurses must safely use invasive and non-invasive procedures, medical devices, and current technological and pharmacological interventions, where relevant, in medical and surgical nursing practice, providing information and taking account of individual needs and preferences.

NMC Essential Skills Clusters

This chapter will address the following ESCs:

Cluster: Care, compassion and communication

3. People can trust the newly registered graduate nurse to respect them as individuals and strive to help them preserve their dignity at all times.

By entry to the register:

v.   Is proactive in promoting and maintaining dignity.

> ## Chapter aims
>
> By the end of this chapter, you should be able to:
>
> - identify why patients may need advanced respiratory (ventilatory) support;
> - demonstrate an awareness of the importance of arterial blood gas analysis in the management of patients with respiratory failure;
> - describe non-invasive ventilation (NIV) and mechanical invasive ventilation (MIV);
> - demonstrate an awareness of the factors influencing the choice of appropriate respiratory support;
> - describe the fundamentals of providing a safe holistic approach to caring for patients receiving NIV and MIV.

Introduction

In this chapter you are introduced to Mrs Jenny Matthews. She is 43 years old and for 20 years has had a history of acute exacerbation of asthma. She had eczema as a child and hay fever but wasn't diagnosed with asthma until she was in her twenties. We will follow her on her journey through healthcare as she experiences an acute exacerbation of asthma. The scenario box below provides a summary of her admission to the emergency department.

> ## Scenario: Jenny Matthews
>
> ### Situation
> *Mrs Jenny Matthews, age 43 years.*
>
> *Admitted to the emergency department with a seven-day history of shortness of breath and productive cough. She had previously been seen by her GP and treated with a combination of broad spectrum antibiotics and an increased dose of salbutamol. She was progressing well at home but a sudden onset of increased shortness of breath at 2 a.m. on the morning of the eighth day prompted a 999 call for help from her husband.*
>
> ### Background
> *History of acute asthma for 20 years. Jenny has been admitted to hospital on five occasions during the last seven years. On the last occasion she required emergency intubation and ventilation, staying in intensive care for 48 hours.*
>
> *She did smoke 30 cigarettes a day for 22 years but has reduced this to ten a day. She has a strong family history of reactive airways disease.*
>
> ### Assessment in the emergency room
> Airway (A):   *Patient is agitated and struggling to breathe.*
> Breathing (B): *Dyspnoea, with use of her accessory muscles.*
>   *Unable to complete a full sentence when responding to questions.*
>
> *(Continued)*

continued . . . .

Chest auscultation indicates an expiratory wheeze and bilateral crackles.

Respiration (R): 36 bpm.

SpO₂ 91%.

Blood gases showed:

PH: 7.42

PaO₂: 8.7 kPa

PaCo₂: 3.6 kPa

HCO₃: 24 mmol/L.

Peak expiratory flow rate (PEF): 120 ml/min (Jenny's normal PEF: 300 ml/min).

Circulation (C): HR: 125/min.

BP: 125/72 mmHg.

Disability (D): Blood glucose: 6.8 mmol/L.

Alert and agitated.

Exposure (E): Temp: 37.4°C.

Recommendation

Humidified high-flow oxygen 60%.

Salbutamol 5 mg nebulisers continuously until improvement in PEF.

Hydrocortisone 100 mg IV.

Aminophylline infusion.

IV antibiotics.

Plan to transfer to high dependency for monitoring and evaluation of her treatment.

Jenny's husband, Brendan, has arrived and when he is informed that she needs to be admitted to the high dependency unit he becomes very angry and starts shouting at his wife 'I told you this would happen, I've had enough of this! Why didn't you just give up smoking! I'm going home, you're on your own now!' Jenny seems not to be listening and Brendan Matthews is asked to leave. The staff invite him to stay in a quiet room and approach him for more information. At this point he refuses to stay and instead gives the GP's address and Jenny's parents' phone number saying that he has had enough and he's leaving her.

Why did Jenny's situation deteriorate at home and lead to an emergency admission to HDU?

Less than 24 hours ago Jenny was seemingly making a good recovery from a chest infection when she experienced a sudden deterioration in her condition. Asthma is a chronic inflammatory disorder of the mucosal lining of the bronchi which is associated with bronchial hyper-responsiveness, reversible airway constriction and variable airflow obstruction (McCance and Huether, 2014). Factors involved in triggering an acute asthma attack can include:

- evidence of a family history of asthma;

- exposure to an allergen;

- urban residence;

- air pollution;

- tobacco smoke;

- recurrent respiratory tract infections;

- psychological factors and anxiety.

In Jenny's case, after seven days of antibiotic treatment, she decided it was time to resume smoking, as this was her main way of coping with the stresses of life. This triggered a long and aggressive argument with her husband that continued over the course of the evening. It was later that night that Jenny developed the acute exacerbation of asthma reported in her story. According to Polosa and Thompson (2013) cigarette smoking in asthma is associated with a higher frequency and severity of exacerbations and a higher risk of mortality than non-smokers. There is also evidence to suggest that anxiety and depression is often associated with smoking and an increased frequency of exacerbations for patients with asthma (Leader et al., 2014). For Jenny, the combination of tobacco smoke, stress, a recent respiratory tract infection and her family history combined to trigger the asthma attack.

When Jenny was admitted to the emergency room she was presenting signs and symptoms of the 'early response' phase. According to McCance and Huether (2014) this phase is initiated by exposure to the inhaled irritant and triggers a cascade of inflammatory events that lead to acute and chronic airway dysfunction. The combined impact of mast cell activation releasing vasoactive mediators with degranulation of their inflammatory mediators and an immune activation, leads to:

- vasodilation and increased capillary permeability;

- vascular congestion;

- bronchospasm;

- increased contractile response of the bronchial smooth muscle;

- mucus secretion;

- thickening of airway walls.

This cascade of events leads to bronchial hyper-responsiveness and airway obstruction.

For Jenny the presence of a PEF of less than 50% of her predicted normal range, a respiratory rate of 36 bpm, a pulse of 125 bpm and an inability to complete a sentence in one breath indicated the presence of acute severe asthma (BTS and SIGN, 2014). With oxygen saturations of 91% and signs of type 1 respiratory failure indicated by her arterial blood gas result of PaO_2 8.7 kPa (see Chapter 2), Jenny's condition was becoming life threatening and she required high dependency (level 2) care (BTS and SIGN, 2014).

Why are the arterial blood gas results significant?

In the body, acids (substances that release hydrogen ions (H^+) in solution) are constantly being produced as by-products of normal cell metabolism. For example, the metabolism of proteins produces acids such as sulphuric acid and hydrochloric acid. During the metabolism of carbohydrates about 15,000 mmol of carbon dioxide (CO_2) is produced each day, and although it is not an acid, it is influential in maintaining pH balance.

Carbon dioxide is transported in the circulation in the following ways.

- 20% of CO_2 is attached to haemoglobin and carried as carbaminohaemoglobin ($HHbCO_2$).
- 10% is dissolved in the plasma as carbonic acid (H_2CO_3).
- 70% of CO_2 is carried as a bicarbonate base (a substance that uses up hydrogen ions). Carbonic acid in the presence of an enzyme called carbonic anhydrase is converted to bicarbonate ions (HCO_3^-) and hydrogen ions (H^+).

The relationship between carbonic acid and bicarbonate is a very important factor in how the body regulates the pH (the calculated acidity of the blood) in the circulation, as well as other buffer systems such as the kidney and renal excretion of hydrogen ions. In order to maintain a pH of 7.4 (normal blood pH) the ratio between carbonic acid and bicarbonate should stay at one part carbonic acid to 20 parts bicarbonate ($1\ H_2CO_3 : 20\ HCO3^- + H^+$). This means that if the amount of $HCO3^-$ in the blood falls so must the amount of H_2CO_3 in order to maintain a ratio of 1:20. The body achieves this by increasing the rate and depth of respiration so that more CO_2 is eliminated through respiration and the ratio is maintained. This is called respiratory compensation and can be seen in patients who are producing an excess of metabolic acids such as lactic acid in shock (Chapters 6 and 7) and ketone acid in diabetic ketoacidosis (Chapters 8 and 12).

Left in the circulation, an imbalance in acids or bases would destroy cells and organs, so it is imperative the body has ways to maintain a pH balance at a pH value of between 7.35 and 7.45 in order to maintain normal cell function (Hall, 2011). Should the pH value fall above or below this range, the impact on the body can be critical and in extreme cases lead to death. The body also needs to maintain acid-base balance inside cells so that cells continue to function effectively and intracellular proteins, such as haemoglobin, help to buffer acids inside cells.

What should we be monitoring?

The results obtained from analysis of arterial blood provides information about a number of factors involved in the process of acid-base balance as well as information about the amount of oxygen available to the cells. These include:

- pH value of arterial blood;
- the amount of O_2 in arterial blood (expressed as the partial pressure of oxygen or PaO_2);

- the amount of CO_2 in arterial blood (expressed as the partial pressure of carbon dioxide or $PaCO_2$);

- the amount of bicarbonate and bases available to buffer acids in arterial blood (expressed as mmol/l);

- arterial blood potassium levels;

- arterial haemoglobin;

- blood urea nitrogen, creatinine and glomerular filtration rate to monitor kidney function.

Why are these values important?

The body has a number of ways of maintaining the acid-base balance in health and we will look at five now.

Buffer systems are control mechanisms that can either increase or decrease the number of hydrogen ions in a solution, thus making the solution more acid if the hydrogen ions increase in number or more alkaline if the hydrogen ions are reduced in number (Mattson Porth and Matfin, 2009). These include:

- inside cells proteins act as buffer systems such as the plasma proteins;

- in the circulation it is the bicarbonate buffer system that converts a strong acid that releases large numbers of H^+ to a weak acid that releases much fewer H^+. For example, hydrochloric acid (HCL: strong acid) can be substituted by carbonic acid (H_2CO_3: weak acid), thus reducing the overall H^+:

$$HCl + NaHCO_3 \rightleftharpoons H_2CO_3 + NaCl$$
(sodium bicarbonate)   (sodium chloride)

This equation is reversible and is accelerated by the presence of the enzyme carbonic anhydrase. The carbonic acid produced dissociates into H^+ and HCO_3^- (bicarbonate ions). The H^+ combines with haemoglobin and the bicarbonate diffuses into plasma where it continues to participate in buffering acids.

Respiratory control mechanisms act as another line of defence against alterations in acid-base balance. An increase in ventilation decreases levels of CO_2 in the circulation and a decrease in ventilation increases CO_2 in the blood. Chemoreceptors in the brain stem, carotid and aortic bodies (see Figure 6.1, page 134) sense changes in CO_2, hydrogen ions and O_2 and alter the respiratory rate accordingly. The respiratory control of pH is rapid and occurs within minutes of a change in pH balance but is only approximately 50–70% effective as a buffer system. It is the second line of defence against large changes in pH.

Renal control mechanisms are slower to react but can continue to function for days until the pH value has returned to the normal range. The mechanisms are:

- reabsorption of bicarbonate ions into the circulation;

- excretion of hydrogen ions from acids produced as a result of protein and fat metabolism.

Buffers are the body's first line of defence	The lungs are the body's second line of defence	The kidneys are the body's third line of defence
They act within seconds	They act within seconds to minutes	They act more slowly, measured in hours and days
They remove or release H^+ to correct acid-base balance	They eliminate or retain CO_2 to maintain the ratio of carbonic acid to bicarbonate at 1:20	The have a number of functions: – retention of carbonate ions – elimination of H^+

Table 3.1: How the body defends against abnormal alterations in acid-base balance

Hydrogen-potassium exchange: when there is excess H^+ in the blood, some is able to move into cells in exchange for potassium ions (K^+), and when there is excess K^+ in the blood, it moves into cells and exchanges with H^+. Thus potassium levels and hydrogen levels can change dramatically in some clinical situations such as a patient with diabetic ketoacidosis (see Chapter 8).

Blood urea nitrogen (BUN), creatinine and glomerular filtration rate through creatinine clearance: the measurement of creatinine and glomerular filtration rate are very important measures of renal function and will give an indication of how efficient the patient's kidney function is. If the patient has impaired kidney function the ability for the kidneys to act as the third line of defence in maintaining acid-base balance is impaired. A metabolic acidosis in the context of other indicators can suggest acute kidney injury or chronic renal disease (see Chapter 9).

What do these values tell us?

The pH value determines the presence of acidaemia and alkalaemia.

- Acidaemia: pH <7.35 (a value below 7.35).
- Alkalaemia: pH >7.45 (a value above 7.45).

The partial pressures of oxygen and carbon dioxide give a measure of respiratory function and the presence of respiratory acidosis/alkalosis.

- **Respiratory acidosis:**
  - pH <7.35 and $PaCO_2$ >6.0 kPa;
  - dyspnoea/increased or decreased respiratory function;
  - headache;
  - restlessness, confusion;
  - drowsiness/unconsciousness;
  - tachycardia and arrhythmias.
- **Respiratory alkalosis:**
  - pH >7.45 and $PaCO_2$ <4.9 kPa;
  - feeling light-headed;

o numbness and tingling in the mouth and peripheries;

o inability to concentrate, confusion;

o palpitations.

The levels of bicarbonate and base excess give a measure of metabolic function and represent either a failure to buffer hydrogen ion concentrations with bases leading to acidosis or a failure to buffer bicarbonate concentrations with acids leading to an alkalosis.

- **Metabolic acidosis:**

  o pH <7.35 and HCO_3 <22 mmol/L;

  o headache;

  o restlessness, confusion;

  o coma;

  o cardiac arrhythmias;

  o Kussmaul respirations (rapid shallow)/**respiratory depression**;

  o skin warm and flushed.

- **Metabolic alkalosis:**

  o pH >7.45 and HCO_3 >27 mmol/L;

  o muscle twitching and cramps;

  o feeling dizzy;

  o confusion;

  o lethargy;

  o seizures/coma;

  o nausea and vomiting.

In Table 3.2 you will find clinical examples of patients who have experienced an acid-base imbalance.

What does Jenny's arterial blood gas result tell us about her condition?

By using the step-by-step guide in Table 3.3, an analysis of Jenny's arterial blood gas results and general condition indicate the following.

- **Step 1: Assess oxygenation**

  PaO2 – 8.7 kPa: there is evidence of hypoxaemia with SpO_2 91% with supplemental oxygen of 60%.

- **Step 2: Assess pH level**

  pH – 7.42: there is no evidence of respiratory acidosis or alkalosis.

- **Step 3: Assess respiratory component**

  $PaCo_2$ – 3.6 kPa: this indicates that Jenny has been hyperventilating and expiring CO_2 in an attempt to cope with reduced volumes of air movement in her lungs due to bronchospasm. This is supported by her reduced peak expiratory flow rate (PEF) of 120 ml/min (her normal PEF: 300 ml/min).

Arterial blood gas analysis	Patient examples
Respiratory acidosis: pH <7.35 $PaCO_2$ >6.0 kPa	Gladys Cabrera (62 years) suffers from COPD and she is admitted to hospital with an acute exacerbation of her condition. She is unable to talk due to her breathlessness, rate of 40 bpm, SpO_2 is 72%, she is centrally cyanosed and she is unable to respond to commands. The results of an arterial blood sample are: pH 7.29, PaO_2 4.8 kPa, $PaCO_2$ 8.4 kPa, HCO_3 28.5 mmol/L. Following a rapid assessment of Gladys's condition she was admitted to intensive care for respiratory support and intensive treatment for type II respiratory failure (see Chapter 2).
Respiratory alkalosis: pH >7.45 $PaCO_2$ <4.9 kPa	Joan Butcher (50 years) suffers from anxiety attacks, and these have become worse since progressing to the menopause. On this occasion she has been involved in a minor road traffic collision and she has no obvious injuries. However, when the paramedics arrived at the scene they found her to be breathless and disorientated. She was complaining of pins and needles in her hands and arms, and she felt she couldn't get her breath. Joan was taken to accident and emergency where her arterial blood gas result following admission was: pH: 7.49; $PaCO_2$: 3.2 kPa; HCO_3: 24.2 mmol/L; BE (base excess): −1.0. Joan was hyperventilating and needed to be encouraged to reduce her respiratory rate and allow her carbon dioxide levels to rise back to normal levels.
Metabolic acidosis: pH <7.3 HCO_3 <22 mmol/L	Mary Bevan (58 years) was found by her neighbour lying at the front door in a drowsy and confused state. Mary has type 2 diabetes and has recently developed a severe infection on her leg. Mary's neighbour called the emergency services and Mary was admitted to accident and emergency. Her arterial blood gas following admission was: pH: 7.24; $PaCO_2$: 3.8 kPa; HCO_3: 15.1 mmol/L; BE: −13.7. Mary had Kussmaul respirations at a rate of 35 bpm and a blood glucose of 22 mmol/L. Mary had developed a metabolic acidosis secondary to infection that triggered an increase in blood glucose that necessitated management with insulin.

| Metabolic alkalosis:

pH >7.45
HCO$_3$ >26 mmol/L | Gary Smith (54 years) has been suffering from indigestion-type pain for several days. Rather than go to the GP he has been treating himself with large doses of antacids such as bicarbonate of soda. That afternoon he felt nauseated, weak and tired and still had the persistent indigestion. He visited the GP who decided to admit him to hospital for an assessment of his chest pain. His arterial blood gas following admission was:

pH: 7.49; PaCO$_2$: 5.6 kPa; HCO$_3$: 29.7 mmol/L; BE: +9.0. |
| Respiratory and metabolic acidosis:

pH <7.35
PaCO$_2$ >6.0 kPa
HCO$_3$ <22 mmol/L | Peter Baker (41 years) was admitted to an acute ward with a history of abdominal pain, nausea and vomiting. Peter's condition deteriorated during the first 24 hours, and that evening he had a cardiac arrest. He was resuscitated and transferred to ICU for respiratory support and management of acute pancreatitis. His arterial blood gas following admission was:

pH: 7.15; PaCO$_2$: 7.6 kPa; HCO$_3$: 16.7 mmol/L; BE: −9.8.

Peter has developed a combined acidosis as a result of his cardiac arrest (failed respiration) and severe sepsis associated with pancreatitis and lactic acidosis (see Chapter 7). |

Table 3.2: Clinical examples of patients with changes in acid-base balance

- **Step 4: Assess the metabolic component**

HCO_3- 24 mmol/L: this indicates that Jenny has no evidence of metabolic acidosis or alkalosis.

- **Step 5: Combine your findings**

Jenny is not experiencing any form of acidosis or alkalosis based on these blood gas results, however, the presence of a $PaCo_2$ of 3.6 kPa indicates that Jenny's hyperventilation and lower than normal $PaCo_2$ is correcting any potential for acidosis.

- **Step 6: Clinical interpretation and recommendation**

Clinically Jenny is showing signs of type I respiratory failure (see Chapter 2), she is experiencing increased work of breathing and a reducing peak expiratory flow. The combination of salbutamol (bronchodilation) nebulisers and hydrocortisone will have a direct anti-inflammatory effect on her hypersensitive bronchi and should relieve her symptoms. Jenny, however, continues to be at risk of an escalation of her condition due to a secondary or late response to the initial trigger and requires close monitoring and support during this critical stage (BTS and SIGN, 2014; McCance and Huether, 2014).

Always risk assess	Look: Listen: Feel: Measure
ABG: Step 1 Assess oxygenation. • Normal: PaO_2 11.5–13.5 kPa	• Is there evidence of hypoxaemia? • Is there evidence of high levels of oxygenation? • Is the patient receiving supplemental oxygen?
ABG: Step 2 Assess pH level. • Normal: 7.35–7.45	• Is there evidence of acidosis? pH <7.35 • Is there evidence of alkalosis? pH >7.45
ABG: Step 3 Assess the respiratory component. • $PaCO_2$: 4.5–6.0 kPa	• Is the $PaCO_2$ <4.5 kPa? • Is the $PaCO_2$ >6.0 kPa?
ABG: Step 4 Assess the metabolic component. • HCO_3_-: 22–27 mmol/L	• Is the HCO_3 <22 mmol/L? • Is the HCO_3 >27 mmol/L? • The base excess level (BE) is the quantity of acid or base required to restore the pH to 7.4. Base excess will mirror the bicarbonate level and simply reinforces evidence of a metabolic component (Jevon and Ewens, 2007).

ABG: Step 5
Combine your findings
	• Combine your findings from steps 2/3/4 and identify if there is evidence of:
	   ○ respiratory acidosis;
	   ○ respiratory alkalosis;
	   ○ metabolic acidosis;
	   ○ metabolic alkalosis;

	• signs that the respiratory system has compensated for a metabolic acidosis by increasing the respiratory rate and reducing the CO_2 level; • signs that the renal system has compensated for chronic respiratory acidosis by increasing the level of HCO_3.
ABG: Step 6 Clinical interpretation and recommendation	• Interpret the ABGs in the context of all available patient data.

Table 3.3: A step-by-step approach to assessing arterial blood gas results (ABG)

Activity 3.1   *Decision making*

Read the scenario below and think about the significance of the arterial blood gas results.

Joseph Baglio (age 68 years) has smoked 40 cigarettes a day since his twenties and has experienced angina on exertion for the last five years although this has been managed by the use of beta blockers and GTN. He was admitted to the medical ward six hours ago following a diagnosis of pneumonia. Following his admission he seemed to be responding well to the oxygen therapy and IV antibiotics when he pressed the buzzer and fell forward clutching his chest. When the nurse arrived she found that Joseph was unresponsive with absent respirations and pulse. A cardiac arrest call was placed and he was resuscitated successfully. His arterial blood gas results 30 minutes after his resuscitation were:

pH: 7.05
PaO_2: 8.5 kPa on 60% high-flow oxygen (SpO_2 82%)
$PaCO_2$: 14.1 kPa
HCO_3: 20.5 mmol/L
BE: −3.0
Joseph was conscious, flushed and anxious. His vital signs were T: 38.0°C, R: 32/min, P: 95, BP: 110/70 mmHg.

• Using the step-by-step guide in Table 3.3, what can you interpret from the arterial blood gas result?

One hour later Joseph was conscious but confused. His skin was cold and clammy to touch and his vital signs were T: 38.0°C, R: 32/min, P: 94, BP: 110/70 mmHg. He was receiving 60% humidified high-flow oxygen and diagnosed with acute coronary

(Continued)

continued . . . . •

syndrome with evidence of ST elevation myocardial infarction (STEMI). As well as his beta blockers, he has been prescribed statins for reducing cholesterol (he had previously refused to commence statins when prescribed before), clopidogrel to reduce the risk of another thrombotic event and morphine and nitrates for chest pain. Joseph was not considered a suitable candidate for percutaneous coronary angiography because of his pneumonia and was assessed as a candidate for thrombolysis instead but this was also decided against in light of his traumatic resuscitation. He now had two acute morbidities affecting his respiratory and cardiac system. A second arterial blood gas result was:

pH: 7.20
PaO_2: 9.4k Pa (SpO_2 89%)
$PaCO_2$: 6.70 kPa
HCO_3: 21.4 mmol/L

- Using the step-by-step guide in Table 3.3, what can you interpret from the arterial blood gas result?
- What are your priorities of care for this patient?

Answers are given at the end of the chapter.

With reference to Jenny's story we can see the importance of using a holistic approach to rapid assessment. There are a number of factors that now become significant when monitoring Jenny's condition. For example we know that:

- Jenny has now been awake and fighting for breath since 2 a.m. and it is now 4 a.m.;
- she is emotionally distressed after her husband appears to have left her;
- she is still recovering from an acute respiratory infection and is presenting with type I respiratory failure and about to be transferred to high dependency care.

Case study: Jenny's transfer to HDU

Following her assessment in the emergency room, Jenny was considered to be a level 2 patient requiring high dependency care for assessment and monitoring of her respiratory system. Following admission to HDU the results of her assessment were as follows.

A: *Responding to commands and maintaining her airway.*
B: *SpO_2: 91%*
    60% high-flow humidified O_2
    R: 36/min
    ABGs:
    pH 7.36

> *PaO₂ 8.8 kPa*
>
> *PaCo₂ 4.2 kPa*
>
> C: *HR: 128/min*
>
>   *BP: 130/72 mmHg*
>
> D: *Blood glucose 6.7 mmol/L*
>
>   *Agitated but disorientated*
>
> E: *Temp: 37.5°C*

According to BTS and SIGN (2014), the evidence of a severe hypoxia in the presence of a normalizing $PaCO_2$, and persistent disorientation following intensive treatment, indicates Jenny is having a life-threatening attack. She has been prescribed a once only dose of intravenous magnesium sulphate in an attempt to produce further bronchodilation (Blitz et al., 2005). When her current situation is assessed in the context of her previous admission to ICU, Jenny is referred to the ICU specialist who suggests that she meets the criteria for non-invasive ventilation (NIV) and that commencement of NIV could prevent her from needing intubation and invasive ventilation (Lim et al., 2012). The plan for Jenny is to commence her on NIV and monitor her ABCDE continuously for signs of improvement or deterioration.

What is NIV and why is it appropriate to use this respiratory support for Jenny?

Pulmonary ventilation, or breathing, is essential for life, and the purpose of NIV is to provide varying levels of positive pressure air flow through a tight-fitting mask in order to improve the patient's levels of PaO_2 and $PaCO_2$. Breathing involves the inhalation of gases in air into the lungs and exhalation of gases from the lungs into the atmosphere. All gases in air collectively exert a pressure known as atmospheric pressure. The gases in the lungs also exert a pressure known as alveolar pressure. In air, gases always flow from an area of high pressure to an area of low pressure. During inspiration the thoracic space expands as a result of contraction of the intercostal muscles and diaphragm. This increase in space reduces the overall alveolar pressure in the lungs and air flows into the airways in order to equalise the pressure. Expiration involves relaxation of the respiratory muscles and natural elastic recoil of the lung tissue so that air flows back into the atmosphere. Normal breathing therefore relies on negative pressure ventilation.

For 120 years the principal method of supporting ventilation for patients with respiratory failure was based on the principle of negative pressure ventilation. For example, the **iron lung** was used successfully for patients with respiratory failure caused by neuromuscular diseases such as polio. In the 1950s, during the polio epidemic in Europe, the demand for iron lungs outstripped supply and alternative methods for providing respiratory support were attempted (Lassen et al., 1954). This led to the development of mechanical **invasive ventilation** (MIV), which involved air being forced under pressure into patients' lungs via a tracheostomy tube or endotracheal tube at a rate of between 10 and 20 per minute in order to mimic normal respiration. This dramatically reduced the mortality rate of patients suffering from respiratory failure and became the mainstay treatment (Borthwick et al., 2003).

In the last 25 years the use of non-invasive positive pressure ventilation (NIV) techniques that supply air through a tight-fitting face mask rather than a tube have escalated, and this method has now become the first-line therapy for adult patients with:

- sleep apnoea;
- acute exacerbations of COPD;
- pulmonary oedema;
- neuromuscular disease;
- pneumonia;
- weaning from MIV (BTS, 2000; BTS, 2008; NICE, 2010c).

In Jenny's case the use of NIV to manage an acute severe asthma attack does not have such a strong evidence base (Medoff, 2008). However, BTS and SIGN (2014) recommend that it should be considered as an option to prevent the risk of intubation in patients with acute severe asthma but should be based on skilled clinical assessment and knowledge of the patient's condition. Jenny's respiratory function is compromised but not so impaired that she is in imminent danger of complete respiratory collapse. She is able to protect her own airway, has only mild disorientation and there is no evidence of a pneumothorax on chest X-ray (Medoff, 2008). The types of NIV and their use are explained in Table 3.4.

Activity 3.2   *Reflection*

Reflect back on patients you have nursed and ask yourself the following questions.

- Have I looked after patients with acute respiratory failure either in hospital or the community?
- If so, how did I assess and document the patient care?
- Did the patient need support with oxygen therapy or NIV?
- Did the patient have support from the physiotherapist, dietitian and respiratory nurse?

Hint: This reflection is meant to encourage you to think critically about assessing and managing care and should help you to identify good practice and areas for improvement.

As this answer is based on your own reflection, there is no outline answer at the end of the chapter.

Contraindications for using NIV

The success of NIV techniques in the support of respiratory function relies on effective patient selection. For Jenny, CPAP (can also be referred to as pressure support when given through some ventilators) was chosen as the optimum treatment regime, but this does not mean that the use of NIV will always lead to a successful outcome for every patient. Patients need to be risk assessed

Type of NIV	Benefits	Risks	Patient examples
Continuous positive airways pressure: CPAP. This method provides a continuous flow of positive pressure even at the end of expiration so that some air always remains trapped in the alveoli. This enables oxygen exchange to continue during the whole respiratory cycle and prevents alveolar collapse (atelectasis).	• Improves oxygenation in patients with type I respiratory failure. • Reduces the risk of atelectasis.	• There is reduced clearance of CO_2 due to air being trapped in the alveoli. Not suitable for patients with type II respiratory failure where there are increased levels of CO_2. • The airway is not protected so patients must be able to maintain their own airway.	• Mrs Smith is admitted with severe breathlessness and is producing excessive amounts of pink frothy secretions from her airways. She is diagnosed with acute pulmonary oedema and is commenced on CPAP starting at 5 cm H_2O as part of her ongoing treatment to reduce pulmonary secretions by increasing alveolar pressure to above capillary hydrostatic pressure. • Chao Chan is diagnosed with pneumonia and type I respiratory failure. His PaO_2 is 6.2 kPa and his $PaCO_2$ is 3.6 kPa. He is commenced on CPAP at 5 and then 10 cm H_2O. • Bryn Jones has been diagnosed with **obstructive sleep apnoea**. He suffers from morbid obesity, snoring and daytime fatigue. He has now been fitted with a face mask and CPAP machine for home use. The equipment delivers CPAP at 10 cm H_2O, to be used at night while sleeping.

(Continued)

Table 3.4   (Continued)

Type of NIV	Benefits	Risks	Patient examples
Bilevel NIV or bilevel positive airways pressure ventilation: BiPAP. This method provides two alternating levels of positive pressure during respiration. During inspiration, there is an inspired pressure level (IPAP) and during expiration, an expired pressure level (EPAP).	• Improves oxygenation and CO_2 clearance in patients with type II respiratory failure. • IPAP reduces the work of breathing and conserves the use of oxygen by the body. • A lower EPAP pressure reduces air trapping but still allows continuous gas exchange during respiration while preventing atelactasis.	• The airway is not protected so patients must be able to maintain their own airway.	• Henry Jones has pneumonia. His PaO_2 is 6.8 kPa and his $PaCO_2$ is 6.5 kPa. He is breathless and agitated. He is commenced on BiPAP with an inspiratory pressure of 10 cm H_2O and an expiratory pressure of 4 cm H_2O. • Gladys Cabrera (62 years) suffers from COPD and she is admitted to hospital with an acute exacerbation of her condition. She was commenced on BiPAP at an inspiration pressure (IPAP) of 12 cm H_2O and an expired pressure (EPAP) of 5 cm H_2O with 40% oxygen. She didn't like the face mask but was prepared to give it a try as long as the nurse reminded her.

Table 3.4: Types of non-invasive ventilation and their use

for any contraindications before commencing the therapy and then risk assessed for evidence of any change or deterioration in their condition. This is illustrated in Table 3.5. The contraindications of NIV rarely exist in isolation: often patients will present with one or more of these factors. Knowing the patient and their medical history is an essential part of the rapid decision-making process required when determining a patient's suitability for NIV and relies on good communication between all the carers involved (RCP et al., 2008). Contraindications include:

- life-threatening hypoxaemia;
- severe confusion/agitation/cognitive impairment;
- unconscious patient;
- airway obstruction due to vomiting or a foreign object;
- facial trauma/burns/surgery;
- **pneumothorax**;
- patient unable to protect their own airway;
- copious amounts of respiratory secretions/sputum;
- recent surgery in the upper gastro-intestinal tract;
- severe co-morbidity;
- haemodynamic instability;
- presence of bowel obstruction.

Table 3.5 offers a summary of the risk assessment and nursing interventions required to care for patients receiving NIV.

Risk assessment	Nursing interventions
Contraindications for use of NIV	• Rapid assessment of ABCDE using 'Look: Listen: Feel: Measure' is important to measure the risk of contraindications to treatment with NIV. In particular, the risk of pneumothorax should be ruled out by reviewing the patient's chest X-ray following their admission. • A patient may decide to refuse treatment.
Preparation of the patient and technology	• If the patient has consented and is able to proceed, ensure the equipment has been prepared and checked to ensure it is in working order. • Sit the patient upright and, with their cooperation, attach the face mask. The patient will need a few minutes to get used to the mask. Often NIV is commenced at a low level and increased according to the clinical state of the patient (RCP et al., 2008). • Document baseline clinical data. • Agree and document a treatment plan for escalating and identifying a ceiling of treatment.

(Continued)

Table 3.5   (Continued)

Risk assessment	Nursing interventions

Airway and respirations	• Monitor the patient's airway and respiratory rate, look for signs of respiratory distress and air entry as illustrated in Figure 2.1, page 36.
	• Monitor SpO_2 for evidence of improvement or deterioration.
	• Monitor the patient's arterial blood gas results after:
	  ○ one hour: if there is no change in the patient's condition or a slight improvement, then monitor again in four hours;
	  ○ one hour: if there is a deterioration in the patient's condition:
	    ○ assess patient and check the equipment;
	    ○ consider either increasing the oxygen or pressures;
	    ○ consider a change to mechanical ventilation.

Haemodynamic state	• The increase in pulmonary airway pressure from NIV can cause a rebound reduction in the patient's blood pressure, particularly with CPAP pressures above 10 cm H_2O. • Monitor the patient's blood pressure every five minutes during the first 30 minutes and then at 30 minutes to hourly as the patient's blood pressure stabilises. Continuous arterial monitoring of blood pressure provides an effective way to monitor BP as well as obtaining arterial samples for blood gas analysis.
Mental state and level of consciousness	• Monitor for signs of increased confusion or agitation. Any deterioration in level of consciousness is an indication that the NIV should be discontinued and the treatment plan utilised. • Patients on NIV should not normally be sedated as this can compromise their airway and compliance with treatment.
Fluid balance and gastro-intestinal function	• There is a risk of fluid retention triggered by the stress response (Chapter 6). Look for evidence of reduced urine output and interstitial oedema. • There is a risk of increased air swallowing and gastric distension associated with the air flow. This may be reduced by inserting a nasogastric tube.
Psychological distress	• Patients receiving NIV experience discomfort and distress due to the tight-fitting mask and side effects of the treatment. Communication is difficult with the face mask in place, although this may be resolved for some patients by using a nasal mask. Alternative techniques for delivering the air under pressure include a mouth piece and a helmet. • The role of the nurse in providing support and reassurance is essential. Frequent removal of the mask is counterproductive, and it is important to encourage the patient to keep the mask in situ for at least 30 minutes if any benefit is to be achieved.

- If a patient is becoming very distressed, this will impact on their physiological state and is often an indication to discontinue the NIV and refer to the treatment plan (Jarvis, 2006).
- Optimum management of patients with acute respiratory failure and NIV is achieved in ICU. However, patients can be nursed in acute wards and accident and emergency provided there is an appropriate skill mix and staff ratios of 1 or 2 patients to 1 nurse.

Table 3.5: Risk assessment and management of patients receiving NIV

Case study: Jenny's condition changes

Jenny consented to the use of NIV and commenced the support at a low level of positive pressure (5 cm) and this was gradually increased to 10 cm with support and encouragement from the nursing staff. There seemed to be an initial improvement with an increase in SpO_2 (94%). However, two hours after commencing the NIV Jenny's condition rapidly deteriorated as illustrated in the following assessment.

A: *Difficult to rouse but still able to maintain her airway.*

B: *SpO_2 91% on O_2 60% high-flow humidified O_2*
R 39/min, with shallow respirations
Blood gases showed:
pH 7.20
PaO_2 8.2 kPa
$PaCo_2$ 9.8 kPa
HCO_3 24 mmol/L

C: *HR: 128/min*
BP: 110/72 mmHg

D: *Blood glucose 6.7 mmol/L*
GCS had dropped to 9 (eyes opening to pain 2, inappropriate words 3 and flexion to pain 4).

E: *Temp: 37.5°C*

ABG analysis

- *Jenny has persistent hypoxaemia.*
- *She is acidotic.*
- *The high CO_2 indicates a respiratory acidosis.*
- *No sign of a metabolic acidosis.*

(Continued)

continued . . . .

- *Jenny has hypoxia and a respiratory acidosis.*
- *Her worsening clinical condition of a high respiratory rate, reduction in her level of consciousness and increasing heart rate, combined with hypoxia and respiratory acidosis, indicates severe type II respiratory failure. Immediate intervention with intubation and mechanical ventilation is now required.*

What happens when NIV is not suitable: the case for mechanical invasive ventilation (MIV)

The benefits of supporting patients with respiratory failure with NIV include the following (RCP et al., 2008).

- There is reduced risk of ventilator-acquired pneumonia.
- The patient is fully awake and an active partner in their care.
- The patient may be nursed in an acute care setting.
- The use of NIV may prevent the requirement for invasive respiratory support.

There are, however, a number of reasons why patients may require an escalation of treatment to MIV or direct intervention with MIV without NIV (Brainard and Deutschman, 2010). These include:

- life-threatening hypoxic (PaO_2 below 8.0 kPa) respiratory failure accompanied by patient confusion and/or exhaustion;
- life-threatening hypercarbic ($PaCO_2$ above 6.0 kPa) respiratory failure accompanied by patient confusion and/or exhaustion;
- impaired consciousness and/or the patient's inability to protect their airway.

For patients in these situations, clinical assessment, combined with medical and nursing experience, is the most important tool for judging when invasive support with intubation and mechanical ventilation is required. Based on Jenny's assessment following her deterioration, she meets all of the three criteria above for intubation and mechanical ventilation. Jenny's sudden deterioration may have been related to the combined effects of physical exhaustion and the latent release of inflammatory mediators triggered by the initial inflammatory response several hours before. This can lead to further bronchospasm, oedema, mucus secretion and obstruction of air flow, an increase in variable and uneven airway obstruction and air trapping in the alveoli and hyperventilation (McCance and Huether, 2014). According to Medoff (2008) and Brenner et al. (2009) it is the combination of progressive airways obstruction and physical exhaustion caused by the increased work of breathing that leads to a reduction in the patient's respiratory tidal volume, retention of carbon dioxide, respiratory acidosis and deteriorating cardiovascular

Reason for MIV	Look: Listen: Feel: Measure	Patient examples
Hypoxaemic respiratory failure. • Pneumonia. • Lung consolidation. • Atelectasis. • Pulmonary oedema. • Acute respiratory distress syndrome (ARDS). • **Pulmonary embolism.** • **Carbon monoxide poisoning.**	Central cyanosis. Altered respiratory pattern. Agitation/irritability. Confusion. Exhaustion. Seizures. SpO_2 <85%. PaO_2 <8.0 kPa.	Chao Chan (Table 3.4) is diagnosed with pneumonia and type I respiratory failure. His PaO_2 is 6.2 kPa and his $PaCO_2$ is 3.6 kPa. He was commenced on CPAP at 5 cm H_2O then 10 cm H_2O. However, after the first hour he was confused and agitated, pulling off his mask and refusing to put it back on. His ABGs were PaO_2 5.7 kPa and $PaCO_2$ 5.0 kPa. It was agreed that treatment should be escalated to MIV.
Hypercarbic respiratory failure. • COPD. • Asthma. • Airway obstruction/anatomical. • Deformity. • Cervical injury above level C4 and/or damage to the brain stem. • Excessive sedation. • Guillain-Barré syndrome. • Cardiac arrest. • Heart failure. • Pulmonary embolism.	Increased work of breathing. Use of accessory muscles. Shallow breathing. Dyspnoea. Agitation/irritability. Confusion. Exhaustion. Seizures. Cardiovascular collapse and cardiac arrest. $PaCO_2$ >6.0 kPa.	Mariana Banica (27 years) has a severe scoliosis of her spine (the spine is curved from side to side in an S shape). Since childhood she has been prone to respiratory infections due to reduced and uneven lung capacity. Mariana was admitted to ICU after having collapsed at home following a flu-like illness for three days. On admission she was very confused, cyanosed and her breathing was shallow. Her ABGs were pH: 7.19; PaO_2: 12.7 kPa; $PaCO_2$: 10.7 kPa; HCO_3: 24.0 mmol/L; BE: 0.1. Mariana was intubated and commenced on BiPAP at a rate of 15/min, with an IPAP of 20 cm H_2O and EPAP of 5 cm H_2O.

(Continued)

Table 3.6 (Continued)

Reason for MIV	Look: Listen: Feel: Measure	Patient examples

Impaired consciousness and/or the patient's inability to protect his/her airway.
 	
• Glasgow Coma Scale (GCS) score of <8 indicates the potential for further deterioration in consciousness, reduced ventilation and poor airway protection, for example:
 	
  ○ severe brain injury;
  ○ prolonged effects of general anaesthetic;
  ○ traumatic injury of the face and neck.
	Inability to maintain airway. Unconscious.
	
	GCS <8.
		Pete Williams (19 years) was assaulted on his way home from the pub. A witness said that Pete had been kicked repeatedly on the head while he lay on the floor. In ICU he was agitated and unable to communicate except with grunts. He was opening his eyes and flexing his arms to pain, GCS 7. The computerised tomography scan showed evidence of progressive brain swelling. The management plan for Pete in the first 24 hours was to intubate him with an oral endotracheal tube and provide continuous pressure ventilation (IPAP 30 cm H_2O) with a rate of 15/min in order to protect his airway and maintain PaO_2 >8.0 kPa and $PaCO_2$ 4.5–6.0 kPa. Pete developed ventilator-acquired pneumonia on day four and stayed on MIV for seven days.

Table 3.6: Indications for mechanical invasive ventilation in the critically ill patient

and neurological state, as illustrated in Jenny's case study. Other clinical examples of situations when MIV is required are included in Table 3.6.

Mechanical invasive ventilation in adults can only take place when a patient is intubated with a cuffed endotracheal or tracheostomy tube. The cuff provides a seal around the tube and prevents leaks. The purpose of MIV is to push air under pressure into the patient's lungs to ensure there is effective movement of oxygen and carbon dioxide in and out of the lungs (pulmonary ventilation). There are increasing numbers of types and modes of MIV, but for the purposes of this chapter we will limit discussion to two core modes: pressure-controlled ventilation and volume-controlled ventilation (Carbery, 2008; Grossbach et al., 2011). In Table 3.7 you will find an explanation of these modes together with the advantages and disadvantages of both.

In both pressure-controlled and volume-controlled ventilation the patient's respiratory rate can be managed in one of three ways.

- The patient breathes spontaneously and controls their own rate.
- The patient's respiratory rate is set and controlled by the machine.
- The patient's respiratory rate is supported by a minimum respiratory rate set by the machine and supplemented by the patient's own respiratory rate.

The option of as much or as little respiratory support through MIV allows the patients to be involved in the process of respiratory support and aids their readiness to wean from MIV as they improve.

Case study: Jenny's intubation and ventilation with MIV

Jenny now required immediate intubation and mechanical ventilation and she was induced into anaesthesia with ketamine and alfentanil (short-acting anaesthetic agents) and paralysed with suxamethonium (a fast-acting muscle relaxant) to facilitate safe tracheal intubation with an oral endotracheal tube. Because of the combination of risks related to hyperinflation of the lungs, air trapping and increased airways resistance caused by bronchospasm, inflammation and mucus production, it was decided that the best clinical intervention for Jenny was controlled ventilation with SIMV (Table 3.7), with an inspired tidal volume set at 400 ml and a rate of 16 breaths per minute and a plateau airways pressure of 30 cm. The respiratory rate was set to give Jenny a short inspiration time and a prolonged expiratory time to reduce the risks of further air trapping and barotrauma (Brenner et al., 2009). In order to achieve this type of controlled ventilation it was necessary to fully sedate and paralyse Jenny with neuromuscular blockade and this was achieved by the use of propofol (a short-acting anaesthetic) and cisatracrium (a short-acting neuromuscular blocking agent). Jenny's airway resistance was reduced by suctioning of the airways to remove secretions. A chest X-ray was performed to check the position of the endotracheal tube.

MIV mode	Risks	Benefits
Pressure-controlled/pressure-support ventilation: air is pushed into the lungs until a preset alveolar pressure is reached. For example: • bilevel positive airways pressure (BiPAP) (see NIV). • continuous positive airways pressure (CPAP) (see NIV). • pressure-support ventilation (PS). • positive end expiratory pressure (PEEP).	Ineffective ventilation. Hypo ventilation and variable tidal volumes triggered by reduced lung compliance in the presence of acute lung injury, sputum and/or bronchospasm. Compliance measures the 'ease of stretch' ability in the lungs. The more compliant the lungs are, the less pressure is required to open the airways during MIV.	Reduces the risk of ventilator-associated lung injury.
Volume-controlled ventilation: a preset volume of air is delivered to the lungs with each breath. For example: • synchronised intermittent mandatory ventilation (SIMV).	Ventilator-associated lung injury: • barotrauma: over-distension of some alveoli; • volutrauma: over-distension of the alveoli caused by large tidal volumes; • biotrauma: the release of inflammatory mediators that may increase patient mortality.	The machine delivers a set tidal volume with each breath, thus improving overall ventilation.
Modes that deliver a combination of both. For example: • pressure-regulated volume-controlled ventilation.		Reduces the risk of ventilator-associated lung injury. Ensures effective tidal volumes and pulmonary ventilation.

Table 3.7: A comparison of pressure-controlled and volume-controlled ventilation modes

Research summary: Sedation

The aim of using drugs to sedate patients during MIV is to promote comfort, relieve distress and anxiety, and facilitate effective respiratory function. The majority of drugs used for this purpose, however, can cause side effects, including: depression of the cardiovascular system leading to reduced BP; respiratory depression and delayed weaning from respiratory support; reduced motility of the gastro-intestinal tract with delayed absorption of nutrients and poor quality sleep (Whitehouse et al., 2014). The use of sedation assessment scales and sedation protocols have been recommended as a method for getting the balance right between the advantages and disadvantages of using sedation. The Ramsay scale, Riker Sedation-Agitation scale and Richmond Agitation and Sedation scale are examples of tools adapted for patients on MIV (Ramsay et al., 1974; Riker et al., 2001; Ely et al., 2003). There is limited evidence, however, that such scales and protocols can improve patient outcomes (O'Connor et al., 2010; Williams et al., 2008; Whitehouse et al., 2014). There is evidence, however, that daily sedation interruption combined with patient assessment can improve patient outcome (Chen et al., 2014). There is also evidence that healthcare staff do not always follow sedation recommendations due to lack of awareness, lack of conceptual agreement with the guidance, poor strength of evidence in their use and lack of clarity over who is responsible for prescribing the guidance (Sneyers et al., 2014; Miller et al., 2012). In summary, the use of sedation protocols and daily sedation interruption while seen to be clinically effective continue to be areas that require further research and should always be used in the context of the patient's clinical condition.

Why are tidal volume, respiratory rate and airway pressure important in promoting optimum ventilation?

The tidal volume (TV) is the volume of air in each breath and can be measured as inspired (ITV) and expired (ETV) tidal volume. The respiratory rate (R) describes the total number of respirations in a minute. If a patient is on MIV this may include set ventilator breaths and the patient's own breaths. Minute volume is the total volume of air either inspired (IMV) or expired (EMV) in one minute and is equal to tidal volume times respiratory rate (Hall, 2011). Airway pressure is the same as alveolar pressure and is the pressure required or allowed to push air into the patient's lungs.

When assessing and monitoring a patient receiving MIV, tidal volume, rate, minute volume and airway pressure are some of the important indicators for measuring effective ventilation. For example, increasing ITV, R or IMV can improve the elimination of CO_2. If, however, by doing this the inspired airway pressure goes above 30–35 cm H_2O, then the patient becomes at risk of acute lung injury. Patients such as Jenny often have high airway resistance and it becomes harder to push air into the lungs. In this situation it is important to reduce the risks of barotrauma and pneumothorax caused by high inflation pressures by balancing the controlled respiratory rate and ITV to ensure inspired airway pressure does not exceed 30–35 cm H_2O. Promoting effective patient ventilation therefore requires assessment, monitoring, communication and collaboration with the patient, nurse, intensivist (anaesthetist) and physiotherapist to promote optimum lung function, and with the dietitian to promote optimum nutrition to support the patient's metabolic requirements and promote recovery (Woodrow, 2012). A summary of the risk assessment and management of patients such as Jenny is illustrated in Table 3.8.

Risk assessment	Nursing interventions

Airway
 	
• Risk of the endotracheal tube/tracheostomy (tube) occluding due to poor humidification, the patient biting down on the tube and/or secretions.
• Risk of airway irritation.
• Risk of the tube becoming dislodged.
• Risk of unplanned extubation.
	• Look for evidence of distress and agitation such as coughing and biting on the tube, assess the patient's sedation score and reassure. If the patient continues to be distressed, there is a higher risk of unplanned extubation and/or trauma to the patient's airways. If necessary, increase the sedation according to the prescribed guideline until the patient is comfortable.
	• Humidification of the airways can be achieved by:
	  o heat/moisture exchange (HME) filters that are attached to the ventilator circuit close to the endotracheal tube;
	  o hot water humidifiers (37°C);
	  o cold water humidifiers.

Breathing • Risk of airways becoming partially occluded leading to a rise in airway pressure and ineffective ventilation. • Risk of air leak due to poor connections. • Risk of inappropriately set alarm parameters. • Risk of ventilator-associated lung injury and ventilator-associated pneumonia (VAP).	• Narrowing or occlusion of the patient's airway can be identified by an increase in the inspired airway pressure and evidence of patient agitation, rattling/bubbling on chest auscultation. • Endotracheal suction is used to remove secretions in the trachea but should only be performed when there is evidence of the above. Suction can be painful, distressing and increase the risk of infection and trauma to the airways. • A loose connection can be identified by a reduction in inspired airway pressure, tidal volume and reduction in SpO_2. • Assess respirations, inspired and expired tidal volumes and airway pressure, SpO_2 and ABG analysis if the patient's condition changes. • Set alarm limits to between 5 and 10 marks above and below the prescribed range and assess the patient hourly. • Adhere to the ventilator bundle (see Concept summary: Care bundles).

Circulation

- Risk of impaired circulation and cardiac function: MIV increases venous return pressure because the right side of the heart has to pump against a higher alveolar pressure, thus raising the patient's CVP. Left ventricular cardiac output is reduced due to more blood staying in the venous circulation. Thus the patient is at risk of hypotension and oedema.
- Risk of liver dysfunction leading to clotting disorders, immunosuppression and reduced albumin production.

- Assess the patient's vital signs for evidence of impaired circulation using continuous monitoring: heart rate and rhythm; BP; CVP; chest X-ray; signs of venous thrombosis; urine output, which should be ≥0.5 ml/kg/hr (> about 30 ml/hr).
- Adhere to the ventilator bundle to reduce the risk of VAP.
- Assess the patient for signs of peripheral oedema, bruising.
- Assess blood results including: serum electrolytes; urea and creatinine; liver function tests; clotting.
- Assess and screen for sepsis daily (Chapter 7).

Disability

- Inability to communicate verbally due to the endotracheal tube and sedation.
- Risk of pain.
- Risk of poor skin integrity, dry eyes and mouth.
- Risk of anxiety, delirium and/or boredom.

- When appropriate, encourage the patient to use non-verbal means of communication, picture cards and alphabet cards. Use eye contact and explain all procedures before they are attempted.
- Assess the patient's pain using non-verbal cues and pain scores and manage appropriately.
- Assess the integrity of the patient's eyes and mouth hourly and manage appropriately according to each patient's needs.
- Adopt the Institute for Healthcare Improvement (IHI, 2009) care bundle for pressure ulcer prevention: risk assess on admission; reassess daily: inspect skin, manage moisture on the skin, optimise nutrition and hydration, minimise pressure through positioning.
- Help the patient to be orientated to night and day, and assess for signs of delirium (Chapter 8).
- Encourage family-centred care and patient-focused care.
- Encourage the patient to be involved in decisions and, where possible, life outside the unit.

(Continued)

Table 3.8   (Continued)

Risk assessment	Nursing interventions
Exposure and safe environment • Risk of infection associated with the use of invasive procedures. • Risk of noise and the environment disturbing sleep and rest.	• Risk assess and manage the patient with due regard to the ventilator bundle and risk assessment for sepsis. • Assess noise levels and reduce noise pollution where possible. Reorientate the patient to their environment and offer reassurance when appropriate.

Table 3.8: Risk assessment and plan of care for a ventilated patient

Concept summary: Care bundles

Evidence-based practice is concerned with ensuring that the best available evidence is applied to practice. One method for achieving this is through the use of care bundles. Care bundles are a group of evidence-based interventions that, when combined, provide the most clinically effective method for reducing risk and improving patient outcome (Fulbrook and Mooney, 2003). The ventilator care bundle is an example of how combining selective interventions appears to have reduced the incidence of ventilator-acquired pneumonia (Lawrence and Fullbrook, 2011; Eom et al., 2014). The bundle recommended by the IHI (2014) combines the following five elements.

• Elevation of the head of the bed to 30–45%.
• Periodic interruption of the patient's sedation and daily assessment of the patient's readiness for extubation.
• Peptic ulcer disease prophylaxis.
• Venous thromboembolism prophylaxis.
• Daily oral care with chlorhexidine.

Case study: Jenny's ventilation with MIV

Jenny continued to be ventilated, sedated and paralysed for a further 12 hours until her clinical condition improved and her neuromuscular blocking agent was discontinued. Jenny's sedation was ceased and she was assessed:

A: Airway maintained through an oral endotracheal tube.
Responding to commands.

B: SpO$_2$: 95%

    O$_2$ 60%

    Ventilation mode: SIMV

    ITV: 400 ml

    Controlled R: 16/min

    Blood gases showed:

       pH 7.32

       PaO$_2$ 11 kPa

       PaCO$_2$ 6.0 kPa

C: HR: 120/min

    BP: 110/70 mmHg

D: *Blood glucose 6.7 mmol/L*

    Sedated with reducing levels of propofol according to protocol

E: *Temp: 37.5°C*

ABG analysis

- *Jenny's oxygen levels have improved and are now within the accepted safe range.*
- *She is slightly acidotic but considerably improved from her results prior to MIV.*
- *The high CO$_2$ indicates the upper limit of normal.*
- *No sign of a metabolic acidosis.*
- *Jenny no longer has hypoxia or hypercapnia.*
- *Her clinical condition has improved and she no longer has evidence of respiratory failure. The recommendation is to continue to reduce her sedation and encourage her to trigger her own breaths while reducing the preset ventilator rate. Once she is breathing without the help of the MIV the plan is to extubate her and monitor her condition.*

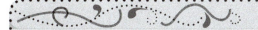

Chapter summary

In this chapter you have been introduced to patients who need advanced respiratory support. The technology and assessment strategies for patients in these situations are often complex and the patient's condition can change suddenly. We have seen how Jenny's condition initially deteriorated but continuous assessment of her condition alerted staff to changes in her condition and she received intensive care. To complete her story, Jenny's condition improved sufficiently for her to be transferred to a general ward and she was discharged from hospital five days later. She decided to separate from her husband and has managed to give up smoking and make a new life for herself. She can still remember her time in the intensive care unit and is determined to improve how she manages her asthma in order to reduce the risk of readmission.

(Continued)

Chapter 3

continued . . . .• •

The important messages to gain from this chapter are as follows.

- Always begin by assessing the patient's airway, breathing and circulation, disability and environment, and you will always be able to prioritise care and communicate your concerns.
- Interpretation of the patient's condition through blood gas analysis means much more if the results are assessed in the context of the patient's story.

Activities: brief outline answers

Activity 3.1: Decision making (pages 63–4)

Using the step-by-step guide in Table 3.3, what can you interpret from the arterial blood gas result?

These are the first set of ABG results.

- Joseph was showing signs of hypoxaemia on 60% oxygen.
- pH 7.07: shows evidence of acidosis.
- $PaCO_2$: 14.1 kPa shows evidence of respiratory acidosis.
- HCO_3: 20.5 mmol/L shows evidence of metabolic acidosis also.
- Joseph shows signs of both a respiratory and metabolic acidosis.
- This result in the context of his clinical situation are consistent with a period of inadequate oxygenation and tissue perfusion related to his cardiac arrest. Re-establishment and maintenance of Joseph's respiration and circulation will provide an opportunity for acid-base balance to be restored.

Using the step-by-step guide in Table 3.3, what can you interpret from Joseph's second arterial blood gas result?

- Joseph's oxygen levels had improved however his PaO_2 and SpO_2 are still below the accepted level.
- His pH of 7.20 is still showing signs of acidaemia.
- $PaCO_2$: 6.70 kPa still shows evidence of respiratory acidosis but has improved from his previous results.
- HCO_3: 22.5 mmol/L shows evidence of a resolving metabolic acidosis compared to the previous result.
- Joseph still shows signs of both a respiratory and metabolic acidosis, however, this is not as severe as his post cardiac arrest results.
- Joseph's ABGs still indicate evidence of type II respiratory failure which has now been complicated by a diagnosis of a STEMI.

What are your priorities of care for this patient?

- Joseph needs to receive support for his respiratory failure and should be assessed to determine the most suitable treatment plan. This may be a combination of nebulised short-acting **beta agonist**, short-acting **muscarinic antagonist** and intravenous antibiotics. He should be encouraged to sit up in the most comfortable breathing position and be assessed for NIV. Following an assessment from the critical care outreach team, Joseph was transferred to ICU for NIV and was commenced on bilevel positive airways pressure.
- Your role is to risk assess the patient and reassure him, and if he is commenced on NIV, to support him to promote his comfort.
- Joseph will require continuous assessment of his respiratory and cardiac function with a view to reducing the NIV support over the next few hours if his condition continues to improve.
- He will need continued support and reassurance to maximise the effect of the respiratory support and his cardiovascular status should be monitored to assess for signs of deterioration following his cardiac event.

Further reading

Moore, T and Woodrow, P (2009) *High Dependency Nursing Care: Observation, Intervention and Support for Level 2 Patients.* Second edition. London: Routledge.

This book offers practical help with learning how to use the technology when involved in the care of level 2 patients.

San Diego Patient Safety Council (2009) *Tool Kit: ICU Sedation Guidelines of Care.* San Diego: San Diego Patient Safety Council. http://www.carefusion.com/pdf/The_Center/2008-PCA-toolkit-disclaimer-updated-may-30-2014.pdf

This document gives you a helpful introduction to some of the drugs used to promote safety and pain relief for patients with mechanical ventilation. It also gives you examples of some of the assessment tools available for monitoring pain and sedation.

Useful websites

http://www.ics.ac.uk/ics-homepage/guidelines-and-standards

The Intensive Care Society site provides access to relevant innovations and standards that relate to the care of patients who are critically ill. The website is multidisciplinary and offers information to patients and relatives in user-friendly guides. A revised edition of sedation guidance is now available on this website.

www.ihi.org

The Institute for Healthcare Improvement website offers evidence-based and practical ways in which to provide safe and effective care for patients with acute and critical care needs.

Chapter 4
The patient with chest pain

Thomas C. Barton and David Barton

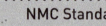

NMC Standards for Pre-registration Nursing Education

This chapter will address the following competencies:

Domain 3: Nursing practice and decision-making

3.1. Adult nurses must safely use a range of diagnostic skills, employing appropriate technology, to assess the needs of service users.

4.1. Adult nurses must safely use invasive and non-invasive procedures, medical devices, and current technological and pharmacological interventions, where relevant, in medical and surgical nursing practice, providing information and taking account of individual needs and preferences.

7.1. Adult nurses must recognise the early signs of illness in people of all ages. They must make accurate assessments and start appropriate and timely management of those who are acutely ill, at risk of clinical deterioration, or require emergency care.

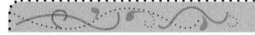

NMC Essential Skills Clusters

This chapter will address the following ESCs:

Cluster: Medicines management

34. People can trust the newly registered graduate nurse to work within legal and ethical frameworks that underpin safe and effective medicines management.

35. People can trust the newly registered graduate nurse to work as part of a team to offer holistic care and a range of treatment options of which medicines may form a part.

Chapter aims

By the end of this chapter, you should be able to:

- identify common causes of chest pain;
- distinguish symptom complexes in different kinds of chest pain;

- critically examine vital signs and understand other related investigations;
- identify and prioritise the most appropriate clinical nursing interventions;
- identify patient concerns and needs wider than those of the presenting chest pain.

Introduction

As a nurse, you will often work with patients who present with chest pain. Despite being a common symptom, it is also one of the most alarming for the patient and their family because most people associate chest pain with having a heart attack. The heart is the most vital of organs: we can feel it beating and hear its activity, and we all know that if it stops, this will quickly lead to death. However, a nurse must understand a great deal more about the causes of chest pain, as these can be many, commonly of cardiovascular, musculoskeletal, gastric or respiratory origin. A key aim of this chapter is to provide some insights on the more common causes of chest pain, how they may be identified and how they may be appropriately managed (ICSI, 2009). This chapter also explores the crucial part that the nurse, and teams of nurses, play in prioritising and managing interventions and care that enable recovery.

We will look at four patient scenarios that are typical of chest pain presentations. While the scenarios are condition based, you can follow the logical prioritisation of nursing interventions that are vital in managing such presentations. This will include those interventions required from the onset of the patient's chest pain through to those interventions that will enable a full recovery. In order to do this you will need to develop and apply your knowledge of nursing assessment, your ability to identify clinical signs and to formulate a reasonable nursing diagnosis based on symptom complexes and underlying pathophysiology. As well as your professional responsibilities of care, your identification of patients' physiological, psychological and wider social needs, and collaborative working when planning and implementing interventions and care, will be essential.

The nature of acute care is that often complete patient notes are not always immediately available or patients themselves give incomplete or varying histories. As you work through each scenario you will note that we have not necessarily given comprehensive information on every aspect of the patient's needs, or all the information that may have been gleaned by the nursing assessments. We hope that you will pick up on these omissions, as there are activities where you will be able reflect on this. It will be you (the nurse) who should be seeking out and identifying these 'wider' concerns that extend beyond the patient's immediate presenting symptoms. Each of the scenarios is divided into three sections.

- The case history.

- The assessment of the presenting condition.

- Immediate and ongoing management of the presenting condition.

Possible causes of chest pain

The most common causes of chest pain are:

- cardiovascular disease (ischaemic coronary artery disease, conduction and rhythm disorders, congenital disorder);
- respiratory disease (chronic obstructive pulmonary disease, infection, asthma, cancer, pneumothorax);
- musculoskeletal disorder or injury (mechanical injury, trauma);
- gastro-intestinal disease (gastritis, infection, herniation, pancreatitis and gall bladder disease);
- psychological causation (emotional disturbance, mental health disorder).

How do you assess and prioritise care for patients with chest pain?

Assessment of the patient experiencing chest pain, and the crucial information that arises from this, is vital in enabling the nurse to prioritise nursing interventions. It is undertaken using the normal tools and criteria that are used in any patient assessment: an initial primary assessment, followed by a comprehensive patient health history, including medications and symptom presentation, all coupled with baseline vital signs. It is important to remember that information may be gained from several sources: from the patient and their family and from other members of the care team such as doctors, nurses, healthcare assistants and physiotherapists. What is crucial is that all this information is properly collated and acted on in an appropriate way by all members of that multidisciplinary team (MDT).

This assessment (shown in the box 'Taking the patient history') will enable the nurse to prioritise the most immediate acute presentation of chest pain. Significant interventions will almost always include ongoing monitoring of vital signs (see the box 'Vital signs'), undertaking electrocardiographs (ECGs), administering prescribed medication and ensuring a high standard of information and communication with the patient and all members of the MDT.

Taking the patient history

The primary nursing assessment is always 'Look: Listen: Feel: Measure'.

Taking a full patient history is a structured and systematic process. You should follow a format to ensure you gain as full a picture of the patient as possible.

- The presenting complaint – what is the problem? What are the presenting symptoms as reported by the patient and/or family?
- The history of the presenting complaint – when did it happen? Where did it happen? How did it feel? What happened then?

- Past medical history – a review of the patient's previous medical history.
- Medications/drugs including over-the-counter medication and recreational drugs.
- Social history – a general review of the patient's social background, family, employment, housing, recent foreign travel etc.
- A family history – a review of the patient's family medical history.
- A general systems review – nervous system, musculoskeletal, heart, lungs, bowels, renal – do you have headaches, any aches and pains, any chest or heart problems? How is your appetite? How are your bowels? Are you passing urine?

Vital signs

The primary nursing assessment is always 'Look: Listen: Feel: Measure'.

Recording vital signs is a fundamental aspect of clinical data collection and is a core component of the overall assessment. The core vital signs that are most commonly recorded are:

- respiratory rate;
- pulse;
- blood pressure;
- temperature;
- oxygen saturation;
- significant results – bloods, X-ray, scans.

Also consider pain – quality and severity – and altered levels of consciousness, including confusion.

Taking vital signs is *not* a one-off activity and the regime of further measurements will depend on the patient's condition and the expert judgement of the medical and senior nursing staff.

Chest pain of acute onset of suspected cardiac origin

While there are many different causes of chest pain, many people readily associate chest pain, particularly if the pain is severe and sudden in onset, with a cardiac cause – a heart attack. There is a widespread fear of cardiac events being associated with a high mortality even though other causes of chest pain such as asthma, pneumothorax or gastro-intestinal bleeding can also be potentially deadly. Crucially, however, these can often be entirely reversible or curable; acute asthma can be reversed, pneumothorax and gastro-intestinal bleeds can be cured. Cardiac causes of chest pain can vary in clinical severity but in many cases can be alarming for the patient, whether the cause is angina or full myocardial infarction (MI).

Conversely, from a healthcare professional's point of view, it is entirely appropriate to be concerned about cardiac causes of pain, not just because they can they be fatal, but also because if survived there is a distinct possibility of later significant morbidity. Heart failure arising from myocardial muscle **ischaemia** and subsequent scarring of the myocardium can result in poor cardiac wall function and/or cardiac wall decompensation. This is where the area of muscle that was thick and strong, perhaps in response to years of high blood pressure, stretches out as the now weaker, damaged, scarred myocardium fails to maintain its shape under the pressure the blood exerts on it. In turn, these factors may lead to a poor ejection fraction (the percentage of blood expelled from a ventricle during systole). This may be compounded further if the papillary muscles are affected by the myocardial ischaemia. This can cause dysfunction of the tricuspid and/or mitral valves (depending on the site of the ischaemia). Failure to initiate appropriate treatments, or failure of treatments to fully resolve cardiac ischaemic events, is likely to result in ischaemic heart disease. The person may have reduced exercise tolerance and become easily short of breath. They may develop trouble sleeping at night, waking up breathless. They may be prone to accumulating fluid in their legs or other parts of the body, which may cause complications varying from the very acutely unwell patient with pulmonary oedema or large pleural effusions to more chronic problems such as angina, reduced mobility, palpitations or abnormal heart rhythms. Some patients with pre-existing ischaemic heart disease may indeed already suffer many of these symptoms and be at high risk of further myocardial infarctions. Should these patients survive, their symptoms are likely to worsen.

With so much at stake, the importance of providing high quality care to patients with chest pain that may be cardiac in origin cannot be over-estimated. NICE has produced guidance on treating ischaemic heart conditions. While the guidance is extensive and cannot be reproduced in this chapter, the following crucial points are highlighted.

- Chest pain should be differentiated as either stable or unstable. Factors to consider include whether the pain is brought on by exercise and relieved by rest. If the pain is stable, the patient should be treated for stable angina as advised by the NICE pathway for stable angina (NICE, 2015). If the pain is unstable it is an acute coronary syndrome (ACS) (NICE, 2015) and requires further investigation urgently.

- If the onset of pain was within the last 12 hours, the person still has pain and their ECG is abnormal or unavailable, emergency admission to hospital is needed.

- If onset of the pain was between 12 and 72 hours ago and acute coronary syndrome is suspected, the patient requires urgent same-day referral for review in hospital.

- If onset of the pain was more than 72 hours ago and has completely resolved, but there are signs of complications such as pulmonary oedema, a clinically informed judgement should be made on whether to refer the person as an emergency or urgent same-day assessment. If there are no complications, ECG and blood troponin levels (troponin T is a cardiac enzyme released during damage to the myocardium; it can be used to assess for MI/ACS) should be tested and a clinical judgement made about whether referral is required and, if so, how urgently.

With ACS, 300 mg of aspirin should be given at the earliest opportunity if available, and so long as there is no clear evidence the patient is allergic to it. Written documentation should be sent with the patient that aspirin has been given. Oxygen saturations should be maintained between 94–98% (or 88–92% if the patient has a background of COPD at risk of hypercapnic respiratory failure) with supplementary oxygen if required. If a 12-lead ECG is available this should also be done at the earliest opportunity.

Once an ECG is obtained and it has been interpreted by a suitably competent healthcare professional there are essentially two possible conclusions.

First, there is elevation of the **ST segment** of the patient's ECG. This is the characteristic finding of ST elevation myocardial infarction (**STEMI**). Any troponin T bloods requested will invariably be high and further treatment for the patient should not be delayed while waiting for the results. A symptomatic patient with ST elevation on ECG is diagnostic of STEMI. In this situation, the next step depends on the time of onset of pain and the services available at the hospital or nearby hospitals. If the hospital has a cardiac angiography service, the preferred treatment is cardiac angiography with follow-on primary percutaneous coronary intervention (PCI) to revascularise the ischaemic myocardium. Angiography is a non-surgical technique using an inflatable balloon to widen the coronary arteries; a stent can then also be placed if required.

If a PCI cannot be offered then fibrinolysis using a thrombolytic, 'clot busting', drug may be considered. Administering such a drug will render a patient completely incapable of making clots and as a result they will be at high risk of bleeding. Certain patients will not be eligible for this treatment due to other health problems (recent surgery for example) and careful assessment of the risks versus benefit of administering the drugs must take place. Certain drugs can only be given once, specifically streptokinase, so if the patient has had this before, it is accepted UK practice that they cannot have it again. A thrombolised patient requires close monitoring in hospital. A patient who has recurrent MI will require referral to a specialist cardiologist who may consider follow-up angiography and PCI.

Second, in the absence of the more obvious ST segment elevation, diagnosis of MI is more difficult. ECG should be interpreted by an expert who will look for patterns that may indicate myocardial ischaemia. Blood tests such as troponin T may give an indication of the extent of myocardial damage. If the result is extremely high this, combined with any ECG findings, may lead to a diagnosis of non-ST elevation myocardial infarction (NSTEMI). More subtle findings or results may result in a diagnosis of unstable angina. The management of both conditions is essentially the same.

Initially these patients will all be treated with aspirin, with a loading dose of 300mg aspirin if not given at an earlier point in their care. They will also be anticoagulated using a low molecular weight heparin such as fondaparinux, if angiography is likely within 24 hours. Within the following six months, all patients should be risk assessed as part of a thorough clinical assessment and will be judged as being at a certain level of risk of mortality and risk of adverse cardiac events from their myocardial ischaemia. Patients at lowest or low risk should be offered conservative management, have ischaemia testing and assessment of their left ventricular function by echocardiogram (often called an ECHO). These patients can be discharged home if well prior to outpatient follow-up and possible coronary angiography. Patients with intermediate or higher risks require more urgent assessment and intervention. New generation cardiac CT scanners can offer more information on the extent of a patient's cardiac ischaemia and need for **revascularisation**, but ultimately angiography or CT assessment of ischaemia is indicated within 96 hours of admission so long as there are no contraindications such as bleeding. The results of these investigations will then allow the cardiologists to decide, with the patient, whether PCI or coronary artery bypass grafting (CABG) is the best option for the patient.

Finally, the guidelines crucially advise that patients suffering from ACS/MI should have discharge and follow-up arrangements, a course of cardiac rehabilitation, management of risk factors and secondary prevention measures, i.e. high cholesterol, high blood pressure, aspirin, statins and advice on lifestyle changes such as smoking cessation, diet and weight.

Respiratory causes of chest pain

Case study: Mr Adams

Mr Adams, a 57-year-old man who has retired early, has attended his local GP surgery as he has become increasingly short of breath during a summer heatwave. His wife insisted that he go and see his GP. He tells the receptionist that he is feeling very unwell, that he has chest tightness and a generalised dull pain in his chest. He is asked to wait and told that a doctor will see him very soon. Shortly afterwards, following a spasmodic episode of coughing, he collapses in the waiting room. The receptionist reports to the attending practice nurse that Mr Adams became suddenly very short of breath and was wheezing and that he had attempted to use an inhaler prior to collapsing on his chair.

The practice nurse makes an immediate initial visual and verbal assessment of Mr Adams and finds him to be conscious but clearly in distress. He appears flushed and sweaty, is breathing noticeably quickly and has an audible wheeze. He can speak in short sentences only, but with assistance he can be helped to a wheelchair and moved to another room to be assessed. This immediate assessment informs appropriate interventions and the urgency of the presenting condition.

In a quiet room, Mr Adams manages to take his inhaler himself and appears to settle slightly. The practice nurse records his clinical observations – an important baseline – and they are as follows.

- *Respiratory rate: 28 bpm (audible wheezing).*
- *Pulse: 100 bpm (regular, bounding).*
- *Blood pressure: 140/78 mmHg.*
- *Temperature: 37°C.*

Activity 4.1   *Critical thinking*

Are these observations normal? What do you make of these observations?

An outline answer to this activity is given at the end of the chapter.

The practice nurse undertakes a more detailed assessment of Mr Adams's recent health history – this is important in developing a more detailed picture of the patient. Mr Adams reports that he has chronic bronchitis, having previously been a heavy smoker, and that he has been short of breath and coughing more than normal for a couple of days. He feels the hot weather is making his shortness of breath worse and this in turn is making his chest very tight. He has had to use his inhalers more frequently over the past couple of days. He is also treated for hypertension and high cholesterol and he is overweight. In recent years his chronic bronchitis has become more severe and led to long periods off work before he retired. He is well known to the GP. Due to the sudden collapse of Mr Adams, and his distressed state, the practice nurse makes the decision that he is an immediate priority and that he requires constant observation. She stays with him, monitoring his respiratory status and offering him reassurance.

One of the surgery's GPs arrives and takes a full medical history and performs an examination of Mr Adams. This reveals that, in addition to the practice nurse's observations, Mr Adams has also been coughing up green sputum for the past two days (it is normally a light creamy colour).

The details of the GP's examination of Mr Adams are that:

- he is breathless at rest;
- he is using his accessory muscles to breathe;
- he has poor chest expansion;
- he is peripherally warm;
- he is cyanosed (appears blue);
- when auscultated, he has quiet breath sounds with a wheeze throughout his lung fields. He also has some basal crackles which are worse on the right.

Activity 4.2   *Critical thinking*

Given this information, at this point what do you think is causing Mr Adams's chest pain?

An outline answer to this activity is given at the end of the chapter.

Management of the presenting condition

The GP diagnoses Mr Adams with infective exacerbation of his chronic bronchitis. The immediate action necessary is urgent admission to hospital. Because of his collapse and the severity of his presentation, the GP wants Mr Adams to be admitted to hospital as a priority for initial investigation and treatment of acute exacerbation of chronic bronchitis.

Following admission to hospital, a first nursing priority is to ensure that he remains closely monitored given that he has collapsed as a result of his significant respiratory difficulties. The other clinical findings (green sputum) suggest he may have an infection, and his history suggests it is getting worse – he requires further and immediate investigations (Bridges and Dukes, 2005). The hospital nurses will need to ensure that the interventions listed below are quickly organised and undertaken so that appropriate therapeutic interventions can be commenced as soon as possible. The further investigations needed are:

- chest X-ray;
- sputum sample;
- blood tests – **FBC**, **U&E** and **CRP**.

These investigations will indicate the location of his infection (chest X-ray), the type of infection (sputum) and the severity of the infection (bloods). They may also highlight any other developing problems or otherwise undiagnosed issues. A next priority for nursing care is to initiate and provide the treatments prescribed, to monitor their effects and to oversee the patient's care pathway.

Treatments and care planning

- Antibiotics, broad spectrum as per local health provider policy, which should be reviewed when a positive sputum culture is available.
- Bronchodilators, which will improve the patient's symptom of shortness of breath, wheeziness and hopefully reduce care requirements by allowing independence.
- Corticosteroids, which may be useful in COPD patients whose symptoms are not controlled by bronchodilators but should be stopped if there is no significant clinical improvement.
- Oxygen if clinically required – and only in small concentrations as higher concentrations can disrupt the patient's reverse drive respiratory effort and worsen their condition. If they remain unwell or are deteriorating with low concentration oxygen, then specialist respiratory medicine opinion should be sought.
- Discharge when improving.

Activity 4.3   *Critical thinking and group working*

While Mr Adams was awaiting admission from the GP surgery to hospital, what other wider concerns should the practice nurse be considering?

Write down a list of points, then compare notes with one or more friends or colleagues. Did you think of the same ones or were there differences?

An outline answer to this activity is given at the end of the chapter.

Musculoskeletal causes of chest pain

Case study: Mr Knight

Mr Knight, a frail 82-year-old widower, has been admitted to a clinical decision unit (CDU) for 24 hours' observation and monitoring of chest pain, having fallen at home tripping over his cat. He has fallen onto the left side of his chest and has had excruciating pain since. He was referred to hospital by his GP following a home visit; the GP was subsequently concerned when he noted that Mr Knight was on warfarin.

In CDU the nurses admit and undertake a primary assessment, quickly followed by a full nursing assessment including a systematic patient history and baseline vital signs. The assessment reveals that Mr Knight takes warfarin, bisoprolol, simvastatin and calcium tablets. Mr Knight tells the nurses that he is worried he is having a heart attack as a result of the fright, and he is clearly very anxious. In addition, it is noted that Mr Knight is lying on a bed wincing with pain and guarding the left side of his chest. It is painful for him to move, and he feels better when he is lying still. He is an articulate man, talking in full sentences, and he does not appear to be having problems breathing. He says he has awful pain in the left of his chest; it is constant and sharp, throbbing in nature and made worse on deep inspiration. The nurses noted baseline vital signs. His observations are as follows.

- *Respiratory rate: 18 bpm.*
- *Pulse: 90 bpm (irregular).*
- *Blood pressure: 120/54 mmHg.*
- *Temperature: 36.7°C.*
- *Oxygen saturation: 98%.*

Activity 4.4   *Critical thinking*

Are these observations normal? At this point, what do you make of these observations?

An outline answer to this activity is given at the end of the chapter.

Mr Knight tells the nurses that he knows he has had an irregular heartbeat for some time and this is why he takes warfarin as his GP tells him he could have a stroke.

An on-call junior doctor takes a full medical history and examines Mr Knight. It is ascertained that he has fallen quite accidentally and has not felt dizzy, faint, blacked out, had palpitations or otherwise lost consciousness before or during his fall. He has pain that is isolated to the left side of his chest – it does not radiate anywhere and he does not feel short of breath. He does find it painful to take deep breaths. The medical examination finds that:

- he is a thin, frail man;
- he is pale;
- he has very extensive bruising and some swelling to the left side of his chest;
- the left side of his chest is painful when palpated;
- there is reduced chest expansion on the left.

Activity 4.5   *Critical thinking*

With the information gained from the initial nursing assessment and with this information from the medical assessment, what do you now think is causing his chest pain?

An outline answer to this activity is given at the end of the chapter.

Management of the presenting condition

The doctor diagnoses Mr Knight with a haematoma and suspects possible rib fractures.

The immediate action taken is to:

- give analgesia;
- gain intravenous access.

Now that Mr Knight has been assessed, it is a priority for the nurses to administer suitably strong prescribed analgesia, such as morphine or another opiate-based medication, for his pain before he goes on to have further necessary investigations. The nurses fully assess his pain both before and after administration of analgesia using a pain scale, but also with particular regard for any effect on respiratory effort. In addition, with evidence of bleeding and anaemia, it would be prudent to gain intravenous access early and the nurses should ensure that cannulation is undertaken as soon as possible.

The further investigations undertaken are:

- blood tests – full blood count (FBC), urea & electrolytes (U&E), international normalised ratio (INR), coagulation screen (COAG);
- chest X-ray;
- 12-lead ECG.

These investigations will identify with certainty if Mr Knight is anaemic as a result of his haematoma, or by an as yet unidentified internal bleed (FBC). The COAG and INR tests will identify how thin his blood is and the clinicians may make a decision to actively reverse the effects of his warfarin. The blood tests may also identify evidence of underlying infection (often a precipitating factor of falls in the elderly). The chest X-ray will either confirm or exclude rib fractures, haemothorax or pneumothorax, and may demonstrate the extent of haematoma in the soft tissues of his chest if large. The nurses will need to perform a 12-lead ECG; this is to rule out myocardial injury that may be masked by his musculoskeletal injury symptoms.

Treatments and care planning

- Treatment will depend on the extent of bleeding. If severely anaemic, Mr Knight may require a transfusion of blood; if less anaemic, a course of iron supplements may be prescribed.

- Prompt administration (if required) of drugs such as vitamin K and beriplex will be required to reverse the effects of the warfarin and help cease bleeding.

- Rib fractures tend to be treated conservatively with analgesia and rest.

The CDU nurses will now need to ensure that Mr Knight is admitted to a ward bed as soon as possible where a full care pathway will be instigated. Key parts of that will include close monitoring of vital signs, pain management and appropriate mobilisation to preserve as much of the gentleman's usual physical function as possible. A significant rationale for this is the potential for stroke, a major risk in elderly patients with AF (atrial fibrillation), and this will be exacerbated by the necessity of stopping warfarin in the light of his bleeding. It is crucial that the nurses note that his risk of stroke is high, and that it is therefore important that he is closely monitored. Once his bleeding has stopped and he is stable, the patient's clinicians will need to decide on whether to restart his warfarin dependent on his thromboembolic and bleeding risks. Tools such as CHADSVAS stroke risk assessment and HAS-BLED bleeding risk tool (Lane and Lip, 2012) can assist in this decision by giving one year risk scores of stroke versus bleed, for example, if the bleeding score is greater than the stroke risk score, it is safer not to anticoagulate the patient.

In addition, the ward nurses must note that with elderly patients who start to develop a tendency to fall, the risk of intracranial bleeding with warfarin as a result of a head injury becomes an issue. These situations are difficult clinical dilemmas and the patient should be fully investigated regarding the cause of their falls as current evidence suggests that all but the most prolifically falling patients should be maintained on warfarin as instance of stroke often outweighs that of intracranial haemorrhage.

Mr Knight presents a complex case for nursing management throughout, given his frailty, poly-pharmacy and multiple underlying health problems. Prioritising nursing interventions will be a pivotal part of Mr Knight's care pathway – with a central aim of enabling his eventual discharge. Full and ongoing nursing assessment, coupled with input from the MDT, will ascertain the best time for discharge. Given his age and frailty, he may require temporary support at home, and the nurses will need to be sure that a package of care is ready for implementation on discharge home if he requires the help.

Activity 4.6   *Critical thinking*

Consider what other social and community issues the nurses may have had to think of.

An outline answer to this activity is given at the end of the chapter.

Gastric/abdominal causes of chest pain

Case study: Mrs Thompson

Mrs Thompson is an 81-year-old lady with dementia who lives in a nursing home. She complained of 'very bad' indigestion after her Sunday meal. Although forgetful and unable to live on her own as a result, Mrs Thompson is generally able to express herself well, and she told the nursing staff at the nursing home that she had severe pain in her chest. The nursing home staff called an ambulance to take her to A&E as they were concerned that she might be having a heart attack.

On admission, the A&E nurses assist Mrs Thompson to a trolley in the general waiting area of the emergency department. They carry out an immediate primary nursing assessment and note that she is clearly uncomfortable, sitting upright and burping a lot. She says she feels nauseous and that she has a very uncomfortable spasmodic burning-type chest pain. This pain is not radiating elsewhere. Her vital signs are as follows.

- *Respiratory rate: 22 bpm.*
- *Pulse: 110 bpm (regular).*
- *Blood pressure: 155/100 mmHg.*
- *Temperature: 36.2°C.*
- *Oxygen saturation: 95%.*

Activity 4.7   *Critical thinking*

- Are these observations normal?
- At this stage, what do you make of these observations?

An outline answer to this activity is given at the end of the chapter.

The A&E nurses note that Mrs Thompson is cooperative. She is able to mobilise with nursing assistance. A full nursing assessment (patient history and vital signs) is undertaken, coupled with an A&E doctor's physical examination and history. These reveal that:

- she is an elderly frail woman with mild to moderate cognition deficits;

- she is pale, but sweaty;

- she has a clear chest with normal heart sounds;

- the ECG reveals sinus tachycardia;

- her abdomen is tender on palpation, but no abnormal masses are identified;

- she has had mild diarrhoea for two days;

- she is on regular gaviscon for persistent 'heartburn'.

Activity 4.8   *Evidence-based practice*

With this information, what do you think is causing her chest pain? (You might want to look up some of the web resources given on page 105.)

An outline answer to this activity is given at the end of the chapter.

Management of the presenting condition

Mrs Thompson is experiencing an acute exacerbation of her chronic gastritis. The medical treatment of gastritis and the related prioritisation of nursing intervention will depend on what the underlying cause is: diet, infection, other medications such as aspirin, **non-steroidal anti-inflammatory drugs (NSAIDs)**, steroids. However, a first nursing priority for Mrs Thompson is to alleviate the symptoms; this is undertaken via administration of antacids and H_2 antagonists as prescribed. It is important that the nurses monitor and record the effects of these. Correction of electrolyte and hydration deficits will also be important, and a resultant nursing intervention will focus on administration of prescribed fluids and careful fluid balance monitoring.

Treatments and care planning

As Mrs Thompson is elderly and frail she will be admitted briefly for some investigations to explore possible underlying abnormalities that could be leading to her symptoms. The nursing teams will need to ensure that these investigations are planned and undertaken as soon as possible, and these will include:

- blood tests: blood cell count, presence of *H. pylori*, liver, kidney, gall bladder and pancreas functions;

- urinalysis;

- stool sample, to look for blood in the stool or infections such as *Clostridium difficile*;

- chest and abdominal X-rays;

- repeat 12-lead ECGs.

Activity 4.9	*Reflection*

Reflect on Mrs Thompson's situation and what you might do if she were your patient. What other wider concerns should the nurses caring for Mrs Thompson be thinking of relating to her total care and return to her nursing home?

An outline answer to this activity is given at the end of the chapter.

Cardiac causes of chest pain

Case study: Harry Smith

*Harry Smith is a 58-year-old retired manager. He is married and a grandfather. He was diagnosed with type 2 diabetes when he was 48 years old. Harry began smoking when he was 15 years old and only gave up smoking 40 cigarettes a day when he was diagnosed with diabetes. He had given up completely by the age of 50. Harry also suffers from hypertension and **hyperlipidaemia** and has been prescribed an ACE inhibitor (**angiotensin converting enzyme** inhibitor) to reduce his blood pressure, statins to reduce his blood cholesterol and aspirin to reduce the risk of clot formation. Harry is known to be at high risk of developing acute cardiovascular disease (NICE, 2008).*

Harry generally doesn't enjoy physical exercise, but he does enjoy gardening, and on the morning of his admission he had decided to start the first grass cut of the spring. Halfway through the job he developed central chest pain and he rested until the pain subsided. Not willing to leave a job half done, Harry went back outside to finish the grass. Later that afternoon Harry's wife came home to find him collapsed in the chair with severe central crushing chest pain.

Following an urgent admission by ambulance to A&E, Harry was immediately seen by A&E nurses and doctors and diagnosed with a primary myocardial infarction due to occlusion of a coronary artery. The ECG revealed evidence of ST elevation in the chest leads from V2 to V5, and Harry's troponin levels were elevated above the accepted reference limit.

The A&E nurses quickly assessed Harry's condition on admission. They found the following.

- *Respirations: 22 bpm.*
- *Pulse: 110 bpm, sinus tachycardia.*
- *BP: 110/80 mmHg.*
- *Temperature: 37.5°C.*
- *SpO_2: 96%.*
- *He was pale and anxious.*
- *He had central chest pain and a 'heavy' left arm.*

Activity 4.10   *Critical thinking*

Are these observations normal? What do you make of these observations?

An outline answer to this activity is given at the end of the chapter.

Management of the presenting condition

Harry was compensating for the loss of cardiac output by increasing his heart rate and respirations. A major nursing priority was to relieve his pain, which subsequently would alleviate ongoing stress on the heart. Pain assessment using a pain scale is a nursing priority. Harry was prescribed diamorphine to relieve the chest pain; this was administered by the nurses with measurable good effect. He was also prescribed aspirin to prevent further platelet aggregation and oxygen therapy to support a SpO_2 between 96 and 98%. He was booked for immediate angiography and PCI within 90 minutes of admission to A&E (ICSI, 2009).

Monitoring fluid balance is a crucial nursing intervention in the patient with compromised cardiac function, and it was noted that Harry had not yet passed urine. The nurses inserted a urinary catheter, which drained 90 ml of urine. He had last passed urine while at home before the onset of his symptoms. Renal function is reliant on adequate perfusion of the kidneys. They are therefore sensitive to low blood pressure or poor perfusion resulting from compromised cardiac function and monitoring urine output can give an indication of how well the patient's organs are being perfused. This is crucial information as the other major organ most sensitive to damage from poor perfusion is the brain. Identifying poor perfusion is the first and most important step in being able to enact interventions to protect the patient from further organ damage.

Remember

Always 'Look: Listen: Feel: Measure'.

Ongoing management of the presenting condition

Just prior to transfer for angiography, the A&E nurses reassessed Harry and found the following.

- BP 83/55 mmHg.
- SpO_2 85%.
- His skin was cold and clammy.
- He was confused.
- He had central cyanosis.
- He was nauseated.

Activity 4.11 | *Critical thinking*

Are these observations normal? What do you make of these observations?

An outline answer to this activity is given at the end of the chapter.

Harry was presenting with the clinical features of uncompensated and progressive **cardiogenic shock**. Cardiogenic shock or cardiac shock is a clinical state where the cardiac output (volume of blood ejected from the left ventricle) is reduced, leading to inadequate perfusion of blood to the tissues, triggering the shock response. This can also be described as pump failure.

The most common cause of cardiogenic shock is myocardial infarction, when 40% of the heart muscle in the left ventricle has been damaged and the patient experiences failure of the left ventricle (Gowda et al., 2008). Other causes include severe contusion or bruising to the myocardium or a ventricular septal defect that reduces the efficiency of the left ventricular chamber as a pump. Cardiogenic shock can also occur in patients who develop septic shock and this is discussed in Chapter 7.

Regardless of the cause, the onset of cardiogenic shock triggers a cycle of events that lead to a continuing decline in cardiac function. Patients who develop cardiogenic shock often present with dramatic and distinctive features including:

- being pale and cyanosed;
- being confused and disorientated;
- feeling cold and clammy to touch;
- having increased respiratory rate, tachycardia and hypotension.

Treatments and care planning

It is a priority that the nurses caring for Harry continue with a full systematic regime of ongoing regular assessment from the outset. The rationale for this is that patients such as Harry may be admitted to A&E with clinical features already present, but in many cases the cardiogenic shock may develop between five to seven hours after the onset of chest pain and the initial MI (Babaev et al., 2005).

Harry's presentation and past medical history highlight a number of factors that increase the risk of patients developing cardiogenic shock.

- He has a history of diabetes.
- He has had a large anterior-lateral myocardial infarction, including ST elevation across his chest leads (V2-V5).
- He has an elevated troponin level.

The extent of ST elevation suggests that the damaged area involves both the front (anterior) and side (lateral) sections of his left ventricular myocardium and could involve 40% of his left ventricle.

Harry should remain in the resuscitation unit of A&E until they are ready to receive him in the cardiac catheter suite and/or operating department. He will need to be closely monitored every 15–30 minutes for a change in his condition. Following PCI or additional cardiac surgery, Harry will require support in the coronary care or cardiac intensive care unit. Here nurses will provide continuous highly specialist support.

Further treatments and care planning

For Harry, the large area of ischaemia and inflammation to his heart muscle (myocardium) in the left ventricle caused by the coronary occlusion has led to reduced blood pressure and cardiac output. This has happened because the reduction in blood flow and oxygen available to the heart has led to a reduction in the energy available to support cardiac contraction. As a consequence, Harry has reduced perfusion of vital organs and tissues.

The physiological response to shock in Harry's case would involve the triggering of the flight/fight response, including nervous and hormonal responses. This includes stimulation of the sympathetic nervous system to increase heart rate and peripheral vasoconstriction and the release of epinephrine (adrenaline) and norepinephrine (noradrenaline). However, due to the damage to Harry's heart, his body is unable to compensate for the reduction in cardiac output, and in spite of an increase in heart and respiratory rate, his blood pressure is below the level required to achieve adequate tissue perfusion. With no intervention the progressive reduction in blood pressure will continue, leading to the progressive stages of shock, including a further reduction in cardiac output, metabolic acidosis, further myocardial depression, loss of consciousness and reduced urine output.

The initial clinical priorities of care for patients in Harry's situation are the same as for ACS and that is to restore tissue perfusion in order to stabilise and facilitate recovery of the damaged myocardium. For Harry, restoring the circulation to the muscle damaged by the coronary occlusion will prevent the continual cycle of deterioration into cardiogenic shock.

Heart muscle will begin to die through the process of necrosis and form scar tissue if the blood supply is not restored within four to five hours after injury. The primary treatment for patients in cardiogenic shock, therefore, is PCI and restoration of blood flow. This has been demonstrated to improve the long-term survival rates of patients such as Harry when compared to medical stabilisation alone (Hockman et al., 2006).

In order to stabilise Harry for safe transfer to the operating department, medical stabilisation is first required. The nursing priorities for this will include:

- providing oxygen therapy to restore SpO_2 to 98%;
- instituting and monitoring of prescribed fluid resuscitation to improve vascular circulation;
- administration and monitoring of intravenous drugs to improve cardiac function (**inotropic therapy**) such as **dobutamine**, **dopamine** and milrinone (see Chapter 7).

If Harry's condition does not respond to PCI, or if he is unsuitable for reperfusion therapy with thrombolytic drugs (dissolving the blood clot) or coronary artery bypass surgery, medical support will be the most effective option (Babaev et al., 2005). In this case Harry may need the support of non-invasive ventilation (NIV) and intra-aortic counterpulsation. The nursing management of such complex procedures will be undertaken within high dependency areas.

The provision of intra-aortic counterpulsation involves the insertion of a catheter into the aorta. The catheter has a balloon at the distal end and during cardiac diastole (ventricular relaxation) the balloon will inflate. This creates a back pressure during ventricular relaxation that will improve the blood supply to the coronary arteries that branch off the aorta above the catheter tip. During cardiac systole the balloon deflates and creates a reduction in peripheral resistance, thus reducing the workload of the left ventricle and improving cardiac output.

Harry was commenced on oxygen therapy and received fluid resuscitation. An intravenous anti-emetic was prescribed and administered by the nurses to relieve the nausea. He was transferred immediately to the cardiac catheter suite and underwent PCI with the insertion of two stents to the left anterior descending artery. A stent is a 'stainless' tube that, when inserted and guided into place with a cardiac catheter, expands and pushes against the inner (endothelial) layer of the coronary artery, expanding the diameter of the artery and improving blood flow to the ischaemic myocardium.

The key interventions responsible for Harry's recovery were:

- timely assessment and diagnosis;
- fast and efficient communication;
- the work of the paramedical staff that transferred him to A&E;
- efficient and thorough nursing and medical assessment in A&E, and early recognition and reporting of his deterioration to the cardiology team;
- cardiology intervention;
- critical care support – specialist nursing care.

Activity 4.12   *Reflection*

With appropriate intervention, Harry will be able to return home. What do you think are the main issues that the nurses should consider in enabling the 'journey' to recovery when Harry goes home?

An outline answer to this activity is given at the end of the chapter.

Following the PCI, Harry's condition began to improve. His blood pressure quickly improved to 90/60 mmHg and he became less confused and cyanosed. Over several days his condition continued to improve and he was discharged from hospital eight days after the onset of his chest pain. Prior to discharge Harry was commenced on a rehabilitation programme that focused on reviewing and improving diet, exercise and medication to reduce the risk of further cardiac problems.

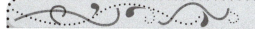

Chapter summary

This chapter has presented four clinical scenarios that have highlighted different causes of chest pain. The first three demonstrate how chest pain may arise as a result of other factors than myocardial infarction. This is not comprehensive and we have not delved into other less common reasons such as adverse drug side effects or anxiety-related issues. The final scenario, however, has presented a classical, and serious, presentation of chest pain that is directly related to cardiac disease.

Key points that must arise from this are:

- the need for rapid and full systematic nursing assessment;
- the need for prioritisation of initial nursing interventions;
- the need for nurses to take immediate and regular ongoing vital signs;
- the need to keep an open mind on the cause of 'chest pain';
- the need for holistic nursing assessment throughout the patient journey.

We hope that you take from this chapter, if nothing else, the knowledge that there may be many causes of chest pain, and many means of assessing and intervention.

Activities: brief outline answers

Activity 4.1: Critical thinking (page 91)

The respiratory rate is very high for a man of this age at rest; the pulse is slightly elevated; the blood pressure is within a normal range for a man of this age; the temperature is on the border of elevation above normal.

Activity 4.2: Critical thinking (page 91)

This symptom complex is highly suggestive of a chest infection that is exacerbating ongoing lung disease.

Activity 4.3: Critical thinking and group working (pages 92–3)

Mr Adams's wife will need to be contacted and given information regarding his prospective admission, and an opportunity to ask questions or attend the surgery to be with her husband. The nurse should be responsive to her expected concern and anxiety. In addition the nurse should be able to provide information as to where Mr Adams will be first admitted – most likely to a medical admissions unit.

Activity 4.4: Critical thinking (page 93)

The respiratory rate is slightly elevated; his pulse would not be considered abnormal in a man of his age – later investigation revealed underlying atrial fibrillation treated with bisoprolol and warfarin; blood pressure is slightly low for a man of his age and review of his bisoprolol dose should be considered; temperature is within a normal range; oxygen saturation is normal.

Activity 4.5: Critical thinking (page 94)

With a history of a fall, this information is highly suggestive of trauma – a potential haematoma – and could point to rib fractures. The nurse should be aware of the potential for pneumothorax and monitor respiratory function closely.

Activity 4.6: Critical thinking (page 96)

You should have picked up on two key issues – the first leading you to the second. First, Mr. Knight tripped over his cat: who would be available to care for the cat while he was in hospital? Second, the scenario does not provide any information on his social status. Does he live alone? Does he have family? How accessible is his accommodation for the shops? Does he have friendly neighbours? What is his financial situation? Does his accommodation need modification to make it safer for him? Will there be a requirement for community nursing or community healthcare support? Your reflection on Mr Knight should have taken in these wider holistic concerns.

Activity 4.7: Critical thinking (page 96)

The respiratory rate is elevated; the pulse is elevated – tachycardia; the blood pressure is moderately high – particularly the diastolic; the temperature is normal; the oxygen saturation is acceptable for the patient's age.

It would be difficult in isolation to make any conclusion from these readings. However, in conjunction with other findings they would evidence a patient experiencing pain.

Activity 4.8: Evidence-based practice (page 97)

These findings are highly suggestive of acute or chronic gastritis – and further enquiry would reveal that Mrs Thompson has a history of persistent heartburn.

Activity 4.9: Reflection (page 98)

A significant issue for this woman is her dementia. The scenario presents her as very cooperative – but as increasingly forgetful. There is also a real possibility that dementia may worsen in future. An important issue that arises from nurses planning discharge to the nursing home will be ensuring that the nursing home understands her problems. Dietary advice will need to be given to minimise episodes of gastritis, this coupled with a carefully monitored regime of H_2 antagonists and antacids.

Activity 4.10: Critical thinking (page 99)

The respiratory rate is significantly high; the pulse is elevated – tachycardia at rest; the blood pressure is low, even for a known and treated hypertensive; the temperature is above the normal range; the SpO_2 is acceptable.

Central chest pain radiating to the left arm accompanied with pallor is typically suggestive of myocardial infarction, although this could only be confirmed in the light of other investigations.

The observations point to a physiological state of compensating shock.

Activity 4.11: Critical thinking (page 100)

The blood pressure is significantly low from the previous baseline; the SpO_2 is significantly low; this clinical profile points to a developing physiological state of decompensating shock.

Activity 4.12: Reflection (page 102)

Harry was commenced on a rehabilitation programme while still an inpatient and will continue that programme following discharge home. The key elements to cardiac rehabilitation programmes focus on improving diet, exercise and appropriate medication management. Support and compliance with all of these will help to reduce the risk of further cardiac problems.

Further reading

White, A K and Johnson, M (2000) Men making sense of their chest pain – niggles, doubts and denials. *Journal of Clinical Nursing.* 9(4): 534–41.

An interesting paper that suggests that men's self-concept as 'healthy' may inhibit a speedy response to the signs and symptoms of acute coronary pain.

Albarran, J (2002) The language of chest pain. *Nursing Times.* 98(4): 38–40.

An interesting and easy read on chest pain, nursing assessment and how patients express their pain.

Blanchard, J F and Murnaghan, D A (2010) Nursing patients with acute chest pain: practice guided by the Prince Edward Island conceptual model for nursing. *Nurse Education in Practice.* 10(1): 48–51.

An interesting paper that considers chest pain in relation to nursing models and nursing theory.

O'Shea, L (2010) Differential diagnosis of chest pain. *Practice Nurse.* 40(6): 13.

An informative review of chest pain and related physical examination and patient history taking.

Pope, BB (2006) What's causing your patient's chest pain? *Nursing Management: Critical Care Insider.* Suppl 21–4.

An informative review of chest pain and its management in a critical care nursing environment.

Useful websites

www.nhs.uk/conditions/chest-pain/Pages/Introduction.aspx

NHS Choices is the UK's biggest health website. It provides a comprehensive health information service. NHS Choices includes around 20,000 regularly updated articles. There are also hundreds of thousands of entries in more than 50 directories that you can use to find and choose health services in England.

A useful and easy to read page on chest pain and its causes.

www.patient.co.uk/doctor/Chest-Pain.htm

Patient.co.uk offers comprehensive health information provided by GPs and nurses to patients during consultations. This PatientPlus article is written for healthcare professionals.

www.netdoctor.co.uk/diseases/facts/angina.htm

NetDoctor.co.uk is a collaboration between doctors, healthcare professionals, information specialists and patients. It is a comprehensive web resource. This article is a useful review of angina.

www.familydoctor.org/familydoctor/en/health-tools/search-by-symptom/chest-pain-acute.html

This website is operated by the American Academy of Family Physicians (AAFP), a national medical organisation representing more than 100,300 family physicians, family practice residents and medical students. The following page presents a useful algorithm in chest pain diagnosis.

www.nice.org.uk

The National Institute for Health and Care Excellence website offers guidance, advice, quality standards and information services for health, public health and social care. Also contains resources to help maximise use of evidence and guidance.

Chapter 5
The patient in pain

Catherine Williams

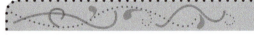

NMC Standards for Pre-registration Nursing Education

This chapter will address the following competencies:

Domain 3: Nursing practice and decision-making
Generic competencies:
3.   All nurses must carry out comprehensive, systematic nursing assessments that take account of relevant physical, social, cultural, psychological, spiritual, genetic and environmental factors, in partnership with service users and others through interaction, observation and measurement.
6.   All nurses must practise safely by being aware of the correct use, limitations and hazards of common interventions, including nursing activities, treatments, and the use of medical devices and equipment. The nurse must be able to evaluate their use, report any concerns promptly through appropriate channels and modify care where necessary to maintain safety. They must contribute to the collection of local and national data and formulation of policy on risks, hazards and adverse outcomes.

Field-specific competencies:
3.1.   Adult nurses must safely use a range of diagnostic skills, employing appropriate technology, to assess the needs of service users.

NMC Essential Skills Clusters

This chapter will address the following ESCs:

Cluster: Organisational aspects of care
9.   People can trust the newly registered graduate nurse to treat them as partners and work with them to make a holistic and systematic assessment of their needs; to develop a personalised plan that is based on mutual understanding and respect for their individual situation, promoting health and well-being, minimising risk of harm and promoting their safety at all times.
10.   People can trust the newly registered graduate nurse to deliver nursing interventions and evaluate their effectiveness against the agreed assessment and care plan.

Cluster: Medicines management

36. People can trust the newly registered graduate nurse to ensure safe and effective practice in medicines management through comprehensive knowledge of medicines, their actions, risks and benefits.

38. People can trust the newly registered graduate nurse to administer medicines safely and in a timely manner, including controlled drugs.

39. People can trust a newly registered graduate nurse to keep and maintain accurate records using information technology, where appropriate, within a multi-disciplinary framework as a leader and as part of a team and in a variety of care settings including at home

41. People can trust the newly registered graduate nurse to use and evaluate up-to-date information on medicines management and work within national and local policy guidelines.

Chapter aims

By the end of this chapter, you should be able to:

- discuss the anatomy and physiology of pain transmission;
- define acute and chronic pain;
- effectively assess pain using a variety of assessment tools;
- reflect on clinical examples in the chapter and apply this to your own clinical situation.

Introduction

This chapter is about the physical and psychological impact of pain, and will explain how you perform an accurate pain assessment. It will explain the importance of monitoring patients using clinical assessment skills and procedures.

Traditionally pain is considered to be the fifth vital sign after temperature, pulse, respiration and blood pressure (National Confidential Enquiry into Patient Outcome and Death, 2010) and should form an integral component of your nursing assessment. If we can learn to measure a patient's pain as routinely as we take their pulse, blood pressure, temperature and respiration, then we will have taken a huge step towards managing it.

Pain can have harmful physiological, psychological and emotional effects on your patient. Many patients in the clinical environment experience pain, which is usually related to surgery, trauma or some form of organ disease.

> ### Case study: Kate's story
>
> *Maddie, a student nurse, is on a placement in the burns unit and is working with her mentor on admissions. One evening a patient called Kate is transferred for assessment to the burns unit. She has sustained a 13% scald to both legs. She is still in a great deal of discomfort despite receiving a total dose of 30 mg of intravenous morphine (in increments of 10 mg) and paracetamol 1 g intravenously prior to transfer from A&E. The medical staff on call is reluctant to give further opiates at present as she is concerned that this will increase the risk of respiratory depression. However, Kate is asked to assess her pain level on a scale of 0–10 and rates the pain as 11. Maddie's mentor explains that the patient's nerve endings have been left exposed to the air by her injury and that the uncovering of the wound for assessment is contributing to Kate's discomfort. The mentor also explains that the wound will have to be cleaned and debrided prior to dressings being applied and that this is likely to make the pain worse, albeit temporarily. The mentor then becomes an advocate for the patient and suggests to the medical staff that she might benefit from using **nitrous oxide** for pain relief until the wound can be covered. Checks are made with the patient and there are no contraindications for her to receive this form of analgesia. The mentor sets about explaining to Kate how to use the nitrous oxide inhalation system; they are able to proceed with the wound assessment and types of dressings. When the wounds are properly dressed and no longer exposed to the air, Kate's discomfort abates and she is able to breathe normally and no longer requires the nitrous oxide.*

The aetiology of pain

Wilson (2007) describes acute pain as being a physiological response that warns us of a threat or danger to the body. Because of the increase in hormone production and sympathetic output in the body from injury or illness, your patient, when in pain, will experience an increase in heart rate and blood pressure, which increases cardiac work and oxygen consumption. Patients who are not appropriately managed for acute pain are at higher risk of developing chronic pain syndrome (Rivara et al., 2008).

This physiological response comes from the nervous system that directs and manages the functions of all the cells and tissues in our body. In short, the theory is that a stimulus activates the nerve ending pain receptors, and this stimulus is known as a **nociceptor**. For example, if you burn your finger, the tissue damage activates the nociceptors, which in turn transmit impulses to the brain via the spinal cord causing you to experience **nociceptive pain**. Other forms of nociceptive pain are arthritis, sickle cell crisis and post-operative pain.

Another type of pain stimulus is known as **somatic pain**, which is a type of nociceptive pain. The nerves that detect somatic pain are located in the skin and deep tissues and they send impulses to the brain when they detect some kind of tissue damage, for example, if you cut your finger, stretch a muscle too far or exercise for a long period of time. The pain experienced will be sharp due to the tissues being rich in the A delta (A) fibres sending rapid signals to the brain, and this is why you are able to clearly locate the origin of the pain and it usually causes you to cry or scream.

Pain from deeper tissues is known as **visceral pain**. Visceral pain is also a type of nociceptive pain, but it originates from the internal organs. Like somatic pain, the nociceptors send signals to the spinal cord and brain when damage is detected. Visceral pain is often described as generalised aching or squeezing in the body. For example, if you suffer from irritable bowel syndrome or bladder disorders, you will experience visceral pain. The generalised aching or squeezing felt is caused by compression or stretching of the abdominal cavity. Visceral pain can radiate to other areas in the body, which is why pinpointing its exact location can be difficult.

Activity 5.1 **Evidence-based practice and research**

Research nociceptive, visceral and somatic pain in more depth. Try to identify the specific areas of the body that may be affected, what type of injury may cause them in a patient and how the pain for each area may be experienced. As a nurse why it is important to identify the types of pain our patients experience?

What are the contraindications for the use of nitrous oxide?

There is no outline answer provided for this activity.

Types of pain

When treating patients you always need to consider the type of pain that they are suffering so that you can use the appropriate strategy to alleviate it.

Pain is classified as acute or chronic (Dougherty and Lister, 2008). **Acute pain** is normally of sudden onset, usually occurring as a result of tissue damage, injury or disease, and it tends to resolve over time as tissues heal. **Chronic pain** begins with an episode of acute pain, but unlike acute pain, chronic pain does not resolve over time. The most common causes of chronic pain are degenerative conditions such as osteoarthritis or diabetic complications such as neuropathy. Table 5.1 shows some common examples of chronic and acute pain.

Chronic pain	Acute pain
Diabetic neuropathy	Migraine/headache
Back pain	Burns
Osteoarthritis/rheumatoid arthritis	Fractures
Multiple sclerosis	Lacerations
Cancer	Abdominal pain
Neuralgia	Toothache
Post-surgical pain	Post-surgical pain

Table 5.1: Examples of chronic and acute pain

The way in which we experience pain is very complex. All sorts of factors influence our experience, including our thoughts and feelings. You need to be aware that some patients can suffer from both forms of pain (chronic and acute), and a number of nursing interventions that you routinely perform on your patient such as suctioning, line insertion, repositioning and physio-therapy can cause additional pain and discomfort. One way to understand what is happening is what is called the **gate control theory** of pain (Melzack, 1996).

Providing comfort to your patient who is in pain is a vital role of the nurse, and implementing supportive measures will minimise the overall pain and anxiety in your patient. Communication, reassurance, touch and explanations are important skills that you need to incorporate into your practice. Simple measures such as reducing noise levels and light and relieving prolonged pressure or limb placement by turning pillows over may help relieve positioning discomfort in your patient and decrease anxiety levels.

Activity 5.2   *Decision making*

Think about the case study: Kate's story. What type of pain do you think Kate is suffering from and how are these factors opening the pain gate? What is your reasoning for deciding this? What interventions could you introduce to close the pain gate?

An outline answer can be found at the end of the chapter.

Pain assessment

Assessment of pain is an important aspect of your role that requires a number of skills, including observation, interpretation and communication skills. Other interventions that can be used to assess pain include:

- analgesic administration;
- emotional support;
- cognitive techniques;
- comfort measures.

Pain assessment in patients is often poor because pain is an individual experience, but remember that the patient's response to pain can be affected by a multitude of variables such as age or culture, not just the type of pain and its duration.

Activity 5.3   *Reflection*

Think of three or four patients you have cared for who were in considerable pain or whose pain needed careful management. How did they express pain? Did they express their pain in the same way as other patients? If not, what were the differences?

There is no outline answer at the end of the chapter as this activity is based on your own reflections.

What should be covered in your pain assessment?

Your initial assessment of the patient's pain assessment should include:

- the underlying condition;
- whether the pain is acute or chronic;
- whether any medical treatment is being given;
- related symptoms such as vomiting and breathlessness;
- meaning or significance of the pain for the patient.

You can undertake an initial or ongoing assessment using a pain assessment tool. Many assessment tools are available, although the most commonly used pain scale in the healthcare setting is the numerical rating scale. The numerical scale offers the individual in pain an opportunity to rate their pain score. The user rates their scale from 0 to 10 when asked, or places a mark on a line indicating their level of pain. The lowest figure indicates the absence of pain, and the highest figure represents the most intense pain possible.

An advantage of the numerical scale assessment is that it follows the World Health Organization (WHO) analgesic ladder (WHO, 1996). The WHO ladder provides a simple step-by-step guide to increase or decrease analgesics and its advantages include:

- simplicity – in that only a few, widely known drugs are employed;
- applicability – to a wide variety of situations and prescribers worldwide;
- safety – in that the safer drug is used first.

Activity 5.4   *Reflection*

Investigate the pain relief analgesic ladder devised by the WHO. Reflect back on a patient you have cared for who benefited from having their medication linked to the principles of the ladder.

There is no outline answer at the end of the chapter as this activity is based on your own reflections.

Another pain assessment method that is easy to remember is the PQRST mnemonic, which stands for Provokes, Quality, Radiates, Severity and Time (Skaer, 1998), shown in the box 'Pain recognition and assessment'. This method has five simple characteristics to help you in the questioning of the patient's pain assessment, but remember that you must let the patient describe the pain, as sometimes they say what they think you would like to hear.

Pain recognition and assessment

P = Provokes

- What causes pain?
- What makes it better?
- What makes it worse?

Q = Quality

- What does it feel like? Can you describe the pain? Is it:
  - sharp?
  - dull?
  - stabbing?
  - burning?
  - crushing?

R = Radiates

- Where does the pain radiate?
- Is it in one place?
- Does it move around?
- Did it start elsewhere and is now localised to one spot?

S = Severity

- How severe is the pain on a scale of 1–10? This can be a difficult one as the rating will differ from patient to patient.

T = Time

- Time pain started?
- How long did it last?
- Is it constant or does it come and go?

In the absence of patients being unable to self-report pain due to mechanical ventilation, altered level of consciousness or cognitive status, current recommendations advocate the use of a valid behaviour pain scale such as the Critical-Care Pain Observation Tool (CPOT) (Arbour et al., 2011). The Behavioural Pain Scale (BPS) is very useful in the assessment of pain in critically ill patients as it works by evaluating facial expressions, upper limb movements and compliance with mechanical ventilation. Although not the ideal assessment, when used alongside other non-verbal signs such as blood pressure, heart rate and vasoconstriction, it can help indicate pain in your patient.

It is vital that you regard the patient's pain as an assessment priority. Unless pain is assessed regularly and effectively, your patient will continue to suffer unnecessarily.

Assessment in the very young, the cognitively impaired (such as the sedated patient or those with dementia) and those with communication problems can pose problems, but there are suitable pain assessment tools such as verbal rating, visual analogue, body diagrams, questionnaires and pain diaries.

Effective pain assessment is a fundamental part of your nursing care, and the accountability of pain assessment lies firmly within the domain of nursing. To enable you to do this effectively, keep in mind the following.

- Seek to establish a relationship with your patient.
- Use open questions.
- Observe your patient for clues regarding pain.
- Avoid jumping to conclusions.

Activity 5.5   *Critical thinking*

Consider our case study patient, Kate. Of the assessments scales that have been discussed, which one do you think would be most appropriate for her, and why? Would Kate benefit from the CPOT assessment? What other factors will you observe in your assessment?

An outline answer to this activity is at the end of the chapter.

Managing your patient's pain

The choice of drug used to alleviate your patient's pain depends upon the nature and severity of the pain, and many other factors that the doctor will consider.

The three main classes of drugs that are commonly used within the hospital care environment are:

- non-opioids;
- opioids;
- anti-emetics.

We will now go on to look at each of these classes of drugs in more detail.

Non-opioids

This class of analgesics is better suited to treating musculoskeletal pain or mild to moderate pain generally associated with inflammation. Non-opioids are widely used and include aspirin, paracetamol, ibuprofen and diclofenac. Paracctamol is included in this group but has very weak anti-inflammatory effects. The route of administration will depend on your patient's condition. Take care to bear in mind your patient's renal clearance as **nephrotoxic** medication such as NSAIDs increase the risk of kidney failure. Non-opioid analgesics such as paracetamol and aspirin are readily available over the counter, though many stronger forms may require a doctor's prescription.

For further information and guidance on pharmacology and therapeutics of this group of drugs, you should refer to the *British National Formulary* (**www.bnf.org**).

Opioids

Some prescription medicines contain drugs that are controlled under the Misuse of Drugs legislation. These medicines are called controlled drugs. Examples include: **benzodiazepine**, morphine, pethidine and methadone. Opioids originate from the opium poppy and are generally suitable for treating moderate to severe pain. They work by interfering with the transmission of the pain signal to the brain and changing the way the brain perceives pain. However, potentially lethal side effects such as respiratory depression and changes in consciousness level mean that they must be appropriately selected, prescribed, administered and monitored. Opioids can be short-acting or long-acting, depending on how they are manufactured. Morphine is recognised as one of the strongest of opioid therapy; it relieves dull, prolonged pain and is long-acting, making it a good choice of drug for bolus administration. Bolus administration is when a relatively large dose of medication is administered into a vein in a short period, usually within 1–30 minutes.

Diamorphine is synthesised from morphine and works by mimicking the action of naturally occurring pain-reducing chemicals called endorphins. Pethidine is a synthetic form of morphine and has muscle relaxant properties, but due to its very short-acting properties it is rarely used in the ICU setting and more frequently used within a ward setting. Fentanyl is a synthetic opioid that is more potent than morphine and is not appropriate for general pain management due to its strength. Because it does not cause histamine release in your patients there is less risk of hypotension. Fentanyl derivatives include remifentanyl and alfentanyl.

Ketamine is a co-analgesic, and is most effective when used alongside a low-dose opioid. It has analgesic effects in itself, although high doses can cause disorienting side effects, and it tends to increase heart rate and blood pressure.

Opioids can be administered via multiple routes but have many side effects such as respiratory depression, cough suppression, constipation, urinary retention, and nausea and vomiting, with the additional potential to depress the gag reflex, causing aspiration; hence, close observation and documentation is vital to prevent complications occurring.

For further information and guidance on the pharmacology and therapeutics on this group of drugs, please refer to the *British National Formulary* (**www.bnf.org**).

Anti-emetics

You can buy some anti-emetics that help relieve nausea and vomiting over the counter without a doctor's prescription, but generally anti-emetics are prescription-only drugs.

Many different types of drugs are used to control nausea and vomiting. Some affect brain function by preventing the stimulation of the vomiting centre, and others work on the gut by speeding up motility. The most commonly used anti-emetics such as ondansetron, prochlorperazine and cyclizine affect the vomiting centre, whereas metoclopramide increases gut motility. The patient's symptoms will affect the choice of anti-emetic.

For further information and guidance on the pharmacology and therapeutics on this group of drugs, please refer to the *British National Formulary* (**www.bnf.org**).

Activity 5.6   *Critical thinking*

Research the main analgesics previously discussed, using the *British National Formulary* (*BNF*) at **www.bnf.org** and ascertain the contraindications, interactions and side effects of these drugs.

Identify whether each of the drugs are mild, moderate or severe analgesics in line with the WHO (1996) pain ladder.

Think about the burns patient, Kate. How effective are these drugs likely to be for her? Why is the analgesia not working effectively? Is this to do with the type of injury, the choice of drug or the individual?

An outline answer is given at the end of the chapter.

Epidurals

An epidural anaesthetic works by blocking the nerve roots that lead to the uterus and lower part of the body. The nerve roots are located in a space near the spinal cord called the epidural space. The epidural space extends from the base of the skull to the sacrum and the space is identified by feeling for bony landmarks on the spine and pelvis. A fine-bore catheter is inserted into the epidural space and the ligaments and bones of the spinal cord; the catheter is secured to the patient's back and then attached to the infusion device.

The area of analgesic effect is dependent on the site of insertion in relation to the surgery. Epidural location sites are:

- T6–T9 abdominal surgery – exploratory laparotomy;
- T7–T10 upper abdominal surgery – repair of abdominal aortic aneurysm;
- T9–L1 lower abdominal surgery – repair of inguinal hernias;
- L1–L4 hip and knee surgery (Dougherty and Lister, 2008).

The drugs most commonly used for epidural analgesia are opioids such as fentanyl and bupivacaine. Bupivacaine can be used on its own (usually for a bolus dose) and dosage will depend on the size of the catheter and the type of surgery. Remember that epidural analgesia is contraindicated in patients who have:

- local or systemic infection;
- known neurological disease;
- coagulation disorders or who are undergoing anticoagulant therapy;

- spinal arthritis/spinal deformities;

- hypotension;

- marked hypertension (Hastings, 2009).

Activity 5.7   *Critical thinking*

What is epidural analgesia? Where is it administered? What do you think might be the specific nursing care associated with administering drugs via this route?

An outline answer can be found at the end of the chapter.

You always need to observe the epidural site for any signs of infection, inflammation and **phlebitis** during your assessment. When removing the epidural line, ensure you use a strict aseptic technique to reduce the risk of infection and haematoma. As a matter of good practice you should always check **clotting time** (PT 10–14 seconds) before removal and always check the catheter tip is intact after removal. Because of the risk of bleeding, avoid prophylactic heparin administration before and after removal of the line (times will be identified in your local policy); many clinical areas have specific step-down analgesia protocols that are implemented to avoid premature discontinuation – see your local policy for further guidance. Epidural use is usually limited to a maximum of four days because of the significant risk of infection after this period of time. Any concern you may have about the epidural site or infusion should be discussed immediately with the pain team or the anaesthetist.

As with all controlled drugs you must prepare, administer and document the drugs according to your hospital policy. For further information and guidance with regard to pharmacology and therapeutics, please refer to the *British National Formulary* (**www.bng.org**).

Patient-controlled analgesia

Patient-controlled analgesia (PCA) is widely used for the treatment of pain in the ICU environment. The PCA offers on-demand, intermittent, IV administration of opioids under patient control (with or without a continuous background infusion). This technique is based on the use of a sophisticated microprocessor-controlled infusion pump that delivers a pre-programmed dose of opioid when the patient pushes a demand button; lock-out controls are set to prevent excessive administration or overdose.

Activity 5.8   *Critical thinking*

Research PCA – what is it? What are the main advantages and disadvantages of its use in patients experiencing pain in hospital or in the community?

There is no answer to this activity at the end of the chapter. The issues are discussed below.

Using a PCA system allows your patient more immediate relief of incidental (breakthrough) pain and can provide a greater sense of personal control over pain. It can be reassuring to your patient to know that an analgesic is quickly available and that they are in control of the administration.

As the opioid analgesia is not administered unless the patient presses the control, it is important that they are able to operate it properly. The PCA system will be unsuitable for a patient who does not have the cognitive ability to understand how to use the PCA device, or who is unable or unwilling to operate the handset.

Because a strong opioid is being administered, you will need to have a clear understanding of the contraindications and therapeutics of the drug being administered and its side effects. As with epidurals, hourly checks of the following must be completed and documented:

- heart rate;
- blood pressure;
- respiratory rate;
- oxygen saturations;
- pain score;
- sedation score;
- nausea/vomiting;
- dose used.

In addition to your patient checks, pump checks need to be completed to enable continuing assessment. Pump checks include:

- programme check;
- amount delivered;
- successful attempts;
- unsuccessful attempts – *this will indicate that analgesic needs are not being met and the regime needs to be urgently reviewed*;
- lock-out time – the lock-out interval is designed to prevent overdose. Ideally, it should be long enough for the patient to experience the maximal effect of one dose before another is permitted.

A PCA is usually needed for a few days after surgery/medical interventions, and many ICUs have specific step-down analgesia protocols to prevent premature discontinuation and ensure patients remain pain free during the step down from intravenous to oral medication. Any concern you may have about the PCA infusion should be discussed immediately with the pain team or the anaesthetist.

As with all controlled drugs you must prepare, administer and document the drugs according to your local policy. For further information and guidance with regard to pharmacology and therapeutics, please refer to the *British National Formulary* (**www.bng.org**).

Recognising deterioration in your patient

When you have a critically ill patient who has difficulty communicating their pain due to altered levels of consciousness or endotracheal intubation, they may have a continuous infusion to prevent exacerbation of pain. Unfortunately, there are risks of over-dosage, especially in patients with kidney or liver dysfunction. You must report any changes in your patient's pain or overall condition. You will need to make frequent observations and assessments so that you spot any change in their condition or adverse effects caused by treatment. Be aware of patients receiving strong opiates and sedation for post-operative pain as they could be at risk of respiratory depression. You will need to assess pain and sedation hourly. When caring for a patient in pain, it is useful to remember the following.

- Think of pain as the fifth vital sign – any increase in your patient's pain may mean deterioration in your patient's condition.

- Always report any new sources for pain identified by your patient – this could be a sign of surgical and/or medical complications.

- Opioids have strong side effects. Your patient will require specific and close monitoring and you may need to administer other drugs to overcome the side effects.

- Never focus solely on the one aspect of your patient's pain – take into account all possible factors that may be affecting their pain management.

Non-pharmacological pain management

Non-pharmacological approaches may contribute to effective analgesia, are often well accepted by patients and are a useful adjunct in managing pain. The role of non-pharmacological approaches to pain management is evolving and it is likely that some non-pharmacological and complementary therapies may make an important contribution to holistic patient care. The goals of non-pharmacological interventions are to:

- minimise fear and distress;
- make pain more tolerable;
- give the patient a sense of control over the situation and their behaviour;
- teach and enhance coping strategies.

Common non-pharmacological pain-control methods widely used in hospitals and in the community are distraction, music therapy, hypnosis, cold and heat application, transcutaneous electrical nerve stimulators (TENS) and massage therapy. You need to be familiar with each of these methods. It is also important that you develop a therapeutic nurse–patient relationship and pay attention to comfort measures, as these will aid pain control in your patient. Fear and anxiety make pain worse, so your nursing care should aim to alleviate these feelings.

Scenario

Kate is now at home recovering from her burns and being visited by Seeta, who is the community nurse responsible for her continuing care. Seeta is accompanied by Jaimie who is on clinical experience in the community.

Jaimie has been learning about pain management and is interested to see how Seeta will be approaching the problem in Kate's case.

Seeta asks Kate how she is coping with the pain and, rather to Jaimie's surprise, asks whether she finds listening to music helpful. Seeta explores with Kate whether adjusting the lighting in her room might help and discusses with her how best to make her as comfortable as possible. She then suggests playing some of Kate's favourite CDs in a relaxed atmosphere.

Seeta goes on to suggest to Kate that she might benefit from one or more of the following: music therapy, hypnosis or cognitive behavioural therapy (CBT). She has leaflets about all of these she is able to leave with Kate.

Seeta then gives Kate a leaflet about transcutaneous electrical nerve stimulators and explains how this works. She explains to Kate how she might access any of these therapies.

As they leave Kate's house, Jaimie realises her understanding of how pain can be managed has been broadened by watching and listening to Seeta at work.

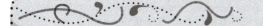

Chapter summary

Pain can be triggered by many medical conditions, including ischaemia, infections, inflammation, oedema, distension, immobilisation, incisions and wounds. The use of invasive and non-invasive medical devices can also cause pain in your patient. In addition, many commonly performed nursing procedures such as suctioning, turning, dressing changes, and the insertion and removal of catheters may be a source of pain for your patient, and these need to be taken into consideration when assessing pain.

Preventing pain will improve your patient's physiological and psychological outcomes, enabling earlier discharge. Remember that pain is individual to each patient (McCaffery and Pasero, 1999) and will always require regular individual assessment. Pain is usually a symptom of a problem, and even though analgesia will be provided, the cause of your patient's pain will still need to be investigated. Unless pain is assessed regularly and effectively, the patient will continue to suffer unnecessarily.

(Continued)

continued . . . . ●

Pain management has to be one of your top nursing priorities and you must continue to monitor outcomes related to pain management. Some patients may be able to verbally or non-verbally communicate their pain-control needs; the critically ill intubated patient may not be able to communicate their level of pain adequately, and this needs to be recognised in the care plan. To fulfil the above you will need to have a thorough understanding of the actions of analgesics, their side effects, dosages and differing methods of administration and appropriate use within the ICU setting to ensure a positive outcome for your patient.

Activities: brief outline answers

Activity 5.2: Decision making (page 110)

Kate is suffering from acute pain. Burn pain is one of the most difficult forms of acute pain to treat. The type of tissue damage with a burn injury is likely to generate unusually high levels of pain. The gate is opened by the activity in the small diameter nerve fibres being exposed due to the burn injury. Interventions used to close the gate can include relaxation/mental factors/activity and other physical factors.

Activity 5.5: Critical thinking (page 113)

Assessment tools are essential to the diagnosis of underlying burn pain syndromes and the effectiveness of their treatment. The better tool to use with this patient is one of the verbal self-report instruments that measure pain intensity, such as the '0–10' numeric rating scale. This is the most appropriate tool as assessing pain in the burn-injured patient is complex and as she is able to communicate well; this assessment tool will give you a clear picture of her pain status.

Activity 5.6: Critical thinking (page 115)

Burn pain is difficult to control because of its unique characteristics, its multiple components and its changing patterns over time. Cleansing wounds, changing dressings and providing physical therapy involve repeated manipulations of painful sites. Understanding the mechanisms that contribute to the intensity and variability of burn injury pain over time is crucial to its proper management.

Activity 5.7: Critical thinking (page 116)

An epidural is a form of regional analgesia involving an infusion of drugs through a catheter placed into the epidural space. Epidural analgesia may be administered either as a continuous infusion, as patient-controlled epidural analgesia (PCEA), or as a combination of the two. The injection can cause both a loss of sensation and a loss of pain by blocking the transmission of signals through nerves in or near the spinal cord. A comprehensive assessment should include: vital signs, pain and sedation levels, level of consciousness, ability to void, sensation and motor function, presence of potential adverse side effects and complications, and evaluation of insertion site.

Your patient will require vital signs monitoring throughout its use for signs of hypotension (due to **vasodilation** of the vessels) and respiratory depression (due to opioid analgesia). Most clinical areas advocate an hourly protocol check of:

- heart rate;
- blood pressure – hypertension should not be managed by tilting the patient's head down as this will allow the drug to travel up to T4 and cause paralysis of the respiratory muscles;
- respiratory rate;
- oxygen saturations;
- pain score;
- dose delivered;
- sedation score;

- nausea/vomiting – if your patient is complaining of a headache and nausea/vomiting, this may be a sign of a dural puncture;
- level of sensory/motor block – the block should be high enough to provide effective analgesia but not to paralyse the respiratory muscles. If this occurs, you must stop the infusion immediately;
- the dressing.

Further reading

Caudill, M (2008) *Managing Pain Before It Manages You.* Third edition. New York: Guilford Press.

This book continues to be the gold standard for the self-management of pain. It is informative and easy to read, focusing on what people can do on their own to manage persistent pain.

Herndon, D N (2007) *Total Burn Care.* Third edition. London: W B Saunders.

This book will give you a comprehensive overview of the assessment and management of a patient with moderate and severe thermal burns.

Mann, E and Carr, E (2006) *Pain Management: Essential Clinical Skills for Nurses.* London: Blackwell Publishing.

Pain management is a practical guide to current best practice, providing students and newly qualified nurses with the knowledge and skills required to care for a person experiencing, or at risk of experiencing, pain.

Useful websites

www.ncepod.org.uk

National Confidential Enquiry into Patient Outcome and Death. This is a useful site when looking at promoting improvements in healthcare.

www.bnf.org

BNF. Compiled with the advice of clinical experts, this essential reference provides up-to-date guidance on prescribing, dispensing and administering medicines.

www.britishpainsociety.org

The British Pain Society. This is a useful website for current information on all matters relating to pain.

www.nice.org.uk

Website of the National Institute for Health and Care Excellence. This website allows you to access a series of national clinical guidelines to secure consistent, high quality, evidence-based care for patients using the NHS.

Chapter 6
The patient in shock

Desiree Tait

NMC Standards for Pre-registration Nursing Education

This chapter will address the following competencies:

Domain 3: Nursing practice and decision-making

3.1. Adult nurses must safely use a range of diagnostic skills, employing appropriate technology, to assess the needs of service users.

7.1. Adult nurses must recognise the early signs of illness in people of all ages. They must make accurate assessments and start appropriate and timely management of those who are acutely ill, at risk of clinical deterioration, or require emergency care.

Chapter aims

By the end of this chapter, you should be able to:

- describe and identify the causes of shock;
- describe clinical features of shock and the clinical implications for the patient;
- differentiate between and diagnose possible causes of the patient's deterioration;
- demonstrate how to assess, record and respond to patients at risk of shock;
- demonstrate an awareness of risk assessment in the context of holistic care;
- reflect on clinical examples illustrated in the chapter and apply this to your own clinical situation.

Introduction

This chapter provides an overview of the general causes and manifestations of shock and examines in detail the care of a patient with **hypovolaemic shock**. The underlying physiology, social psychology and ethical implications of the patient's care will be discussed in the context of risk assessment and collaborative management of care. The chapter proceeds with an overview of the knowledge and skills required to assess, differentiate and manage the care of patients who progress to clinical shock. The assessment and management of patients with cardiogenic shock are discussed in Chapter 4, and patients with distributive shock, including sepsis and **septic shock**, are discussed in detail in Chapter 7.

What is shock and why does it occur?

Shock is best defined as a life-threatening, generalized form of acute circulatory failure associated with inadequate oxygen utilization by the cells. It is a state in which the circulation is unable to deliver sufficient oxygen to meet the demands of the tissues, resulting in cellular dysfunction.

(Cecconi et al., 2014, p1796)

For example, if a patient has a haemorrhage and loses 30% of their total blood volume, the patient will have reduced levels of circulating blood to transport oxygen and nutrients to the body's cells leading to a very low oxygen concentration in the tissues (**dysoxia**). Without the oxygen and nutrients required for normal cell function, the body's organs and tissues will start to fail. Initially, the patient's physiological systems will try to compensate by triggering the sympathetic nervous system and the flight/fight response.

We tend to see the flight/fight response as a biological response that is triggered in situations of perceived stress when the body will focus on providing energy and resources to the brain, heart and muscles to aid either running away from danger or standing and fighting. In the case of a haemorrhaging patient, the response is designed to keep the blood supply flowing to the vital organs. If the cause of blood loss is not diagnosed and treated, the patient will continue to deteriorate and move to the progressive stage of shock, or uncompensated shock, when the patient is no longer able to compensate for the amount of blood lost (the key stages are set out in Table 6.3 later in this chapter). At this stage the body is using all its reserves to try to maintain homeostasis, and if left untreated, the refractory stage of shock will be reached – the point when the body organs start to malfunction due to tissue hypoxia. You will come across shock in many clinical situations and different locations. A person may go into shock for a number of reasons, for example, physical trauma, dehydration, sepsis, anaphylaxis and haemorrhage. Such situations can occur in the person's home, outside, and in any hospital or care setting. The types of shock are classified in four categories according to the underlying cause.

- **Hypovolaemic shock** due to decreased circulating blood volume.
- **Cardiogenic shock** due to impaired cardiac function.
- **Obstructive shock** caused by an obstruction to the circulating blood flow.
- **Distributive shock** caused by altered distribution of blood in the central and peripheral circulation and includes:

  o septic shock associated with systemic inflammatory response syndrome (see Chapter 7);

  o anaphylactic shock that occurs as a consequence of hypersensitivity to an allergen;

  o neurogenic shock due to widespread vasodilation associated with autonomic dysfunction (McCance and Huether, 2014).

All of these situations will result in insufficient blood, and therefore oxygen and nutrients, to the cells. Table 6.1 lists the categories and common causes of shock in each category, with some clinical examples. Table 6.2 provides a summary of the clinical features that are present when patients are diagnosed with a particular type of shock.

Categories of shock	Causes of shock	Clinical examples
Hypovolaemic	Decreased blood/plasma/extra cellular fluid volume due to the following. • External haemorrhage. • Internal haemorrhage. • Trauma and fractures. • Severe vomiting and diarrhoea. • Dehydration. • Major burns. • Peritonitis/**acute pancreatitis** – inflammation in the peritoneal cavity or the pancreas.	• Tom was stabbed in the leg and sustained an estimated blood loss of 750 ml. • Terry Jones was admitted with haematemesis and melaena. • Bill Holland sustained a fractured shaft of femur in a road traffic collision. • Meera has food poisoning. • Betty slipped and fell and has been lying on her kitchen floor for two days with no food or water. • Jane was trapped in her car as it caught fire and she sustained 80% burns. • Henry was admitted with acute abdominal pain, gallstones and pancreatitis.
Cardiogenic	Impaired cardiac function leading to reduced cardiac output and blood pressure due to the following. • Myocardial infarction (MI) – blocking of a coronary artery. • Myocardial contusion – bruising of the heart muscle. • Structural defects such as a ventricular septal defect – a hole in the wall of the septum between the right and left ventricles. • Cardiac arrhythmias – narrow and broad complex tachycardia.	• Harry Smith is diagnosed with a large myocardial infarction and develops cardiogenic shock (see case study in Chapter 4 on page 98). • Bill Holland sustained severe trauma to his sternum and myocardial contusion from the seat belt during the collision. • Fred recovered well from acute coronary syndrome until two weeks after treatment when he collapsed and was diagnosed with a ventricular septal defect secondary to an MI. • Jane was experiencing repeated episodes of broad complex tachycardia and her blood pressure had fallen to 80/35 mmHg.
Obstructive	Obstruction to the circulating blood flow due to the following.	• Bert was one hour into his post-operative care following cardiac surgery when he suddenly collapsed, becoming breathless and disorientated.

	• Cardiac tamponade – bleeding or fluid between the myocardial and pericardial layers of the heart, causing the heart to be squashed. • Pulmonary embolus – obstruction of oxygenated blood back to the left side of the heart. • Tension pneumothorax – air leaking and trapped between the pleural layers of the lungs causing the lungs and heart to become squashed in the thoracic cavity.	• Jamila had been complaining at home of a red and swollen leg for two days when she suddenly collapsed with chest pain and breathlessness. A deep vein thrombosis in her leg had travelled in the circulation to the lungs causing an obstruction in blood flow. • Sarah was a passenger on a flight from London to Florida when she suddenly experienced severe difficulty with breathing. The change in pressure during the flight had caused a tension pneumothorax in her right lung.	

Distributive	Altered distribution of blood flow to the central and peripheral circulation.
	
	• Septic shock caused by Gram-positive bacteria/ Gram-negative bacteria and systemic inflammatory response syndrome (SIRS) leading to vasodilation and body organ failure.
	• Anaphylaxis following exposure to an antigen.
	• Neurogenic caused by:
	  o cervical spinal cord injury leading to impaired function of the sympathetic nervous system and the flight/ fight response;
	  o anaesthesia/sedation causing depression of the respiratory and circulatory system.
		• Angela had been admitted to the ward in a distressed and confused state, with severe hypotension and a diagnosis of severe sepsis secondary to a urinary tract infection. Within an hour Angela's condition had deteriorated and she was admitted to ITU with septic shock and SIRS (see Chapter 7).
		• Helen was admitted to A&E in a collapsed state after being stung by a bee 20 minutes before.
		• Paul sustained injuries to his cervical spine and spinal cord as the result of his car overturning. His blood pressure was 80/40 mmHg and his pulse 50 bpm.
		• Mary had been given a general anaesthetic for a surgical procedure, following which she had difficulty waking up, her respiratory rate was 10 bpm, pulse 55 bpm and BP 84/52 mmHg.	

Table 6.1: Categories and common causes of shock

Assessment	Hypovolaemic	Cardiogenic	Obstructive	Distributive		
				Septic	Anaphylactic	Neurogenic
Look Skin colour? Trauma/injury? Behaviour? Level of consciousness	Pale Restless, anxious Blood or fluid loss	Grey skin with central and peripheral cyanosis Drowsy and confused	Grey skin with central and peripheral cyanosis Breathless Altered LOC sudden onset	Initially flushed with vasodilation Pale and cynosed later Exhaustion Confusion	Redness and swelling on face and neck Breathless, wheeze Blistering/wheals/pruritis Exposure to an allergen Altered LOC	Pale Faint Altered LOC Post-anaesthesia/head/spinal injury
Listen Patient/relative story Past and recent history	Thirst	Thirst			Fear/anxiety	
Feel Skin Pulse?	Skin cool	Skin cold and clammy	Skin cool and clammy		Skin warm	Skin warm and dry

Measure						
Respiration (R)	Tachypnea	Tachypnea	Tachypnea	Tachypnea	Tachypnea	Bradypnea
Oxygen saturation (SpO$_2$)	Reduced	Reduced	Reduced	Reduced	Reduced	Reduced
Arterial blood gas analysis	Metabolic acidosis (ma)	Hypoxia	Hypoxia	Hypoxia, ma as shock progresses	Hypoxia as shock progresses	Hypoxia as shock progresses
Pulse (P)	Tachycardia	Tachycardia	Tachycardia	Tachycardia	Tachycardia	Bradycardia
Blood pressure (BP)	Hypotension	Normal BP to hypotension	Normal BP to hypotension	Hypotension	Hypotension	Hypotension
ECG		Cardiac arrhythmias	Cardiac arrhythmias			
LOC						
Central venous pressure (CVP)	Reduced CVP	Elevated CVP	Reduced CVP	Reduced CVP	Reduced CVP	
Urine output	Reduced urine output	Reduced urine output	Reduced urine output	Reduced urine output	Reduced urine output	Reduced urine output
Pain score	Pain relative to cause	Pain relative to cause	Pain relative to cause	Fever with white cell count above or below the norm		

Table 6.2: A summary of the clinical features found on assessment of patients with different types of shock

If any of these signs are present the patient is at risk and should be risk assessed using track and trigger, sepsis screening and SBAR.

Activity 6.1   *Reflection*

With reference to Tables 6.1 and 6.2, think back to your experiences in the clinical setting and identify examples of situations where patients have been diagnosed as being in shock.

- Are any of the clinical situations you identified listed in Table 6.1?
- Did the patient deteriorate suddenly or over a period of several hours?
- What clinical signs and features were present to indicate your patient was in shock?

Hint: These reflective questions will help you to practise linking the causes and types of shock to the signs and symptoms present in the patients you have nursed.

There is no outline answer at the end of the chapter as this activity is based on your own reflections.

Shock, regardless of the cause, has a high incidence of morbidity and mortality that increases as the length of time between the onset of clinical deterioration and treatment increases. Early recognition and anticipation of the potential for patients to develop shock is a key nursing activity that can lead to reduced morbidity and mortality of patients in your care (NICE, 2007, 2010d; RCP, 2012).

What are the stages and signs of shock?

In health, the balance between the body's physiological systems is maintained through homeostasis. This process involves the purposeful control and maintenance of the body's organs so that normal body functions can continue efficiently. These integrated systems usually operate through negative feedback systems: physiological control mechanisms that respond to a change in the normal range of a substance by triggering other mechanisms until the uncontrolled substance is back within normal range (Hall, 2011). The effects can be manifested through physical, emotional and behavioural reactions to a stressor, such as haemorrhage. For example, using negative feedback, a fall in blood pressure will be identified by pressure sensors in the aorta and carotid arteries. A message will be sent to the brain via the autonomic nervous system that triggers the body to resist the fall in blood pressure by causing blood vessels in the peripheral circulation to constrict (patient becomes pale). As a consequence, the volume of blood in the central circulation will increase and ensure that the heart, brain and muscles receive oxygen. This can be described as the **initial stage of shock**.

If the underlying cause of inadequate tissue perfusion is not corrected the flight/fight response is able to continue to support and compensate for impaired circulation and uptake of oxygen by increasing the pulse and respiratory rate, preserving body fluids by reducing urine output and attempting to maintain an effective supply of blood and oxygen to the tissues. This is known as the **compensatory stage of shock**. Diagnosis, support and management of the underlying cause can reverse the progression of shock at this stage.

If the underlying cause continues to be left untreated the compensatory mechanisms will be unable to maintain effective circulation, and the patient will collapse. Inadequate circulation leads to ischaemia (decreased blood supply to the tissues) and **tissue dysoxia**. Without an adequate supply of oxygen, the cells will no longer be able to function effectively and will start to fail. This is known as the **progressive stage of shock**. When a patient enters the progressive stage of shock they are critically ill and need intensive support. It is during this stage that organ failure, such as acute renal failure and acute lung injury, is likely to occur. Even with intensive support of the body's systems, the damage to body organs is likely to continue, leading to multiple organ failure. This is known as the **refractory stage** when shock becomes irreversible and the patient is likely to die.

Regardless of the type and cause of shock, if the patient does not receive the appropriate interventions, the ultimate outcome will be the same. However, with timely assessment and intervention, the effects of shock can be reversed before the patient progresses to the final and irreversible stage. The four progressive and interrelated stages of shock are presented in Table 6.3.

Stages of shock	Physiological and clinical progress	Patient example
1. Initial	• The body systems are able to accommodate the clinical trigger or cause. • Clinical features are often not apparent at this stage and the situation can go unrecognised. • Shock is reversible with assessment and intervention.	Mrs Brown has a two-day history of diarrhoea and vomiting. Her GP records her vital signs as: R: 18/min; P: 92/min; BP: 110/65. These are within the normal range; however, if her symptoms persist, she could go into hypovolaemic shock. He prescribes an intramuscular injection of anti-emetic to reduce the vomiting and suggests she contacts the surgery again tomorrow if she feels no better.
2. Compensatory	• If the cause remains active the body's physiological systems will be triggered. • Clinical features include an increase in pulse, respirations	The following day Mrs Brown's vital signs have deteriorated. The vomiting has subsided but the diarrhoea persists. She is anxious, cold to touch and thirsty. Her vital

(Continued)

Table 6.3   (Continued)

Stages of shock	Physiological and clinical progress	Patient example
	and a reduction in BP, and will be evident as the flight/fight response initiates a cascade of physiological responses in an attempt to compensate for the loss of homeostasis. • Shock is reversible with assessment and intervention.	signs are: R: 20/min; P: 100/min; BP: 89/58.
3. Progressive	• The underlying cause and impact persists. • Physiologically the body has used all the compensatory mechanisms available in an attempt to return to homeostasis and has failed to compensate. • This leads to tissue ischaemia and hypoxia. • Shock is reversible in the early stages with appropriate assessment and management.	Mrs Brown was taken to the A&E unit where an assessment shows evidence of further deterioration. She is confused and agitated. She has not passed urine for 24 hours. Her vital signs are: R: 24/min; P: 110/min; BP: 80/50. Mrs Brown receives fluid resuscitation and management of the underlying cause. Her condition improves and within four days she is discharged home.
4. Refractory	• Physiologically the body has been unable to compensate, leading to cell death, tissue death and multiple organ dysfunction syndrome. • Shock is irreversible.	If Mrs Brown had not been referred to A&E in a timely manner by the GP, her condition would have continued to deteriorate and without support she would have become drowsy and eventually lost consciousness. She would have become peripherally and centrally cyanosed (see Chapters 2 and 3), and her vital signs would have been: R: 30/min; P: 120/min; BP: 65/40. She would be suffering from tissue hypoxia and acute kidney injury.

Table 6.3: The stages of shock, illustrated by a clinical example

Hypovolaemic shock

Assessment and management of patients with hypovolaemic shock

As we have seen, hypovolaemic shock occurs as a result of the loss of a critical volume of blood, plasma or extracellular fluid. In a healthy adult male at a weight of 70 kg the total blood volume is an estimated 4,900 ml (70 ml of blood/kg). This is the volume required to maintain an effective circulation (Grossman and Porth, 2013). If a patient loses up to 10% of their circulating volume, the body will respond and compensate so that no obvious clinical signs are evident. However, if the loss continues unabated, clinical signs will become evident when approximately 15% loss is reached. The greater the volume of loss, the more significant the clinical effects become and cardiac output decreases exponentially (Hall, 2011). When cardiac output falls, this means that there is a reduced volume of blood being pumped into the systemic circulation every minute. To try to increase the volume and establish stability, the body will increase the heart rate. However, with a continuing loss of blood or body fluids, the body will find the task of compensating for the loss more difficult. Table 6.4 illustrates the physiological impact of hypovolaemic shock caused by haemorrhage on the patient's clinical features, based on percentage of blood loss (American College of Surgeons, 2008). It is important to note that assessing patients based only on percentage of blood loss provides a limited amount of information and a complete assessment of other factors that affect the patient's oxygen delivery, such as a patient's co-morbidities and medications, should also be completed (Bersten and Soni, 2014). External blood loss leading to hypovolaemia can be measured through visual estimation on examination of the patient and environment. For example, a patient with bleeding oesophageal varices (ruptured blood vessels in the oesophagus) will have a recent history of acute and severe haematemesis. When bleeding is internal, the pattern of evidence is more complex and can only be estimated on the basis of a physiological understanding of the patient's condition and following a clinical assessment and examination of the patient. For example, a patient with a fractured shaft of the femur can have an estimated blood and fluid loss of up to 2,000 ml, while a patient with a traumatic fracture of the tibia can lose an estimated 800ml into the surrounding interstitial tissue around the site of the fracture. In this example both patients have a risk of developing shock, but the patient with a fractured shaft of femur will have a much higher risk of going into shock within 30 minutes of injury than the patient with a fractured tibia. This will be manifested by evidence of patient anxiety, pale cool skin, tachycardia, tachypnea, and reduced blood pressure and pulse pressure (difference measured between the systolic and diastolic BP).

Other causes of hypovolaemic shock are listed in Table 6.1 (page 124) and include a variety of clinical conditions associated with acute loss of blood, plasma or extracellular fluid. Patients with diarrhoea and vomiting, fever and dehydration all experience fluid loss associated with loss of body fluids. Patients with severe burns experience loss of body fluids and plasma, and this is explained in more detail in Chapter 10. Patients who experience third space fluid shift movements experience loss of fluid available to support the circulation. Fluid shifts into a space where it would not normally collect in such large volumes, such as with peritonitis, when fluid shifts into

On assessment	Initial	Compensatory	Progressive	Refractory
Loss of blood or body fluid volume	0–15%, 750 ml	15–30%, 750–1,500 ml	30–40%, 1,500–2,000 ml	>40%, >2,000 ml
Look/Feel	Minimal clinical signs	Cool skin	Pale, cool	Pale, cold to touch
Look/Listen	Anxious	Anxious	Confused and agitated	Loss of consciousness
Measure respiratory rate		Tachypnea	Tachypnea	Increasing tachypnea
Measure heart rate		Tachycardia	Tachycardia	Increasing tachycardia
Measure blood pressure	Unchanged	Reduced BP and pulse pressure	Hypotension below systolic of 90 mmHg	Severe hypotension, with narrow pulse pressure
Measure urine output	No change noticable	Reduced	Oliguria	Oliguria progressing to anuria

Table 6.4: Stages of hypovolaemic shock based on percentage of blood/fluid loss for a 70 kg male with examples of clinical signs at each stage

the peritoneal cavity, and with pancreatitis and ileus, when fluid shifts into the gastro-intestinal cavity (Redden and Wotton 2002a, 2002b).

When assessing patients with a history of excessive fluid loss it is important to assess factors such as evidence of dehydration, including dry mucus membranes, dry furred tongue and sunken eyeballs. Clinical signs can determine the severity of the patient's condition and also the likely cause. Assessing and communicating all the clinical signs and information collated to the care team can improve the patient's potential for recovery and should be undertaken using a comprehensive and systematic approach recommended by NICE (2007) and illustrated in Chapter 1 (page 12).

Your role as a nurse in assessing, anticipating and interpreting the signs of a patient going into shock cannot be overestimated. In the remainder of the chapter we have used the case study of Megan James to explore in detail the pathophysiology of shock and the nurse's role in assessing, recognising and managing a patient as she progresses through each stage of hypovolaemic shock.

Case study: Megan's story

Sophie, a second-year student nurse, was responsible for the management of six patients on a surgical ward under the supervision of her mentor. One of the patients in her care was Megan, a 75-year-old woman who had been admitted that day with acute abdominal pain and nausea. Megan has a history of ischaemic heart disease and is routinely prescribed ACE inhibitors, statins and aspirin 75 mg. She had been assessed by the surgical registrar, and the agreed plan was to withhold oral intake, commence intravenous fluids, manage pain relief and monitor her progress. Megan's blood results on admission were within the normal range and included the following: Na, 135 mmol/L; K, 4.1 mmol/L; creatinine, 75 μmol/L and venous lactate, 1.7 mmol/L. Based on this information and Megan's two-day history of reduced fluid intake, the medical team prescribed sodium chloride 0.18% and glucose 4% at 83 ml/hour. This is consistent with NICE (2013) guidance on fluid therapy and is supported by Frost (2015). Sophie, on the advice of her mentor, commenced four hourly observations of her vital signs but two hours later she went to check on Megan and noticed a change in her condition.

- *Megan seemed to be more restless and said 'I don't feel very well nurse'.*
- *R: increased from 18/min to 20/min.*
- *SpO$_2$: decreased from 97% to 96%.*
- *She looked pale and her hands were cold.*
- *Temp: 36.9°C (no change).*
- *HR: increased from 90/min to 93/min.*
- *BP: decreased from 120/90 mmHg to 115/87 mmHg.*
- *Has passed urine since admission (100 ml).*
- *NEWS: increased from 0 to 1*

Sophie felt concerned and contacted the house officer to tell him of the change in NEWS (National Early Warning Score – see Chapter 1). He suggested that she should keep monitoring Megan and that they would review her on the medical round later that day. Sophie decided (on her own initiative) to increase Megan's observations to hourly even though the NEWS indicated a low risk. She was worried but she didn't know why.

Risk assessment, pathophysiology and priorities of care for patients in the initial stage of shock

In the initial stages of shock patients' physiological responses are influenced by a number of factors. These include the cause and severity of the stressor or trauma (trigger/cause), the age of the patient, their co-morbidities and medications. For example, the physiological effects of ageing can impact negatively on skin integrity, the musculoskeletal system and immune system; this leads to an increased risk of the patient having multiple pathologies and increased susceptibility to the effects of shock (Bersten and Soni, 2014). In Megan's case she had been unwell for several days with abdominal pain, nausea and indigestion and during that time she had only taken sips of water and was potentially dehydrated. Megan had been taking 75 mg aspirin for ten years as part of her routine medication as well as anti-hypertensive drugs and statins to reduce her cholesterol. According to the BNF (2013) the side effects of aspirin include gastro-intestinal haemorrhage (occasionally major) and with Megan's presenting history this should have been identified as a possible cause of her pain although there was no documented evidence of this in her notes.

In the initial stage, any reduction in the volume of circulating blood is detected by pressure-sensitive baroreceptors and chemoreceptors that are sensitive to changes in carbon dioxide and oxygen in the arterial circulation. These receptors are located in the arch of the aorta and carotid sinuses. When the receptors are triggered, impulses are relayed to the respiratory and cardiovascular centre in the medulla oblongata (brain stem), where they effect changes via the sympathetic nervous system: to increase the heart rate and force of cardiac contraction, trigger peripheral vasoconstriction and improve blood pressure. This trigger mechanism is illustrated in Figure 6.1. In Megan's story this response was demonstrated when Sophie noticed a slight reduction in Megan's systolic blood pressure and a corresponding slight increase in her respiratory rate and pulse. Sophie risk assessed her patient using NEWS and identified that all the physiological changes occurred within the normal range, and therefore did not identify Megan as being at risk. At the time Megan had also become more restless and anxious, but Sophie had been unable to connect the subtle changes in her patient's behaviour to clinical deterioration; she was worried but didn't know why.

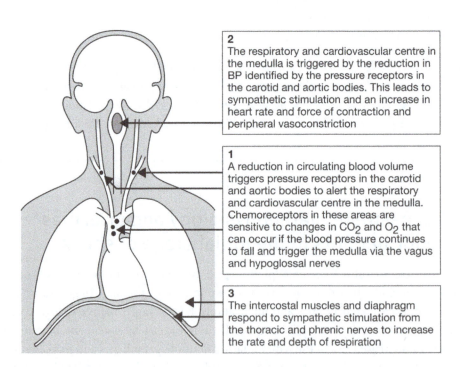

2
The respiratory and cardiovascular centre in the medulla is triggered by the reduction in BP identified by the pressure receptors in the carotid and aortic bodies. This leads to sympathetic stimulation and an increase in heart rate and force of contraction and peripheral vasoconstriction

1
A reduction in circulating blood volume triggers pressure receptors in the carotid and aortic bodies to alert the respiratory and cardiovascular centre in the medulla. Chemoreceptors in these areas are sensitive to changes in CO_2 and O_2 that can occur if the blood pressure continues to fall and trigger the medulla via the vagus and hypoglossal nerves

3
The intercostal muscles and diaphragm respond to sympathetic stimulation from the thoracic and phrenic nerves to increase the rate and depth of respiration

Figure 6.1: The trigger and compensatory feedback mechanisms that occur during the initial stage of shock

This example highlights the importance of undertaking a holistic assessment and clinical interpretation of the patient's situation as well as having an awareness of the risks associated with the patient's illness. According to Cecconi et al. (2014) in their consensus statement on shock: physical assessment of a patient's skin (perfusion); brain (mental status); and kidneys (urine output) will provide evidence of altered tissue perfusion. They also propose that the presence of hypotension as a single indicator should not be required to define shock. If Sophie had contacted the surgeon using the SBAR approach (see Chapter 1) and given a more detailed assessment of the patient at this stage she could have identified changes in Megan's perfusion (pale skin and cold hands), mental state (anxiety and feeling unwell) and subtle changes in her vital signs indicating the initial stage of shock.

What can we learn from Megan's story?

Sophie had identified that Megan's condition was changing and she had taken some correct steps to increase the monitoring of vital signs, but she had not reported that Megan had become more restless, pale and anxious. These signs were all indicative of a patient's deteriorating condition. The very slight increase in Megan's NEWS, without further corroborating clinical information, meant that she was considered to be at a low risk and the surgical team did not attend. As a result, both nursing and medical staff had been unable to interpret, communicate and act on the available clinical evidence effectively. Shock is a complex condition that can manifest in many different ways and although Sophie was concerned, she didn't have the knowledge and experience to act on those concerns. In order to have anticipated Megan's deterioration sooner, Sophie's priorities at this stage should have been to:

- risk assess the patient for the potential to develop shock by reviewing her past and recent medical history;
- identify and understand the signs and symptoms of impending shock;
- be alert to changes in the patient's clinical condition, no matter how small;
- recognise that NEWS is useful when identifying a trend in vital signs but should always be interpreted in the context of the patient's clinical condition;
- prevent significant deterioration in a patient's condition by checking the patient more frequently as illustrated by Sophie above;
- communicate any concerns using an SBAR approach (see Chapter 1);
- act in a timely manner; the patient will continue to deteriorate whether you take action or not.

The key to successful management of patients in hypovolaemic shock is the assessment and early detection of the problem, followed by action to prevent or reduce further fluid loss. The primary aim is to restore circulating volume while attempting to prevent further fluid loss. Fluid resuscitation of patients in hypovolaemic shock is complex and determined by a number of factors that relate to the patient and the primary cause. These include:

- the primary cause and type of fluid lost: blood, plasma, interstitial fluid;
- the age of the patient;

- evidence of co-morbidities such as heart failure, diabetes;

- fluid and electrolyte balance;

- blood glucose (Cecconi et al., 2014).

In Megan's case her recent history indicated that she was dehydrated and had a past medical history of hypertension and possible impaired cardiac function. She had been unable to take her prescribed antihypertensive medication in the last few days and this would have also had an impact on her circulatory system (BNF, 2013). Sophie was correct to feel concerned about Megan and by increasing the frequency of her vital signs assessment to hourly it allowed her to identify when Megan continued to deteriorate as the story reveals.

Compensatory stage of hypovolaemic shock

Case study: Megan James's condition deteriorates

One hour later as Sophie approached Megan to check her vital signs she realised that her condition had changed significantly.

- *Megan appeared pale, peripherally cyanosed and cold to touch.*
- *She was agitated and appeared frightened.*
- *Within minutes Megan vomited 400 ml liquid that tested positive to blood (coffee ground vomit). She also asked for a bedpan and passed 300 ml of a dark liquid stool that indicated positive to blood (melaena).*
- *R: 25/min.*
- *SpO_2: 91%.*
- *Core temperature: 37.5°C.*
- *HR: 115/min.*
- *BP: 90/70 mmHg.*
- *NEWS: 11.*
- *100 ml of urine passed in the last four hours (estimated weight 60 kg).*
- *ABG: pH: 7.40 (n = 7.35–7.45); PaO_2: 8.9 kPa (n = 10.6–13.3); $PaCO_2$: 4.2 kPa (n = 4.7–6.7); HCO_3: 22.0 mmol/L (n = 25–30).*
- *Lactate 2.3 mmol/L.*

Sophie alerted her mentor and called the critical care outreach team immediately.

Risk assessment, pathophysiology and priorities of care for compensatory stage

The early clinical evidence of compensatory mechanisms at work include changes in respiratory rate as a result of increased pulse, changes in skin pallor and temperature as a result of peripheral vasoconstriction, and changes in blood pressure. In Megan's case both her respiratory and heart rate have increased and blood pressure decreased. An estimation of urine output over four hours indicates that she has passed less than 30 ml per hour, signifying oliguria (reduced urine output <0.5 ml/kg/hr). These findings, along with a change in her behaviour and evidence of 700 ml of fluid loss, lead to a diagnosis of hypovolaemic shock with Megan's physiological systems attempting to compensate for the loss of blood volume.

The physiological response that occurs during the compensatory stage is immediate and occurs when adrenergic neurotransmitters stimulate alpha and beta 1 and 2 receptors in the smooth muscle of arterioles, cardiac muscle and skeletal muscle to increase heart rate, cause peripheral vasoconstriction and improve blood pressure. Stimulation of the beta 2 receptors also triggers bronchodilation and an added potential to improve lung ventilation by increasing the rate and depth of respiration, as illustrated in Figure 6.1. The sympathetic nervous system also triggers the adrenal medulla of the adrenal gland to release the catecholamines, adrenaline and noradrenaline (epinephrine and norepinephrine), in order to continue providing the compensatory response, and this is illustrated in Figure 6.2. These are examples of negative feedback mechanisms that are used to restore homeostasis.

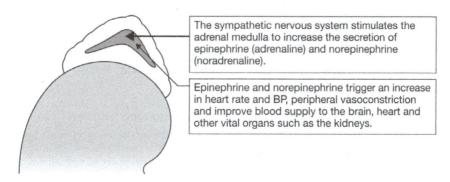

The sympathetic nervous system stimulates the adrenal medulla to increase the secretion of epinephrine (adrenaline) and norepinephrine (noradrenaline).

Epinephrine and norepinephrine trigger an increase in heart rate and BP, peripheral vasoconstriction and improve blood supply to the brain, heart and other vital organs such as the kidneys.

Figure 6.2: The triggering of the adrenal medulla that occurs during the compensatory stage of shock

This stimulation of a sympathetic neural response occurs in most types of shock as part of the flight/fight response explained earlier, apart from distributive shock. For example, in neurogenic shock the sympathetic response may be impaired by spinal injury, nerve injury or drugs such as general anaesthetic (Hammer and McPhee, 2014). In septic shock and anaphylactic shock the sympathetic response is challenged by a severe inflammatory response and systemic vasodilation (Hammer and McPhee, 2014). Table 6.2 (pages 126–7) provides a comparison of the different features of shock found on clinical assessment and illustrates that the cause of shock can influence the early signs and symptoms.

In Megan's case the release of catecholamines, in the form of epinephrine (adrenaline) and norepinephrine (noradrenaline), continue to affect the alpha and beta receptors and thus continue the adrenergic response. The net effect of this is to increase respiratory rate and depth, increase heart rate, and improve blood flow to the coronary arteries, skeletal muscle, heart and brain through stimulation of the beta adrenergic receptors. The stimulation of alpha receptors continues to increase peripheral resistance by causing peripheral vasoconstriction, leading to coolness and pallor of the skin. Figures 6.1 and 6.2 illustrate the mechanisms involved in the initial and compensatory response, and Figure 6.3 illustrates the other mechanisms involved in providing physiological compensation (McCance and Huether, 2014).

The initial fall in blood pressure also triggers a renal and a neural/adrenergic response. This response is described as the **renin-angiotensin-aldosterone mechanism**. Renin is an enzyme that is produced and stored in the juxtaglomerular cells of the kidneys. The juxtaglomerular cells are sensitive to changes in the responses of the sympathetic nervous system, and a reduction in blood flow to the kidneys will release renin into the circulation. Once in the circulation renin triggers the activation of **angiotensin I** from an inactive circulating protein. Angiotensin I is then converted by an enzyme called angiotensin converting enzyme (ACE) that is found in the lungs and kidney endothelial cells to **angiotensin II**, as the blood flows through the pulmonary circulation. Once activated, angiotensin II affects short- and long-term regulation of blood pressure.

- In short-term regulation, angiotensin II:
  - causes a vasoconstrictor effect on arterioles leading to increased peripheral vascular resistance and peripheral shutdown;
  - reduces sodium excretion from the kidneys so that the body retains more sodium and water.

- In long-term regulation, angiotensin II stimulates **aldosterone** secretion from the adrenal cortex. Aldosterone increases sodium and water retention by the kidneys. This increases the volume of extracellular fluid and circulating volume.

Another hormonal response triggered by reduced circulating volume and increased plasma **osmolarity** (increased concentration of salts) is **antidiuretic hormone (ADH)** or **vasopressin**. When triggered, vasopressin is released from the posterior pituitary gland and has a powerful vasoconstrictor effect on arterioles in the systemic circulation. Vasopressin also has an antidiuretic effect and increases absorption of water from the kidneys in response to increased plasma osmolarity. These mechanisms are summarised in Figure 6.3.

For Megan this meant that her peripheral temperature was cold, and there was evidence of peripheral shutdown and peripheral cyanosis (blue-tinged nails on her hands and feet). Her reduction in oxygen saturation suggests reduced perfusion and oxygenation of the peripheral circulation due to loss of circulating blood volume, and her reduced urine output is indicative of the renin-angiotensin-aldosterone mechanism and antidiuretic hormone (vasopressin). The triggering of the stress response also led to an increase in her metabolic rate manifested by an increase in her blood lactate levels. According to Marik (2015), as the amount of epinephrine released by the adrenal gland as part of the stress response in shock continues so the amount of lactate produced, as a by-product of metabolism, will increase.

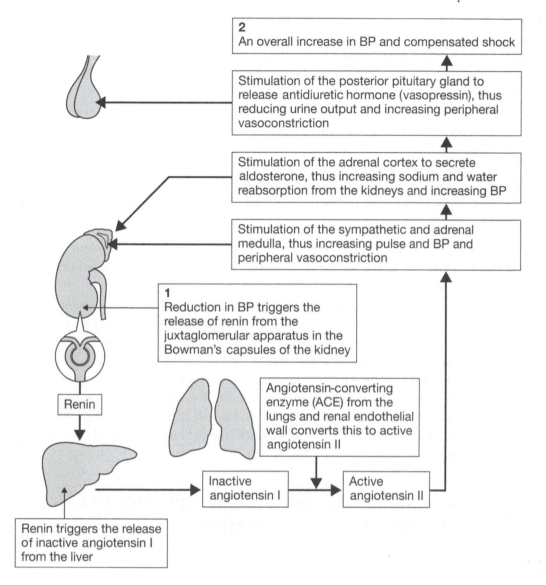

Figure 6.3: The compensatory mechanisms that occur as a physiological response to compensated shock

---

Case study: Risk assessing Megan at the compensatory stage of shock

The outreach team was called and following an assessment they concluded that Megan was only just compensating for her fluid loss but because of her age and cardiac history they are concerned that without more physiological support she will move to the progressive stage of shock. The following treatment regime was recommended.

(Continued)

continued . . .

- *High-flow oxygen 60%, with the aim of increasing SpO$_2$ to 94–96%.*
- *Fluid resuscitation with 500 ml of 0.9% sodium chloride to be given over 15 minutes. This was to be followed by a second ABCDE assessment and further fluid boluses up to a total volume of 2000 ml. Based on blood lost she was also prescribed two units of blood.*
- *Blood samples were taken for a full blood count (FBC) to determine haemoglobin level (Hb) and group and cross matching; urea and electrolytes (U&E) to look for evidence of changes indicative of acute renal failure and an imbalance in electrolytes; liver function tests (LFT), **prothrombin time (PT)** and **activated partial thromboplastin (APPT)** to assess for evidence of deranged clotting.*
- *A urinary catheter was inserted and a further 50 ml of urine is collected, confirming oliguria.*

An emergency endoscopy carried out once Megan had stabilised revealed an actively bleeding duodenal ulcer that was beginning to clot. The location of the bleeding site on the posterior wall of the duodenum made it difficult to clip and the medical team were concerned that there was a 30–40% chance of the site bleeding again based on previous clinical evidence (Sung, 2014). It was agreed that Megan should be transferred to level 2 (high dependency care) for monitoring and stabilisation of her condition. She was commenced on a proton pump inhibitor via the intravenous route to reduce gastric acidity and the risk of further bleeding, and continued to have nothing by mouth. Proton pump inhibitors such as omeprazole block the production of stomach acid by shutting down a system in the stomach cells known as the proton pump, which is responsible for the production of stomach acid (Rang et al., 2012). Should Megan's condition deteriorate further with evidence of a further bleed she would require a second endoscopy and possibly surgery.

Risk assessment, pathophysiology and priorities of care following fluid resuscitation

Case study: Initial improvement in Megan's condition

During the first two hours of Megan's admission to the high dependency unit her condition began to stabilise. On assessment:

- *she looked pale, and her hands and feet were still cool to touch;*
- *she described feeling very tired;*
- *R: 22/min;*
- *SpO$_2$: 94%;*
- *HR: 105/min;*
- *BP: 105/75 mmHg;*
- *core temp: 37.8°C;*

- urine output: 35 ml/hr;
- she has received fluid resuscitation with saline and blood and is now in a positive balance of two litres;
- ABG: pH: 7.32 (n = 7.35–7.45); PaO_2: 9.8 kPa (n = 10.6–13.3); $PaCO_2$: 5.0 kPa (n = 4.7–6.7); HCO_3: 22.0 mmol/L (n = 25–30);
- Lactate: 2.3 mmol/L (n = 0.5–2.0).

The improvement in Megan's condition following her episode of haematemesis and melaena suggests that her peptic ulcer is no longer actively bleeding and that endoscopic haemostasis has led to her condition becoming more stable.

Activity 6.2   *Decision making*

1. How frequently would you assess Megan's vital signs now that she is feeling better?
2. What clinical signs would indicate that Megan's condition was getting worse?
3. What information would you give Megan at this stage about her condition?

There are answers to this activity at the end of the chapter.

Progressive stage of hypovolaemic shock

Case study: Megan's condition deteriorates

One hour later Megan's condition deteriorated and an ABCDE assessment revealed the following.

- She is pale, peripherally cyanosed and cold to touch.
- She is confused and drowsy.
- R: 28/min with fast shallow respirations.
- SpO_2: 88%.
- Pulse: 120/min, sinus tachycardia.
- BP: 70/48 mmHg.
- Vomited 500 ml of altered blood.
- Passed 500ml of liquid, melaena stools.
- Urine output: 25 ml/hr.
- ABG: pH: 7.23 (n = 7.35–7.45); PaO_2: 7.8 kPa (n = 10.6–13.3); $PaCO_2$: 3.8 kPa (n = 4.7–6.7); HCO_3: 15.5 mmol/L (n = 25–30).
- Urea is 11.5 mmol/L (n = 2.5–6.5).
- Creatinine is 155 μmol/L (n = 55–105).
- Lactate is 4.0 mmol/L (n = 0.5–2.0).

Risk assessment, pathophysiology and priorities of care for a patient in the progressive stage of shock

The clinical evidence suggests that Megan has had another bleed and is now in the progressive stage of shock. Megan is also showing signs of type I respiratory failure (see Chapter 2). The clinical signs for this include: confusion and drowsiness, increased respiratory rate accompanied by oxygen saturations (SpO_2) of less than 90% and partial pressure of arterial oxygen (PaO_2) levels of less than 8 kPa (O'Driscoll et al., 2008). Megan also has clinical evidence of a metabolic acidosis indicated by the reduced level of pH and bicarbonate in her arterial blood sample. The critical care team concludes that Megan has developed type I respiratory failure secondary to massive blood loss, hypoperfusion and subsequent metabolic acidosis. The primary cause of her condition is progressive shock induced by a severe gastro-intestinal bleed. This has led to inadequate tissue perfusion of vital organs such as the brain, causing confusion and drowsiness, and the kidneys, leading to acute kidney injury evidenced by reduced urine output and an increasing blood level of creatinine (see Chapter 9 on acute kidney injury).

At this stage the compensatory mechanisms that the body normally recruits as short-term measures to maintain circulation have continued and are becoming detrimental to Megan's well-being in a number of ways.

1. Intense prolonged vasoconstriction causes a reduction in the perfusion of tissues and reduced access to oxygen leading to ischaemia. Megan is peripherally cold and showing signs of peripheral cyanosis.

2. The continued stimulation of the stress response leads to an increased metabolic demand for oxygen.

3. With a marked reduction in oxygen, cells are starved of **adenosine triphosphate (ATP)** production through the aerobic pathway and lack the energy to function effectively.

4. The cells have to rely on a less efficient process of energy production through the anaerobic pathway that produces about 20% of the energy that is normally acquired through aerobic metabolism.

5. The anaerobic pathway produces lactic acid as a by-product of metabolism and this leads to increased acidity in cells and a lactic acidosis. This is evidenced by a raised lactate level and a metabolic acidosis. Megan's respiratory effort has increased in response to the metabolic acidosis in an attempt to compensate for the acidity of the blood. By increasing her respiratory rate she is breathing out more carbon dioxide and water in an attempt to eliminate hydrogen ions (a measure of acidity; see Chapter 3).

6. The inflammatory response is triggered as a result of the ischaemia and damage caused by anaerobic metabolism. As a consequence, tissues in body organs become damaged and inflamed, leading to an increased risk of acute respiratory distress and impaired renal function.

7. Without energy the normal cell function cannot be maintained, and the cells swell due to the failure of the sodium/potassium pump to maintain the fluid balance inside the cell and increased cell permeability.

8. As shock progresses, the inflammatory mediators, **histamine** and **bradykinin**, exert their vasodilatory properties, leading to progressive hypotension and cellular hypoxia (insufficient supply of oxygen).

9. A prolonged hypoxia will lead to suppression of the sympathetic nervous response and the cardiac and respiratory centre in the medulla oblongata; as a result, the patient's level of consciousness deteriorates. Megan is already confused and drowsy and if her condition continues to deteriorate, she will become drowsier and lose consciousness.

As the shock becomes more progressive, tachypnea, tachycardia and hypotension will persist, but there will also be evidence of system failure in the form of pulmonary and peripheral oedema, respiratory failure, renal failure and cardiac failure, manifested by increased demand for oxygen, central and peripheral cyanosis, decreased urinary output and confusion. There may also be evidence of paralytic ileus (absence of bowel sounds) and abdominal distension. The patient will have a metabolic acidosis and altered blood clotting as a result of the hypoxia and inflammatory response (Maiden and Peake, 2014).

The extent of cellular and organ damage that occurs in this progressive stage of shock is determined by the severity of the cause and the period of time your patient spends in the progressive stage. If not reversed, this stage will lead to your patient developing overwhelming cellular damage and destruction, leading to the failure of organs and systems. At this stage the progress of shock becomes irreversible, their body will be unable to respond to supportive therapy and death is inevitable. In Megan's situation, due to her age and co-morbidities her condition has become critical and at risk of progression to refractory shock.

> ### Case study: Managing Megan's care while in progressive shock
>
> *Megan's condition is now critical, and as a result the team decides to increase her respiratory support through intubation and mechanical ventilation with biphasic respiratory support (see Chapter 3), and continue with fluid resuscitation and further transfusions. Once haemodynamically stable, Megan will have a repeat endoscopy to review and stabilise the bleeding duodenal ulcer and continue to be risk assessed for acute kidney injury (see Chapter 9).*

Risk assessment, preventing refractory shock

Refractory shock could occur in Megan's case if the critical care team is unable to re-establish haemodynamic stability and prevent the progression of cellular and tissue damage that will ultimately lead to irreversible failure of the respiratory, cardiovascular, hepatic and renal system. It is the effect of decreased oxygenation and nutrition, the inflammatory response and the release of toxins from ischaemic tissue that leads to refractory shock (Hall, 2011). In severe and/or prolonged shock the body is no longer able to compensate for the loss of circulating volume through the negative feedback systems illustrated in Figures 6.1, 6.2 and 6.3 and, instead, reaches a stage where an increase in the degree of shock causes a further increase in the degree of shock (a type of positive feedback) and any supportive therapy becomes incapable of saving a person's life. The priority is always to risk assess patients using the assessment strategies included in this chapter and to prevent the progression of shock before refractory shock can occur.

In Megan's story the critical care team were able to stabilise her haemodynamic state and a second attempt at endoscopic haemostasis was successful. Megan remained in hospital for a further ten days during which her medication was reviewed and her routine antiplatelet prescription discontinued. We have identified the importance of timing, rapid and accurate risk assessment and communication when caring for patients in shock. In Activity 6.3, you have an opportunity to practise risk assessment and decision making.

Activity 6.3   *Decision making*

In your bay you have two patients causing concern.

Mrs Thompson was admitted for day surgery but was later admitted to your surgical ward following a history of post-operative nausea and vomiting. Her nausea and vomiting have continued for 12 hours, with limited relief from anti-emetic medication. The surgical team are reluctant to commence any supportive care, such as an infusion, assuming that the patient's nausea will settle with the medication.

Mrs Jacks has not passed urine since her return from theatre six hours ago following a **laparoscopic cholecystectomy.**

1. What would you look for when undertaking a risk assessment of Mrs Thompson?
2. What would you look for when undertaking a risk assessment of Mrs Jacks?
3. What information would you collect before informing the medical team of any concerns you have?

There are sample answers for this activity at the end of the chapter.

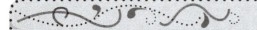

Chapter summary

The aim of this chapter was to help you assess, recognise and respond to patients who go into shock. We have focused on the assessment and management of patients in hypovolaemic shock. In all of the clinical examples illustrated, the key responsibilities of the nurse are the same. They include the following.

- Carry out holistic assessment and monitoring of your patients.
- Know your patients and notice when the situation changes, even when the change is small.

- Ensure timely diagnosis and reporting of changes in the patient's condition: time is of the essence. Any patient who shows a change in their condition that is indicative of hypovolaemic, cardiogenic, obstructive or distributive shock should be risk assessed.
- Ensure there is continual monitoring and reporting of the patient's condition to the appropriate team.
- If unsure, act and express concern about your patient rather than hesitate and lose valuable time.

In Chapter 7 we continue to focus on assessing, recognising and responding to patients who go into shock, and we discuss the priorities of assessment and screening patients for sepsis and septic shock.

Activities: brief outline answers

Activity 6.2: Decision making (page 141)

1. As Megan has improved and has appeared to stabilise, the temptation is to reduce her observations to two hourly. However, Megan is still at risk of further deterioration and given her co-morbidities it would be advisable to continue to monitor her hourly. If you are concerned, increase the frequency of observation to half hourly or every 15 minutes and communicate your concern.
2. Look: Listen: Feel: Measure: the patient is pale, cool to touch, anxious; has increased respiratory rate, increased heart rate and reduced blood pressure; the patient is complaining of nausea, vomiting, diarrhoea, haematemesis and melaena.
3. At this stage in Megan's condition it is important to ask her what she understands about what has happened and explain what has happened and why. She will need reassurance that she is being monitored and being given treatment to promote healing and recovery. You should advise Megan to contact her nurse should she feel nauseated, unwell, faint or wanting to have her bowels open. These are all signs that the ulcer may be actively bleeding.

Activity 6.3: Decision making (page 144)

1. Mrs Thompson has undergone minor surgery but has received nothing by mouth for an estimated 24 hours. She was probably asked to starve from midnight the night before her admission for minor surgery and has been suffering from nausea and vomiting ever since. She is in danger of developing hypovolaemic shock associated with dehydration. You need to assess the following using ABCDE and 'Look: Listen: Feel: Measure'.

   - Look, listen, feel for signs of dehydration: dry mouth, sunken eyes, thirst, anxiety, confusion, cool skin, evidence of pain.
   - Measure: respiratory rate, pulse, BP, urine output and loss through vomiting, signs of negative fluid balance, time period without fluid intake and evidence of improvement following treatment with anti-emetic medication. Is there evidence of tachypnea, tachycardia, and hypotension, NEWS?
   - Mrs Thompson is dehydrated and this is evidenced by tachypnea, tachycardia and hypotension (respirations: 24, pulse: 98, BP: 88/58). She is reviewed based on the nurse's assessment and communication of findings and commenced on an intravenous infusion; she receives a fluid challenge of 500 ml of 0.9% saline in 15 minutes, following which Mrs Thompson's vital signs improve to: respirations: 18; pulse: 90; BP: 95/58. She continues on 125 ml/hour of intravenous saline and is encouraged to drink oral fluids as her nausea begins to subside. She feels much better the following morning and is discharged home that afternoon.

2. Mrs Jacks has not passed urine in the six hours post-operation. There could be a simple explanation in that no one has asked her or helped her to perform this activity. It could also be related to dehydration/ blood or fluid loss, or post-operative pain. You need to assess the following using ABCDE and 'Look: Listen: Feel: Measure'.

- Look, listen and feel for signs of blood/fluid loss and/or dehydration: dry mouth, sunken eyes, thirst, anxiety, cool skin, evidence of pain.
- Measure: respiratory rate, pulse, BP, urine output and loss through vomiting, signs of negative fluid balance, time period without fluid intake. Is there evidence of tachypnea, tachycardia and hypotension?

Following an assessment of her condition Mrs Jacks reveals that she wants to pass urine but was too afraid to ask because everyone looked so busy! After some support and nursing care this patient is able to pass urine and begins to feel much more comfortable. Her vital signs are within the normal range and her pain is well managed.

3. Using SBAR you would collate the information you have collected above into:

- the *situation*: reason for your call;
- the clinical *background*: reason for patient's admission;
- the changes that have occurred in the patient *assessment*: now or over time;
- your *recommendation*: what you want the clinical team to do.

The patient causing concern was Mrs Thompson, and your prompt review has prevented this patient's condition from deteriorating and going into hypovolaemic shock.

Further reading

Edwards, S and Sabato, M (2009) *A Nurse's Survival Guide to Critical Care.* Edinburgh: Churchill Livingstone.

This textbook provides a pocket-sized reference for practical aspects of caring for patients in critical care settings and provides factual and accessible information.

Higgins, C (2013) *Understanding Laboratory Investigations for Nurses and Health Care Professionals.* Third edition. London: Blackwell Publishing.

This textbook provides a user friendly approach to understanding laboratory investigations.

Peate, I and Dutton, H (2012) *Acute Nursing Care: Recognising and Responding to Medical Emergencies.* Harlow: Pearson.

This textbook adopts a systematic approach to managing body systems during medical emergencies.

Useful websites

www.youtube.com/watch?v=Wo90bqiI5BQ and www.youtube.com/watch?v=59uO-8UVC2A

These YouTube videos demonstrate examples of endoscopic management of a person with bleeding peptic ulcers and will help to put Megan's care into context.

Chapter 7
The patient with sepsis and distributive shock

Desiree Tait

NMC Standards for Pre-registration Nursing Education

This chapter will address the following competencies:

Domain 3: Nursing practice and decision-making

Generic competencies:

7. All nurses must be able to recognise and interpret signs of normal and deteriorating mental and physical health and respond promptly to maintain or improve the health and comfort of the service user, acting to keep them and others safe.

Field-specific competencies:

7.1. Adult nurses must recognise the early signs of illness in people of all ages. They must make accurate assessments and start appropriate and timely management of those who are acutely ill, at risk of clinical deterioration, or require emergency care.

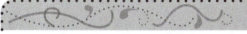

NMC Essential Skills Clusters

This chapter will address the following ESCs:

Cluster: Infection prevention and control

21. People can trust the newly registered graduate nurse to identify and take effective measures to prevent and control infection in accordance with local and national policy.

By entry to the register:

viii. In partnership with people and their carers, plans, delivers and documents care that demonstrates effective risk assessment, infection prevention and control.

Introduction: what is sepsis?

Sepsis can be described as the systemic inflammatory response to a recognised infection (Patrozou and Opal, 2010). An infection occurs when the body has been exposed to pathogenic organisms that have invaded and damaged body tissues. When this happens the body's immune system is able to recognise harmful invaders and provide a defence against the attack; containing and destroying the invader. This process is called the inflammatory response, and when it occurs locally in a particular body region – e.g. a tooth abscess, wound infection, a urinary tract infection – it can be contained, managed and lead to recovery. In some instances recovery requires the help of prescribed antibiotic therapy in order to assist the body's defences. For the majority of people, the infection will be resolved without hospitalisation and the person will make a full recovery. For some patients, however, the disease can progress from an infection to sepsis (blood poisoning/septicaemia) and in some cases, severe sepsis – the body's response to severe infection.

Severe infection can be a trigger for the onset of systemic inflammatory response syndrome (SIRS). This occurs when we trigger a systemic, non-specific inflammatory response to an insult on the body. In the case of sepsis the insult is infection. However, it is important to recognise that other insults are also likely to lead to SIRS and these include:

- mechanical invasive ventilation (MIV);
- aspiration;
- major surgery;
- burns;
- pancreatitis;
- trauma.

SIRS is therefore associated with any situation that places severe trauma or stress on the body, including sepsis and severe sepsis. The relationship between sepsis and SIRS is illustrated in Figure 7.1.

The patient with sepsis and distributive shock

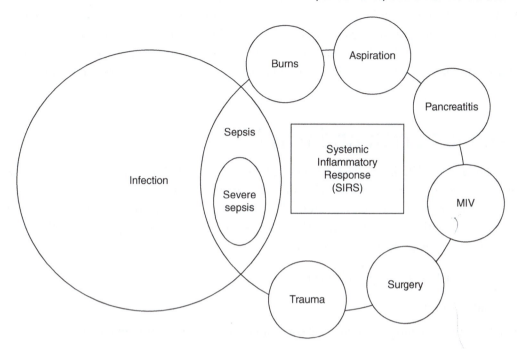

Figure 7.1: The relationships between infection, SIRS, sepsis and severe sepsis

Source: adapted from Bone et al. (1992).

Once sepsis is established the patient's situation, in some cases, can escalate to severe sepsis and septic shock in a matter of hours or days. Both sepsis and severe sepsis are life-threatening conditions and are described as a clinical emergency. Severe sepsis is defined as sepsis plus the failure of at least one organ. The organs affected include:

- respiratory system: acute respiratory distress syndrome (ARDS);
- cardiovascular system: septic cardiomyopathy (depression of myocardial function);
- renal: acute kidney injury;
- hepatic: septic hepatic dysfunction;
- haematological: coagulopathy and disseminated intravascular coagulation (DIC);
- central nervous system: sepsis associated encephalopathy (De Gaudio, 2014).

Severe sepsis can also be complicated by 'septic shock', and this is defined as severe sepsis with hypotension that has not responded to fluid resuscitation (Levy et al., 2003). Table 7.1 illustrates the clinical definitions of these terms and provides clinical examples of patients with those conditions.

According to De Gaudio (2014), the mortality rate for sepsis is 10–15%, for severe sepsis mortality increases to 17–20% and if a patient develops septic shock the mortality rate increases to 43–54%. The important message, therefore, is to risk assess and recognise sepsis early in order to save lives. The Surviving Sepsis Campaign (SSC) (2015) is a global collaboration that was established in 2002 to raise awareness and improve the evidence-based management of sepsis. In the 13 years since their inception, they have raised awareness worldwide of sepsis; developed international evidence-based guidelines and care bundles; supported service improvement and continue to review and update evidence-based care for the management of sepsis, severe sepsis and septic shock. Their continued commitment is to reduce mortality from sepsis worldwide (SSC, 2015).

Who is at risk and why?

According to the UK Sepsis Trust (Daniels, 2013), it is estimated that in the UK 37,000 people die each year as a result of sepsis. When this is compared with other conditions such as lung cancer (the biggest killer after cardiovascular disease) with a mortality rate of less than 35,000, bowel cancer with a mortality of 15,000 and breast cancer with a mortality of 6,000, the extent and severity of the problem begins to become clear.

Sepsis does not discriminate and affects:

- all age groups;
- all healthcare settings including the community, pre-hospital and secondary care;
- a full range of lifestyles from healthy to unhealthy.

Sepsis can no longer be regarded as a condition found mainly in critical care; it is the business of every healthcare worker. There is growing evidence that poor diagnosis of community-acquired sepsis is playing a large part in the morbidity and mortality of patients (McPherson et al., 2013; Daniels, 2013).

Although it is recognised that sepsis can strike anyone, there are groups of people with a higher degree of risk (Sepsis Alliance, 2014). These include:

- the very young and the very old, who are more likely to be immunocompromised;
- people with co-morbidities;
- people with a weakened immune system due to treatments such as immunosuppressant drugs used in inflammatory disorders and cancer treatment;
- people with traumatic injuries;
- people with addictions such as alcohol, smoking and drugs who potentially are already immunocompromised or have damaged organs;
- people who have invasive interventions such as intravenous catheters, urinary catheters or mechanical invasive ventilation;
- people who have a disorder that increases their risk of developing sepsis, such as cystic fibrosis or human immunodeficiency virus (HIV).

Finally, the widespread use of antibiotics has led to an increasing incidence of drug-resistant microorganisms that make treating people in the higher risk categories even more difficult.

Terminology	Definition	Clinical examples
Infection	A local inflammatory response to pathogenic organisms that have invaded and damaged body tissues.	Holly Jackson has been complaining of toothache and a swollen hot left cheek for several days. A visit to the dentist confirmed the presence of a tooth abscess.
Systemic inflammatory response syndrome (SIRS)	A systemic inflammatory response that has been triggered by a severe trauma such as: infection, pancreatitis, burns, aspiration into the lungs, manual invasive ventilation (MIV), major surgery and trauma. SIRS is diagnosed in the presence of at least two of the following. • Respiratory rate >20/min or $PaCO_2$ <4.3 kPa. • Heart rate (pulse) >90/min. • Temperature >38°C or <36°C. • White blood cell count (WBC) >12×10^9/L or <4×10^9/L. • Acutely altered mental state. • Hyperglycaemia >7 mmol/L in the absence of diabetes.	Paul Smith was involved in a road traffic collision that resulted in him sustaining crush injuries to his chest and upper abdomen. Within 24 hours he had evidence of: • T: 38.5°C; • P: 98/min; • R: 36/min. This indicated clinical evidence of SIRS.
Sepsis	SIRS + infection.	Tom Parkin, 71 years old, had been discharged from ICU to the ward eight hours ago after receiving treatment for pneumonia. He had required MIV, invasive haemodynamic monitoring and urinary catheterisation. On assessment: • R: 30/min, dyspnoeic; • SpO_2: 84%; • confused; • skin hot and dry; • centrally cyanosed;

(Continued)

Table 7.1   (Continued)

Terminology	Definition	Clinical examples
		• P: 110/min; • BP: 95/65 mmHg; • T: 38.8°C; • urine output in the last six hours 100 ml; • urinary tract infection diagnosed. This indicated clinical evidence of sepsis.
Severe sepsis	A diagnosis of sepsis accompanied by the failure of at least one body organ such as: acute respiratory distress syndrome (ARDS), acute kidney injury (AKI).	Tom Parkin was re-admitted to ICU where his condition progressed to severe sepsis within an hour of admission. This was evidenced by the development of ARDS. ABGs on 90% O_2: • *pH: 7.166 (acidosis);* • *PaO_2: 7.8 kPa (hypoxia);* • *$PaCO_2$: 6.61 kPa (hypercapnia and respiratory acidosis);* • *HCO_3: 16.0 mmol/L (< bicarbonate and metabolic acidosis);* • *BE: −9 (metabolic acidosis).*
Septic shock	A diagnosis of severe sepsis with hypotension that cannot be corrected by fluid resuscitation.	Sarah Clark (aged 70 years) was admitted to the emergency unit with a two-day history of back and abdominal pain and vomiting. Sarah has chronic renal failure for which she receives dialysis twice a week. On assessment: • R: 38/min; • SpO_2: 87% on 60% oxygen; • P: 136/min; • BP: 75/50 (fluid resuscitation failed); • skin warm and flushed; • lethargic and drowsy; • T: 38.5°C; • urine output 10 ml/hr. Sarah is showing signs of septic shock accompanied by acute respiratory failure together with existing renal failure.

Multiple organ dysfunction (MOD)	Severe sepsis may progress to the failure of more body systems leading to multiple organ failure. This progression may begin with respiratory failure and progress through cardiovascular failure, renal failure and liver failure. Mortality rate for patients with MOD is high.	James Green (38 years) was diagnosed as HIV positive ten years ago. He was admitted to ICU with pneumonia. Within 24 hours of admission, James had the following problems: • R: respiratory support; • SpO$_2$: 80% on 100% oxygen; • deeply unconscious (GCS: 4); • P: 136/min; • BP: 75/50 (failed fluid resuscitation); • T: 38.8°C; • urine output 20 ml/hr with elevated urea and creatinine levels. James is showing signs of septic shock and MOD, with evidence of respiratory, renal, neurological and cardiovascular failure.

Table 7.1: Patient examples and clinical definitions of sepsis according to degree of progression

Identifying the septic patient: what are we looking for?

Sepsis usually originates from a localised infection that leads to an uncontrolled systemic response (Identifying Sepsis Early Group, 2006). The person will present with a deterioration in their clinical condition and, as recommended in Chapter 1, any patient who becomes unwell should be assessed using the ABCDE approach. This approach will help the healthcare team or carer to identify any life-threatening conditions and seek help. Once the assessment has been completed and data collected then risk assessment and management specific to the septic patient should be commenced immediately. Identifying the septic patient includes.

1. ABCDE assessment.
2. Use of the sepsis screening tool:
   • look for SIRS;
   • look for sepsis.
3. If sepsis is diagnosed commence the Sepsis Six Pathway.

When risk assessment and sepsis screening are used to identify sepsis as soon as it begins to emerge and appropriate interventions are initiated, there is evidence that survival rates can improve and patients can be prevented from progressing to the more severe forms of the disease (Levy et al., 2010; Rivers et al., 2001). A screening tool for sepsis should therefore have guidance

If an infection is suspected or the patient has an elevated NEWS score then:

STEP 1: SCREEN FOR SIRS

Does your patient have 2 or more of the following signs and symptoms present?

Temperature: <36 or >38.3°C	YES/NO
Respiratory rate: >20/min	YES/NO
Heart rate: >90/min	YES/NO
Acutely altered mental state	YES/NO
White blood cell count <4 or >12x10⁹/L	YES/NO
Neutrophils <1.0x10⁹/L	YES/NO
Hyperglycaemia >7 mmol/L in the absence of diabetes	YES/NO

If YES your patient has evidence of SIRS THINK SEPSIS

If YES: your patient has SEPSIS:

- **Ensure doctor is present within 30 mins**
- **Commence Sepsis Six Pathway within one hour of diagnosis:**

  1. Oxygen therapy >SpO$_2$ 92%
  2. Take blood cultures
  3. Commence antibiotics
  4. Give fluid
  5. Take Hb/lactate
  6. Monitor hourly urine output

Does your patient have a history or signs of a new infection?

Cough/sputum/chest pain	YES/NO
Abdominal pain/distension/diarrhoea	YES/NO
Dysuria/pain on passing urine	YES/NO
Headache with neck stiffness	YES/NO
Cellulitis/wound infection/septic arthritis	YES/NO
Infusion line/catheter infection	YES/NO
Endocarditis (inflammation of the endocardium)	YES/NO

STEP 2: SCREEN FOR SEVERE SEPSIS AND SEPTIC SHOCK

• Systolic BP <90 mmHg or mean arterial pressure (MAP) <65 mmHg	YES/NO
• Urine output <0.5 ml/kg/hr for 2 hrs	YES/NO
• International normalised ratio for clotting (INR) >1.5	YES/NO
• Activated partial thromboplastin time (APTT) >60 seconds	YES/NO
• Platelets <100 x10⁹/L	YES/NO
• Lactate >2 mmol/L	YES/NO
• Creatinine >177 µmol/L	YES/NO
• Bilirubin >34 µmol/L	YES/NO
• New need for oxygen to keep SpO$_2$ >90%	YES/NO
• Chest X-ray with evidence of bilateral pulmonary infiltrates	YES/NO
• PaO$_2$/fraction of inspired O$_2$ <39.9 kPa	YES/NO

Are any 1 of the above signs of organ dysfunction present?
Including:
Heart rate >131/minute
Respiratory rate >25/minute
AVPU = V, P or U
(UK Sepsis Trust, 2014)

If YES: your patient has **SEVERE SEPSIS/SEPTIC SHOCK:**

- If not already done: commence Sepsis Six Pathway
- Call registrar/consultant
- Call for the critical care outreach team

Figure 7.2: Sepsis and severe sepsis screening, a multidisciplinary assessment

Source: adapted with permission from Dr R Daniels.

on how to assess for evidence of SIRS and infection. An example of how a screening tool might look is illustrated in Figure 7.2 and follows guidance from the UK Sepsis Trust (2014). The progression from sepsis to severe sepsis can take place in a matter of hours. Therefore sepsis screening should not end with the initiation of evidence-based treatment for sepsis but should also include the continued risk assessment for severe sepsis (illustrated in Figure 7.2).

Why is it so important to get it right?

In 2013 the Health Service Ombudsman for England (Mellor, 2013) published a report called 'Time to Act'. The report highlights the death of patients in the NHS after there had been a failure to diagnose and rapidly treat severe sepsis. They found that failings in care occurred mainly in the first few hours of illness when the patient could have been saved by rapid diagnosis and simple treatment. Standards to reduce the risk of untimely death are multidisciplinary and should include the following.

- Clinical factors:
  o take a timely history and clinical examination of the patient;
  o initiate the tests required to identify the source of infection;
  o continued monitoring;
  o commencement of treatment.
- Organisational factors:
  o staff education and training;
  o timely senior nursing and medical support;
  o timely referral to ICU;
  o the use of a clear management plan;
  o effective handover (using SBAR).

The report also found that national audits of standards for the timely use of sepsis protocols continued to show that they were not being met. Following the publication of the Ombudsman's report, the UK Sepsis Trust (2014) in association with NHS England launched 'Red Flag Sepsis'. They propose that sepsis screening should be performed as a two-step process.

- Step 1: screening for SIRS/with evidence of a history of or a new infection.
- Step 2: screening for severe sepsis/septic shock (Figure 7.2).

If severe sepsis or septic shock is confirmed by just one of the criteria listed, escalate the urgency of the situation, call the critical care outreach team and the registrar/consultant. If Sepsis Six interventions have not been commenced at that time, commence them immediately. The launch of 'Red Flag Sepsis' and associated information is designed to encourage all clinical staff to avoid unnecessary delay when assessing and managing a patient with sepsis.

The role of the nurse is critical in relation to both the clinical and organisational factors that can improve patient outcomes. As a nurse you have direct responsibility for assessing and monitoring the patient's condition, even when you may have delegated the task to others. Your role when risk assessing for sepsis includes the following activities and these activities apply wherever you come into contact with a person who is unwell, in the community or a hospital setting.

- Adopt a patient-centred approach to care and know your patient.
- Listen to your patient.
- Risk assess and monitor the patient using the principles of 'Look: Listen: Feel: Measure' and ABCDE assessment.
- Interpret the patient's clinical signs and symptoms in the context of screening for SIRS, sepsis and severe sepsis.
- Communicate and collaborate effectively with the healthcare team.
- Use the agreed clinical pathways and guidance to recognise and respond to clinical signs of deterioration in a timely manner.

Activity 7.1 gives you an opportunity to practise assessing patients for evidence of sepsis.

Activity 7.1 *Decision making*

With the aid of the sepsis screening tool in Figure 7.2, review the scenarios below and determine if any of the patients meet the criteria for either SIRS, sepsis or severe sepsis.

Edward Morris
Edward Morris (69 years) has been diagnosed with inoperable carcinoma of the ascending colon. He underwent two laparoscopic bowel biopsies in a period of two weeks and finally had his diagnosis confirmed. Edward was commenced on chemotherapy one week later and completed the first 14-day cycle of treatment as an outpatient. Seven days later he began to experience acute abdominal pain in the right side of his abdomen and began to feel hot, shivery and unwell. The guidance on his chemotherapy care pathway directed him to monitor his temperature and contact the ward if his temperature was above 38°C. His temperature was 38.6°C and his pulse, taken by his daughter, was 95/min. He contacted the ward staff for advice.

1. Did Edward meet any of the screening criteria?
2. What advice would you give Edward?

Molly Taylor
Molly Taylor (73 years) has been admitted to an acute medical ward with a history of falls. On this occasion she had been found by the milkman who heard her calling for help through the bathroom window. She had got up to go to the toilet at 02.00 hours and had lost consciousness for several hours. Molly had not broken any bones, and apart from a bloodied nose, there appeared to be no clear reason for her loss of consciousness.

Nine hours after admission to hospital she became short of breath and disorientated. Her daughter was visiting at the time and said that Molly did not normally suffer from confusion and that the only relevant thing that had happened in the last few weeks was they had all been suffering from a heavy cold and that Molly had taken to her bed for three days.

Using the principles of 'Look: Listen: Feel: Measure' Molly presented with:

- confusion;
- R: 28/min;
- P: 95/min;
- T: 37.9°C;
- BP: 100/60;
- SpO$_2$: 88%.

1. Did Molly meet any of the screening criteria?
2. How would you respond to Molly's condition?

There are answers to this activity at the end of the chapter.

Why are changes in vital signs important?

In this section we will explore in more detail the significance of clinical signs and focus particularly on temperature, respiration, heart rate, systolic blood pressure (SBP), mental state and signs of infection by exploring the story of Cathy Price. Figure 7.3 provides a summary of the relationship between physiological factors and clinical signs, and Table 7.2 provides a summary of the clinical signs of infection for body systems most likely to be associated with the development of sepsis.

Scenario: Cathy Price

Catherine Price, aged 41 years, has been admitted to hospital via the emergency department (ED) at 20.00 hours on Friday evening. She has been complaining of a three-week history of general malaise, lethargy, nausea, vomiting, and some abdominal discomfort with three episodes of vomiting and diarrhoea in the last 12 hours. Catherine was finding it increasingly difficult to breathe and cough over the last couple of hours, she was fevered and breathless. Her husband had become extremely worried about his wife and had made the decision to not bother with the out-of-hours service, deciding instead to take her straight to ED.

(Continued)

continued . . . •

Background

Three weeks prior to this event she had visited her GP complaining of lower abdominal discomfort, loin pain and feeling generally unwell. Her GP had given her antibiotics, trimethoprim for a urinary tract infection and requested a urine specimen. The specimen proved to be negative. Despite this she remained unwell and returned to her GP a week later with a high temperature, shortness of breath and a chesty cough. She was diagnosed with a chest infection and was given a different antibiotic: amoxicillin. Since then Cathy (as she had asked to be called) had been at home, feeling tired and nauseous, which she had put down to possible side effects of the antibiotics and as the week went on she felt increasing discomfort in her central abdomen. The vomiting and diarrhoea had commenced on the day of admission together with increasing dyspnoea. Cathy had no significant past medical history apart from two normal pregnancies (two daughters aged 10 and 13 years). She had no previous medication history, was not allergic to anything, did not smoke and only drank alcohol on social occasions. In summary she had been a relatively fit housewife and mother of two.

Assessment

A:

- *airway was patent with bilateral chest movements.*

B:

- *R 32/min, regular but high;*
- *on auscultation she had shallow breaths with widespread crackles;*
- *SpO_2 91%;*
- *oxygen was administered at 15 L/min via a non-rebreathing mask;*
- *chest X-Ray showed pulmonary infiltrates.*

C:

- *HR 136/min;*
- *BP 108/46 mmHg;*
- *core temp 38.9°C;*
- *cool peripheries but all her pulses were present;*
- *her skin was pale and clammy;*
- *capillary refill time was four seconds;*
- *an ECG was recorded which revealed a sinus tachycardia;*
- *urinary catheter inserted and 150 ml of residual urine was obtained, an hourly urometer attached following catheterisation;*
- *catheter specimen of urine was sent for culture;*
- *blood was also obtained for culture;*
- *arterial blood gases (ABGs):*

  - *pH: 7.24;*
  - *$PaCO_2$: 6.39 kPa;*

- PaO_2: 8.59 kPa;
- HCO_3: 17 mmol/L;
- oxygen saturations: 91%;
- BE: 3.9 mmol/L.
- lactic acid: 4.7 mmol/L;
- white blood cell (WBC) count: 14×10^9/L;
- haemoglobin (Hb): 8.7 g/dL^{-1};
- platelets: 70×10^9/L;
- potassium (K): 3.2 mmol/L;
- calcium: 4 mmol/L;
- urea: 14.1 mmol/L;
- creatinine: 190 mmol/L.

D:

- AVPU was 'A' – alert, able to answer all questions appropriately.
- Blood sugar 6.4 mmol/L.

E:

- On examination Cathy was tender over her mid abdominal area with some distension felt.

Following an ABCDE assessment, Cathy was screened for SIRS and she met more than two of the diagnostic criteria. These were:

- temperature: <36 or >38.3°C;
- respiratory rate: >20/min;
- heart rate: >90/min;
- WBC count >12 × 10^9/L.

When assessed for a history of infection and signs of a new infection, Cathy had a three week history of infection and had received two courses of antibiotics. She was now presenting with abdominal pain, distention and diarrhoea consistent with an abdominal infection (see Table 7.2). She now met the criteria for sepsis. In the following section we interpret Cathy's clinical signs and blood results so that we can begin to understand what is happening to her and what is likely to happen next, starting with respiration.

Respiration

One of the earliest clinical signs of sepsis is an increase in the patient's respiratory rate. This increase may be triggered by a number of factors related to the patient's condition and include:

- pyrexia;

- evidence of respiratory infection or existing disease;

- pulmonary oedema triggered by a systemic inflammatory response leading to increased capillary permeability and leaking of fluid into the alveoli (Daniels and Nutbeam, 2010).

When Cathy was assessed her respiratory rate was 32/minute, her breathing was shallow and on auscultation widespread crackles were heard. She had been treated for a chest infection a week before admission and this may have exacerbated her respiratory problems. The arterial blood gas results revealed evidence of a combined respiratory and metabolic acidosis and potential type II respiratory failure (Chapter 2). The presence of pyrexia indicates the presence of bacterial pathogens (infective organisms) and this triggers the stress response and a corresponding increase in respiratory rate. Evidence of respiratory crackles on auscultation further raised concern and with evidence of pulmonary infiltrates visible on the chest X-ray, Cathy was showing signs of pulmonary oedema due to increased capillary permeability and movement of fluid into the pulmonary interstitial and alveoli spaces (Murray, 2011). Thus with a respiratory rate of more than 25/min, and evidence of bilateral pulmonary infiltrates, Cathy already met the criteria for severe sepsis (Figure 7.2).

Temperature

A fever or pyrexia occurs in response to the release of pyrogens from the infective organism and inflammatory mediators or chemicals that trigger inflammation. These include cytokines (prostaglandin E2), phagocytes and histamine that are triggered by an event that causes damage to body tissues and cells, including infection (Hall, 2011). This process can be initiated within minutes or hours of damage by pathogens. Not all patients with sepsis or SIRS will present with pyrexia; exceptions include patients who have impaired temperature regulation such as patients with cervical spinal injury, people who are taking anti-inflammatory medication and patients where there is evidence of systemic inflammatory response but no evidence of infection. There are benefits from having a fever and these include the creation of a chemical environment that helps to destroy the invading organisms and facilitation of the immune response. This response is part of a negative feedback loop that includes initially peripheral vasoconstriction and elevation of temperature and secondly periods of peripheral vasodilation and sweating (McCance and Huether, 2014). When this response is systemic, however, the impact on the circulation can lead to profound vasodilation and loss of circulating volume. For Cathy, evidence of a fever (38.9°C) and a raised WBC count of 14×10^9/L was evidence of SIRS and an infection.

Heart rate and blood pressure

When a systemic inflammatory response is triggered, key changes triggered by the release of inflammatory mediators include vasodilation, capillary leak, hypovolaemia and hypoxaemia (Daniels and Nutbeam, 2010). This triggers the stress or flight/fight response (Chapter 6) and the heart rate, cardiac output and blood pressure will initially increase in an attempt to compensate for the fall in central circulating volume as blood is redirected to the peripheral circulation and through increased capillary permeability. In spite of meeting the criteria for severe sepsis, Cathy has been able to maintain a BP of 108/46 mmHg and does not yet meet the criteria for

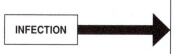 **INFECTION**

Triggers a local inflammatory response

- Inflammatory mediators (histamine, kinins and activation of the **complement system**)
- **Neutrophils** and **phagocytosis** (elevate temperature)
- **Monocytes** and **lymphocytes**
- Containment of infection and repair of damaged tissues

If the infection cannot be contained this will lead to the systemic activation of inflammatory mediators and SYSTEMIC INFLAMMATORY RESPONSE SYNDROME (SIRS)

SIRS triggers a systemic response

- The release of inflammatory mediators (cytokines) including:

  o **interleukins** (increases capillary leak)
  o **tumor necrosis factor** (coagulation, cell death, elevate temperature)
  o **histamine** (increases capillary permeability)
  o **prostaglandins** (elevation of temperature)
  o **nitric oxide** (vasodilation)

- Leading to:

  o vasodilation
  o increased capillary permeability and leaking of fluid out of the circulation
  o the accompanying stress response leads to an increased demand for oxygen and nutrients and increased metabolic rate

    o > respiratory rate
    o > temperature
    o > heart rate

Vasodilation

- Initially leads to an increase in peripheral blood volume and a warm and pink appearance leading to:

  o hypotension
  o increased heart rate
  o core body temperature may fall as a consequence of vasodilation
  o altered mental state as a result of sepsis, shock and hypoxia
  o in the later stages of sepsis the peripheral circulation will shut down and the skin will become cool and mottled

Capillary leak

- Fluid shifts out of the circulation:

  o interstitial oedema
  o hypotension

- Pulmonary oedema:

  o hypoxia
  o increased respiratory rate

- Circulatory failure and distributive shock – **severe sepsis and septic shock**

- Lactic acidosis caused by anaerobic metabolism (Chapter 6)
- Acute respiratory distress syndrome (ARDS) (Chapter 3)
- Single organ dysfunction progressing to multiple organ dysfunction and multiple organ failure
- **Death**

Figure 7.3: Sepsis: how the systemic inflammatory response (SIRS) leads to signs of clinical deterioration

Source: De Gaudio, 2014.

septic shock (Table 7.1). Her heart rate of 136/minute, however, is high and once again meets one of the criteria for severe sepsis (Figure 7.2). When there is loss of central circulating volume the body will continue to try and maintain its homeostatic balance by drawing on fluid reserves in the liver, spleen and mesenteric circulation and if the inflammatory mediators continue unabated, Cathy would be unable to maintain a systolic blood pressure over 90 mmHg and could progress to septic shock. Therefore, vigilance in continuously monitoring her vital signs is required and she needs to be admitted to ICU.

Altered mental state

When a patient presents with an altered mental state, it can include a range of signs such as being:

- lethargic, sleepy, with disorganised movements;
- disorientated, restless;
- bewildered, having difficulty with obeying commands;
- stuporous (having reduced alertness), comatose.

In relation to sepsis and SIRS this altered state may be due to one or more of the following:

- hypoxia;
- hypovolaemia and electrolyte imbalance;
- damage to the neurological system as a direct result of sepsis (Daniels and Nutbeam, 2010).

When Cathy was admitted she was tired but alert and was able to answer questions appropriately. At that stage she was showing no signs of an altered mental state even though her oxygen saturation levels had reduced to 91% and she was dysoxic.

Signs of infection

The changes in clinical signs, together with evidence of infection, provide vital information when screening for sepsis or clinical deterioration. The most common sites for infection that are associated with the development of sepsis are:

- lungs;
- skin;
- abdomen;
- urinary tract.

The clinical signs of infection related to these sites (Daniels, 2013; Daniels and Nutbeam, 2010) are listed in Table 7.2.

Body system	Signs of infection: Look: Listen: Feel: Measure	Clinical examples
Lungs	<ul><li>R: >20/min.</li><li>Dyspnoea.</li><li>Temperature >38°C.</li><li>Yellow/green sputum when expectorating.</li><li>Noisy air entry during auscultation and/or no air entry to some lung quadrants.</li><li>Evidence of consolidation on chest X-ray.</li></ul>	Serena Jones (18 years) works in a busy city centre store. She has had a flu-like illness for eight days and still feels unwell. She returned to work because she is worried that too much time off would reflect badly on her record. Within an hour Serena collapsed on the floor while serving a customer; she was faint, breathless and exhausted. Her respirations were 28/min and her temperature was 38.8°C. Serena was diagnosed with pneumonia (see Chapter 3). *Serena recovered without developing sepsis.*
Skin	<ul><li>Cellulitis: inflamed, red, hot and swollen area of skin that is spreading from a focal point.</li><li>Petechial rash (rash of blood spots).</li><li>Temperature >38°C.</li><li>Wounds: pain, tenderness, inflammation, pus.</li><li>Characteristic smell.</li></ul>	Peter Matthews (70 years) has type 2 diabetes. A week ago he bought new shoes; unfortunately the shoes rubbed and he developed a blister on his left heel. Several days later he noticed his heel, ankle and foot were swollen and red. He made an appointment at the local surgery for the following day. By the time he was assessed by the doctor his leg was red, hot and inflamed up to his knee and he felt hot and tired. His temperature was 39°C. Peter was diagnosed with cellulitis and admitted for 24 hours' observation and intravenous antibiotic therapy. *Peter developed sepsis and required care in ICU.*
Abdomen	<ul><li>Abdominal pain or tenderness.</li><li>Abdominal distention.</li><li>Temperature >38°C.</li><li>Nausea/vomiting.</li><li>Diarrhoea.</li></ul>	Barry Andrews (74 years) enjoyed a party and buffet meal to celebrate his granddaughter's 18th birthday. Two days later he developed acute abdominal pain, nausea, diarrhoea and felt feverish with a temperature of 39.4°C. His symptoms continued for four days before he required admission to hospital for further management. He was diagnosed with a *Campylobacter* infection. *Barry developed severe sepsis and septic shock and is still receiving intensive therapy.*

(Continued)

Table 7.2   (Continued)

Body system	Signs of infection: Look: Listen: Feel: Measure	Clinical examples
Urinary tract	• Cystitis/pain on passing urine (dysuria). • Loin pain. • Frequency and/or urgency when passing urine. • Cloudy urine with a characteristic smell. • Haematuria.	Sandra Brown (18 years) is a first-year undergraduate at university. For the last week she has experienced frequency and urgency when passing urine. Today she awoke with pain in her right loin which increased in severity when she tried to pass urine. Sandra felt nauseated and shivery. She was advised during a visit to the campus medical centre that she had a urinary infection and was asked to provide a specimen of urine for sampling. *Sandra made a complete recovery; she did not develop sepsis.*

Table 7.2: Clinical signs of infection in body systems

Cathy's recent medical history had indicated a history of malaise accompanied initially by lower abdominal and loin pain. The GP had suspected a urinary tract infection, sent a mid-stream urine specimen for culture and sensitivity and prescribed an appropriate antibiotic (Public Health England, 2014). The urine specimen, however, proved negative to bacterial infection and when Cathy returned to her GP a week later he diagnosed a chest infection and prescribed a different antibiotic. The underlying problem of abdominal discomfort, however, remained unresolved but was getting progressively worse. These symptoms now seemed to point to an abdominal infection (Table 7.2) and following an assessment in ED, a computerised tomography (CT) scan was ordered as part of her management recommendations.

What are the priorities of care for a patient diagnosed with sepsis?

So far in this chapter we have focused on risk assessment and diagnosis of a patient with sepsis. We will now continue with Cathy's story and examine if the recommendation and management in ED were evidence-based and timely. During the ABCDE assessment it is important to assess the patient situation, which includes questioning whether there are any limitations of treatment that exist for your patient and whether these limitations are still valid. It is important not to make assumptions about a patient's care and, if possible, always to involve the patient and family in the decision-making process (see Chapter 1). In Cathy's case she was a previously young and fit mother with no limitations on her treatment and she and her husband were actively informed and involved in her management.

When a patient is diagnosed with sepsis the speed of response is critical in order to prevent further deterioration. Dellinger et al. (2013) and Daniels (2013) recommend that resuscitation and diagnosis interventions should be initiated immediately and follow protocolled and goal-directed therapy for initial resuscitation and management. The UK Sepsis Trust (Daniels, 2013) prescribe a set of six tasks that should be completed within the first hour following recognition of sepsis. This group of multidisciplinary interventions is called the Sepsis Six and adopting this plan in a timely manner can reduce patient mortality by preventing the patient's progression towards septic shock. The aim of Sepsis Six is to measure and correct problems with oxygen delivery so that body tissues can maintain adequate tissue perfusion and reduce the likelihood of inadequate tissue perfusion, which will cause shock.

They include the following.

1. *Give high-flow oxygen* (via a non-rebreathing bag if appropriate): according to Daniels (2013) these patients should receive high levels of oxygen regardless of their underlying condition during the resuscitative phase, although he recommends that patients with COPD should be supported by a specialist clinician. Monitoring Hb as well as SpO_2 will identify if the patient is anaemic. A patient with a low Hb may have full oxygen carrying capacity in each haemoglobin molecule but with fewer molecules of haemoglobin available; the patient will experience a decline in the availability of oxygen to the tissues and reduced tissue perfusion leading to fatigue, weakness and shortness of breath, particularly on exertion (Hammer and McPhee, 2014). The use of arterial blood gas analysis, as well as oxygen saturation and Hb, will give a more detailed picture of the underlying condition but waiting for a full set of results should not delay the commencement of high-flow oxygen. Close and continuous monitoring of the patient is critical at this stage but should not prevent the initiation of treatment.

2. *Take blood cultures*: this should be completed before antibiotic therapy has commenced unless this is contraindicated. This is also the time to take samples and swabs of any likely source of infection if appropriate.

3. *Give intravenous antibiotics*: the use of prescribed broad spectrum **empirical antibiotic therapy** can be initiated before the infecting organism is identified and reviewed when more information is available. According to the UK Sepsis Trust, 'each hour's delay in giving antibiotics in septic shock is associated with a 7.6% increase in mortality' (Daniels, 2013, p37).

4. *Start intravenous fluid resuscitation*: a functioning circulation is critical in ensuring body tissues receive oxygen and nutrients. We have already seen that due to SIRS, fluid can be lost to the interstitial spaces and peripheral circulation thus losing valuable central circulating fluid (Figure 7.3). The aims of fluid therapy are to correct hypovolaemia, maintain pulse, keep BP and urine output within agreed parameters and to do so without triggering the symptoms of fluid overload (Chapter 9). If the patient has a systolic BP of >90 mmHg, a reasonable fluid prescription would include 500 ml of Hartmann's solution to be administered over 30–60 minutes. If the patient has a systolic blood pressure of <90 mmHg, then the patient should receive 20 ml/kg/L of Hartmann's solution over 30–60 minutes until they either achieve a BP of >90 mmHg or fail to respond to the fluid challenge.

5. *Check blood levels of haemoglobin and lactate*: a fall in the patient's blood haemoglobin below 7 g/dL^{-1} can adversely affect patient outcome; the patient's haemoglobin should therefore be monitored in order to reduce this risk (Walsh and Ezz-El-Din Saleh, 2006). Cathy's haemoglobin was within an acceptable range at 8.9 g/dL^{-1}. A lactate level of >2 mmol/L in patients

with sepsis is indicative of anaerobic metabolism due to reduced tissue perfusion (shock), particularly if the high level persists over several days. Monitoring lactate over time can provide evidence of the relative success of oxygen therapy and fluid challenges as the lactate level begins to fall. Cathy's lactate was 4.7 mmol/L, which indicated anaerobic metabolism and was consistent with her metabolic acidosis.

6. *Accurately monitor hourly urine output:* a urine output of <0.5 ml/kg/hr for two hours is evidence of reduced perfusion to the kidneys (shock) and can lead to acute renal failure. If the patient does not have a urinary catheter inserted, then it is necessary to organise this. Cathy was catheterised and her urinary output was monitored hourly.

Scenario: Cathy Price – recommendations and management in ED within one hour of admission

- *Commence oxygen therapy to maintain SpO$_2$ above 96% and review on the basis of sepsis screening.*
- *Obtain a sample for blood cultures.*
- *Obtain venous access and a full blood screen including: urea and electrolytes, liver function tests, full blood count, coagulation studies and lactate.*
- *An arterial sample of blood to assess acid/base balance and respiratory function.*
- *Commence intravenous fluids initially at 125 ml/hr and review on the basis of sepsis screening.*
- *Commence fluid resuscitation according to Sepsis Six.*
- *Intubate and commence MIV to support failing respiratory function and manage her pulmonary oedema.*
- *Insert a urinary catheter to monitor hourly urine output.*
- *Commence empirical antibiotics.*
- *CT scan.*
- *To ICU for management of sepsis and newly diagnosed severe sepsis.*

When we return to Cathy's case and review the recommendation and management, we can see that all the Sepsis Six interventions were initiated in the first hour of her admission and at that stage hypotension had been avoided. Cathy is, however, experiencing severe sepsis on the basis of her initial screening criteria and evidence of failing respiratory function.

Case study: Henry Mason

Henry is 71 years old. He used to smoke 20 cigarettes a day but gave up 20 years ago when he was diagnosed with type 2 diabetes. He has very poor eyesight due to bilateral cataracts and is waiting for surgery. He has had hypertension and been on medication for ten years. Henry has already been in hospital for a week. He was originally admitted with pneumonia, and following a respiratory arrest on the medical ward, he spent five days in ICU. During his stay in ICU he required MIV to support his

---

respiratory function as well as intravenous antibiotic therapy, physiotherapy, haemodynamic and nutritional support. In order to monitor and support his condition he had an arterial line, a central line, a urinary catheter and intubation with an endotracheal tube. By the time Henry was discharged from ICU, he was breathing with the support of 40% oxygen, and his urinary catheter, central line and arterial line had been removed. He was making good progress, but 48 hours after his discharge to the ward, Jan, the nurse looking after him, noted that he was reluctant to eat and drink, he was lethargic and his chest sounded noisy. Henry's respiratory rate had increased to 21/min from 18/min but otherwise his vital signs remained unchanged (T: 37.5°C; P: 89/min; BP: 130/85 mmHg). Jan communicated her concerns to the medical team at 18.00 hours and recorded them in the notes.

Activity 7.2   *Decision making*

1. What were Henry's risk factors for developing SIRS and sepsis?
2. With reference to the sepsis screening tool in Figure 7.2, can you identify if Henry met any of the criteria for SIRS and sepsis?
3. Using the screening tool and the recognition and response bundles identified in Chapter 1 (Table 1.2), plan what you would do to support optimum management of Henry from 18.00 hours to 19.00 hours.

There are answers to this activity at the end of the chapter.

How should patients with severe sepsis be managed?

As we have seen, when a patient is diagnosed with sepsis/severe sepsis, it is important to involve the critical care outreach team and transfer the patient to ICU as soon as possible because these patients will need intensive support of their respiratory, cardiovascular and circulatory systems in order to support their body organs, prevent multiple organ dysfunction and improve their chances of survival. In the following sections we will explore how Cathy was managed in relation to the Surviving Sepsis Campaign's international guidance on managing severe sepsis (Dellinger et al., 2013). This guidance recommends that the resuscitation and management bundles for patients with severe sepsis should be completed within 24 hours of diagnosis in order to improve survival. This was achieved for Cathy, although the delay in the early stages of diagnosing the underlying cause of infection by her GP did potentially increase her risk of mortality. A summary of the international guidelines for the management of severe sepsis and septic shock are illustrated in Table 7.3.

When we return to Cathy's story after her transfer to ITU we can see that her condition has been critical and her care complex.

Stages of management	Interventions
Initial resuscitation and infection issues	
Initial resuscitation	Clinical goals during the first six hours. • Central venous pressure (CVP) 8–12 mmHg. • Mean arterial pressure (MAP) ≥65 mmHg. • Urine output ≥0.5 ml/kg/hr. • Central or mixed venous oxygen saturation 70% or 65% respectively (allows you to see how much oxygen is actually being delivered to the tissues). • Reduce lactate to <2 mmol/L.
Screening for sepsis and performance improvement	• Continue with routine screening for severe sepsis and septic shock.
Diagnosis	• Take blood cultures before antibiotic therapy commences where this means there will be no significant delay in commencing antibiotics.
Antimicrobial therapy	• Administer empirical antibiotics within one hour of recognition of severe sepsis and septic shock.
Source control	• Locate/diagnose source of infection.
Infection prevention	• Selective oral and digestive decontamination.
Haemodynamic support and adjunctive therapy	
Fluid therapy for severe sepsis	• Crystalloids are the initial fluid of choice. • Initial fluid challenge in sepsis induced hypotension to achieve a minimum of 30 ml/kg. • The fluid challenge technique should be continued as long as there is haemodynamic improvement.
Vasopressors and inotropic therapy	• Infuse norepinephrine (vasopressor) via a central line in order to maintain a MAP of 65 mmHg. • Vasopressin 0.03 units/minute can be added with norepinephrine when an additional agent is needed to maintain BP. • Dobutamine (inotrope) infusion (up to 20 mcg/kg/min) may be infused to improve cardiac function.
Other supportive therapy	
Blood product administration	• Red blood cell transfusion should occur when Hb <7.0 g/dL^{-1} to target Hb of 7.0–9.0 g/dL^{-1}.
MIV of sepsis-induced acute respiratory distress syndrome (ARDS)	• Target a tidal volume of 6 ml/kg predicted body weight. • Inspiratory plateau pressure should be ≤30 cm H_2O.

	• Add positive end expiratory pressure (PEEP) to avoid alveolar collapse at the end of expiration. • Consider recruitment manoeuvres to re-expand lung tissue in patients with severe unchanged hypoxaemia (prone positioning, high frequency jet ventilation). • Elevate the head of the bed to 30–45 degrees to reduce risk of ventilator associated pneumonia. • Have a weaning protocol in place.
Sedation, analgesia and neuromuscular blockade	• Minimise continuous or intermittent sedation for patients receiving MIV. • Avoid neuromuscular blockade.
Glucose control	• Commence insulin when two consecutive blood sugars are >10 mmol/L.
Renal replacement therapy	• Commence when evidence of acute kidney injury or to manage fluid balance.
DVT prophylaxis	• Commence daily.
Stress ulcer prophylaxis	• Commence on patients with bleeding risk factors.
Nutrition	• Administer oral or enteral feeding as tolerated.
Setting goals of care	• Discuss goals of care with the patient and their family.

Table 7.3: A summary of the international guidelines for the management of severe sepsis and septic shock based on Dellinger et al. (2013)

Scenario: Cathy Price is transferred to ICU for management of severe sepsis

When Cathy was transferred to ICU she continued to be supported on MIV in order to improve her PaO₂ and promote oxygen delivery to the tissues. The SSC guidance for initial resuscitation and supportive therapy for severe sepsis was followed (Dellinger et al., 2013). Initially fluid resuscitation and oxygen therapy improved her BP and urine output but this did not resolve her severe metabolic acidosis and elevated lactate level and she was commenced on renal replacement therapy (Chapter 9). Over the following 24 hours Cathy developed acute respiratory distress syndrome (ARDS) and her condition deteriorated further (Chapter 3). ARDS is associated with inflammation of the lung parenchyma that leads to impaired gas exchange with associated systemic release of inflammatory mediators causing inflammation, reduced lung compliance and hypoxia (Bersten, 2014). Cathy received support in ICU for three weeks before she was transferred to high dependency and eventually to the ward. A year later and Cathy is a sepsis survivor but is still suffering from the effects of severe sepsis in the form of nightmares and panic attacks, poor concentration, memory loss and extreme fatigue consistent with post-sepsis syndrome (Sepsis Alliance, 2015; Winters et al., 2010).

Managing the patient in ICU

The role of the nurse in ICU when supporting patients with sepsis and their families focuses on three key areas.

1. Assessing, monitoring, interpreting and communicating changes in your patient's condition in a timely manner.
2. Providing interventions to support goal-directed therapy.
3. Providing information and reassurance to the patient and family as the disease takes it course.

Airway and breathing

For some patients pneumonia may be the primary cause of sepsis, but this is not the case for all patients. Most patients who develop sepsis will also develop respiratory failure associated with the systemic inflammatory response and, as in Cathy's case, will develop hypoxia, pulmonary oedema and an increased respiratory rate (tachypnea). The aim of management is to support the patient's respiratory function and reduce the risk of any further damage by:

*   providing respiratory support in order to achieve PaO_2 at >8 kPa;
*   adhering to the ventilator bundle explained in Chapter 3;
*   reducing the risk of ventilator associated injury (Chapter 3, Table 3.6).

Cathy developed ARDS and the guidance for mechanical ventilation for sepsis-induced ARDS was followed (Table 7.3).

Cardiac and circulatory system

Patients with sepsis, and particularly septic shock, have hypotension associated with capillary leak (Figure 7.3). The aims of cardiovascular support are to ensure the patient has accurate, safe and continuous monitoring of their heart rate, blood pressure (arterial line), **central venous pressure** (CVP), temperature and urinary catheter in order to manage their fluid requirements. Fluid requirements for patients in septic shock are high during the period of fluid resuscitation but this may change depending on the evidence of fluid volume deficit or overload. Within 24 hours of her admission, Cathy was commenced on renal replacement therapy to manage her severe metabolic acidosis, stabilise her fluid balance and reduce the risk of acute kidney injury (Chapter 9). Goals of early directed therapy for patients with severe sepsis include:

*   CVP >8 mmHg (>12 mmHg if ventilated);
*   systolic blood pressure >90 mmHg (mean arterial pressure (MAP) >65 mmHg);
*   fluid replacement should continue until the patient's systolic blood pressure is above 90 mmHg.

If the patient's blood pressure does not respond to fluid resuscitation they have progressed to septic shock and management in this situation involves the commencement of a group of drugs known as vasopressors, which work by increasing peripheral vasoconstriction and improving blood pressure; many of them occur naturally in the body. They include adrenaline (epinephrine) and noradrenaline (norepinephrine). As a rule these drugs are given intravenously via a central line as they cause peripheral vasoconstriction. They have a half-life of approximately one to two minutes and should not be turned off unless prescribed as the patient will react within minutes with rebound hypotension and bradycardia. It is important, therefore, to assess and monitor your patient's haemodynamic state carefully as these drugs have a virtually instant effect on the cardiac and circulatory system. Noradrenaline (norepinephrine) is the first drug of choice and is infused until the patient is able to maintain a blood pressure above systolic 90 mmHg (MAP 65–85 mmHg) (Dellinger et al., 2013).

Disability and exposure

It is important to assess and review the patient's mental state and level of consciousness hourly as this can be a sign of improvement or deterioration (Chapter 11). In order to reduce the risk of further infection and control existing infections, it is essential to continue with core interventions related to infection prevention and control.

These include:

- hand washing;
- appropriate use of uniforms and personal protective equipment;
- safe disposal of sharps;
- aseptic procedure and adherence to bundles of care such as the central line bundles (IHI, 2015);
- assessment for evidence of developing infection at infusion sites and catheters;
- isolation of patients with healthcare related infection;
- vaccination of healthcare staff.

Finally, when caring for a patient with severe sepsis, it is important to support the patient's mobility, positioning and hygiene in order to reduce the risk of pressure ulcers, impaired circulation and muscle tone. The use of the skin bundle in ICU provides a systematic approach to assessment and management of the patient's skin, nutrition and mobility and can reduce the incidence of pressure ulcers in critically ill patients (Whitlock et al., 2011).

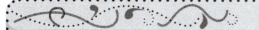

Chapter summary

The aim of this chapter was to help you to assess, recognise and respond in a timely manner to patients who develop sepsis and severe sepsis, including septic shock. The responsibilities of the nurse when caring for patients at risk of sepsis can be summarised as follows.

- Undertake a rigorous assessment and monitoring of the patients in your care.
- Know your patients and recognise that any change in their condition is significant.

(Continued)

continued . . . . •

- Use standard guidelines and protocols to support your decision making.
- Ensure that interventions are timely – they save lives; do not hesitate and lose valuable time.
- Report evidence of change or deterioration in the patient's condition to the relevant medical team and follow up your concerns.
- Anticipate and be prepared to support a patient's deteriorating condition.

Activities: brief outline answers

Activity 7.1: Decision making (pages 156–7)

Edward Morris

1. Edward did meet some of the screening criteria and was clearly showing signs of sepsis.

- T: 38.6°C.
- P: 95/min.
- Completed chemotherapy seven days ago.

2. Advice to give Edward.

- Neutropenic sepsis is a medical emergency, so Edward should be advised to call 999 and ask for the ambulance service. Patients in Edward's situation need an urgent full blood count to determine if neutropenia is present.
- While he is waiting he could collect his overnight bag and a summary of the chemotherapy drugs he has taken.

Molly Taylor

1. Molly did meet some of the screening criteria and was showing signs of sepsis and hypoxia.

- Confusion.
- R: 28/min.
- P: 95/min.
- SpO_2: 88%.

2. Molly is in the high risk range of the response bundle (NICE, 2007).

- Using the SBAR framework, you should contact the outreach team and summarise Molly's current problems, background and most recent vital signs.
- You should respond by anticipating the needs of the patient and outreach team when they arrive. While one person stays with the patient, someone can collect any equipment necessary as illustrated in Henry's story.

Activity 7.2: Decision making (page 167)

1. An examination of Henry's care plan showed that he was at high risk of developing sepsis for the following reasons.

- His age: 71 years.
- He has co-morbidities including diabetes, hypertension and recovering from pneumonia.
- He had required invasive lines and catheters to support his respiratory and cardiovascular function in ICU.
- He is on antibiotic therapy for pneumonia.

2. The increase in Henry's respiratory rate meant that he met one of the criteria for SIRS and evidence of a deterioration in his respiratory function could indicate a new infection. Overall he did not meet the criteria for SIRs and sepsis.

3. Based on Henry's recent medical history and his high risk of developing sepsis, the priorities for care would include:

- contact senior medical staff to ask for a review of Henry's condition using an SBAR approach;
- sit Henry up in the bed and promote a position to support effective respiration, ensure the oxygen mask was fitted securely and encourage him to take deep breaths;
- monitor his observations every 30 minutes and if his condition deteriorates any further then escalate the urgency of the situation;
- continue to screen for SIRS and sepsis.

Further reading

Bersten, A (2014) Acute respiratory distress syndrome, in Bersten, A and Soni, N (2014) *Oh's Intensive Care Manual.* Seventh edition. Oxford: Butterworth Heinemann.

Daniels, R (2013) *Survive Sepsis.* Third edition. Sutton Coldfield: UK Sepsis Trust.

This book offers up-to-date explanations on the risk assessment and pathophysiology of sepsis and would be of interest to those who have placements in critical care areas.

Daniels, R and Nutbeam, T (2010) *ABC of Sepsis (ABC Series).* Oxford: Wiley-Blackwell.

This book offers a more detailed account of how patients with sepsis should be managed in acute and critical care areas and offers a pragmatic guide to the care of these patients.

Useful websites

www.wales.nhs.uk/sitesplus/863/page/65480

This website is linked to Abertawe Bro Morgannwg University Health Board (ABM) and offers you an insight into how one health board was able to reduce the incidence of pressure sores by adopting the Skin Bundle.

www.sepsistrust.org

The UK Sepsis Trust website has information for professionals on sepsis learning resources and information for the public on how to cope with and survive sepsis.

Chapter 8
The patient with delirium

Desiree Tait

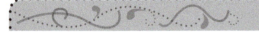

Chapter aims

By the end of this chapter, you should be able to:

- describe the term delirium;
- identify the common causes of delirium;
- demonstrate an awareness of how to risk assess for, and prevent, delirium;
- demonstrate an awareness of how to manage patients with delirium and provide them with a safe environment;
- reflect on, and rehearse, the risk assessment and management of patients with delirium.

Introduction

Case study: Janet's story

My name is Janet and I have been qualified as a nurse for one year. I was working an extra shift one night and I found I had been allocated to work on an acute medical ward. I had never worked on this ward before and didn't know the patients, but after a few hours I began to feel that I was comfortable with the layout and had assessed the patients I had been allocated. That was until midnight when I heard a scream coming from the female section followed by several shouts for help. I rushed down to see what was happening to find that a gentleman from the male section was attempting to get into bed with one of the female patients. The gentleman was pushing Joan (the female patient) out of bed to make room. I pulled her buzzer to call for assistance and tried to calm the situation down. The gentleman's name was Jack Porter (85 years), and at the time I knew nothing about him. I tried to reason with him and explained that he should go back to his bed where he would be more comfortable. He looked at me and nodded, and then walked over to another patient and tried to get into bed with her. I tried to talk to him again and gently held his elbow to steer him away. When I did this he resisted in an aggressive manner, pushing me and pinning me against the wall. The other staff again tried to reason with him, but he began shouting and pushing them away. Someone called for the on-call medical team to attend, and together we were able to calm Jack and persuade him to go back to bed. The medical team prescribed haloperidol and said they would perform a detailed assessment in the morning.

The female patients were terrified by this time and particularly frightened of the fact that it took three nurses and two medics to resolve the situation. No person came to physical harm that night, but the psychological distress felt by the female patients led to a disturbed and sleepless night for them. Jack was also clearly distressed and appeared to believe that we were going to harm him. After Jack had calmed down and I had a chance to reflect, I realised that I needed to understand more about what had just happened.

Janet's story is not uncommon and describes an example of a patient with delirium. The incidence of delirium in acute and critical care settings is high and can increase the risk of morbidity and mortality (European Delirium Association and American Delirium Society, 2014).

According to NICE (2010a), in the UK the prevalence of delirium is 20–30% in medical wards and 10–50% in surgical wards. Similarly, an epidemiological review of the incidence of delirium on medical wards identified that 11–15% of older patients who are admitted will have delirium on admission (prevalent delirium) and a further 29–31% of older patients admitted to medical wards will develop delirium (incident delirium) during their time on the ward (Vasilevskis et al., 2012). In ICU the incidence of delirium in ventilated patients is between 22–83% (Vasilevskis et al., 2012).

According to the National Clinical Guideline Centre (2010) and Morandi et al. (2012), patients who develop delirium have:

- a higher than average incidence of complications such as falls and pressure sores;

- an increased risk of self-extubation and removal of catheters in critical care settings;

- a correspondingly increased length of stay in hospital;

- an increased risk of long-term cognitive impairment associated with critical illness;

- an increased incidence of dementia;

- an increased risk of mortality.

The importance of recognising, responding to and, where possible, preventing delirium cannot be overestimated; in the remainder of the chapter we will explore how delirium can be assessed, diagnosed, prevented and managed.

What is delirium and how should it be described?

Delirium is a term used to describe an altered state of consciousness that is accompanied by a change in cognition or perception. The onset is acute, developing over one to two days and the course of the condition fluctuates according to time and other factors (NICE, 2010a, 2010b). The core features of delirium found in patients include:

- a reduced awareness and understanding of their immediate environment;

- an impaired ability to focus their attention, sustain and change their attention to something else;

- altered cognition, including: memory impairment, disorientation, paranoia, language or perceptual disturbances including hallucinations.

These disturbances develop over several days and tend to fluctuate during the course of the day. For example, acute confusion may only be manifested after dark and can be referred to as sundown syndrome (Beel-Bates and Rogers, 1990). The American Psychiatric Association (2013) updated their classification of delirium in 2013 to focus more on disturbance in attention and awareness although the European Delirium Association and American Delirium Society (2014) argue that the understanding of delirium must extend beyond cognitive testing of attention and that medical assessments must consider both attention and arousal.

For some patients delirium will last a few days; for others it can continue for months, depending on the predisposing and precipitating factors listed in Table 8.2 on pages 181–2. The three subtypes of delirium described by NICE (2010a) are set out in Table 8.1 and are consistent with understanding delirium from a psychomotor behavioural perspective (Morandi et al., 2012).

What causes delirium?

Delirium appears to occur when a single factor, or a combination of factors, leads to a reversible organic mental syndrome. This means that in more than 90% of patients the underlying cause is physiological and related to the impact of the disease and/or the impact of hospitalisation (Aldemir et al., 2001). The pathophysiology of delirium is complex and there are number of theories that have been proposed which ultimately lead to neurotransmitter imbalance in the brain leading to an excess of dopamine (Alce et al., 2014; Borthwick et al., 2006). The main neurotransmitters and receptors that are associated with delirium include (Borthwick et al., 2006):

- *dopamine*: helps to control the brain's reward and pleasure centres, regulate movement and emotional response;
- *acetylcholine*: plays a role in enhancing sensory perceptions when we wake up and in sustaining attention as well as regulating digestion and muscle movement;
- *serotonin*: plays a role in sleep, memory and learning, mood, behaviour and depression;
- *nicotinic and opioid receptors*: neuroreceptors that are associated with addiction;
- *bacterial infection*: endotoxins released as the bacteria breakdown can alter cell function in the brain.

Some factors that trigger delirium are predisposing (patient vulnerability factors), in that some patients have increased risk of developing delirium before they have been admitted to hospital. This may be due to existing dementia, old age, pre-existing illness or functional impairment including vision or hearing loss, malnutrition, drug and/or alcohol abuse and depression (Vasilevskis et al., 2012). Delirium can also be caused by potentially modifiable precipitating factors associated with the severity of the patient's illness, the use of certain drugs, electrolyte and chemical imbalance and sepsis (Vasilevskis et al., 2012). A full list of the predisposing and precipitating factors can be found in Table 8.2, which includes some clinical examples. In the next section we will put these factors into context by returning to Janet's and Jack Porter's story.

Delirium subtype	Clinical signs	Patient examples
Hyperactive	Agitated and restless • Fidgeting. • Pulling at clothes, catheters or tubes. • Moving from side to side. • Shouting and calling out. Disorientated. • Doesn't know who or where they are. • May have difficulty following commands. Paranoia • Sees some members of staff as a threat. • Expresses fear and distress as the environment appears hostile. • May try to escape. • Pain may be expressed as severe. • Evidence of abnormal vital signs and imbalance in fluid and electrolytes.	Charlie Thomas (78 years) was admitted to a cardiac ward after feeling light-headed and dizzy. When he was admitted, his heart rate was 35/min and the ECG showed he had a bradycardia and complete heart block. A temporary pacing wire was inserted and his heart rate and blood pressure improved. Later that night the nurse noticed that his ECG trace had gone flat. She rushed to his bedside to find Charlie out of bed and looking for the exit. He had disconnected himself from the ECG leads but the pacing wire and equipment were still connected. He pushed past the nurse and made his way along the corridor towards the bus stop, wearing only pyjama bottoms. When the nurse caught up with him, he couldn't understand why he had to go with her because he needed to go home – they were expecting him. The nurse sat at the bus stop with Charlie for ten minutes before he agreed to come back to the ward and wait there.
Hypoactive	Disorientated • Doesn't know who or where they are. • May have difficulty following commands. Withdrawn • Lying quietly • Looking away and avoiding opportunities for human contact. • Evidence of abnormal vital signs and imbalance in fluid and electrolytes.	Margaret Adams (83 years) was quiet and withdrawn after her admission yesterday afternoon. She had been found by the postman lying in the hall after having fallen when trying to let the cat out. The door had got stuck open on the carpet so she had been lying in the cold for several hours. Margaret had a fractured neck of femur and was waiting for surgery to stabilise the fracture. She didn't want to talk and when asked about her home arrangements she began to give information that was contradictory to what was in the nursing notes. When Margaret was asked to roll on

	This subtype is often difficult to diagnose and needs careful assessment from advanced assessment tools such as the Confusion Assessment Method for the ICU (CAM-ICU) (Ely, 2014).	her side she didn't move or attempt to help with the procedure and she appeared not to understand simple commands. The nurse noted that this was very different from what she was like on admission when she was alert and keen to know who everyone was.
Mixed	The patient presents with a combination of hyperactive and hypoactive signs, often at different times in the day.	Chester Smith (90 years) was admitted to a surgical ward following an episode of acute abdominal pain; he was diagnosed with appendicitis and had emergency surgery that afternoon. In the post-operative period he appeared vague and withdrawn, and the staff thought that he had dementia. When his granddaughter visited, however, she said that normally he was as 'bright as a button' and that this was unusual behaviour for him. Later that night Chester began to get increasingly agitated, pulling at his urinary catheter and shouting for help. When the nurse tried to assess him, Chester began to shout even louder and pulled his urinary catheter out, throwing it on the floor.

Table 8.1: Subtypes of delirium with clinical examples

Why did Jack Porter develop delirium?

After the incident with Jack, Janet decided to read his notes and try to understand why he behaved the way he did. She found the following predisposing and precipitating factors.

- Predisposing/vulnerability factors
- Age: Jack is 83 years old.
  - He has been married to his wife for 62 years, and during that time they had never been separated for more than a few days and he is lonely and isolated from his family.
  - Jack has type 2 diabetes and hypertension for which he takes a beta blocker (slows the heart rate and reduces cardiac output).
  - Jack had been admitted to hospital with a recent history of blackouts and falls.

- Precipitating
  - ○ Jack has been in hospital for five days.
  - ○ His dose of beta blocker has been reviewed and reduced.
  - ○ He has been diagnosed with a urinary tract infection and prescribed antibiotics.
  - ○ His blood results from earlier today showed a raised sodium and potassium level, and an elevated creatinine level consistent with a risk of acute kidney injury (see Chapter 9).
  - ○ When Jack settled, his respirations were 20/min, his pulse was 58/min and his blood pressure was 110/65 mmHg (lower than normal for Jack); his temperature was 37.5°C and his blood sugar was 7.4 mmol/L.
  - ○ Jack had only passed 500 ml of urine in the last 18 hours, a second risk factor for acute kidney injury (see Chapter 9).

Janet felt concerned for her patient and used the SBAR tool to ask the on-call medical team to review him that night instead of waiting until the morning. He was reviewed and commenced on an infusion of dextrose/saline to improve hydration and was catheterised in order to monitor his urine output. His medication for hypertension was discontinued with a view to assess Jack's renal function in the morning. Jack clearly had a number of predisposing and precipitating factors towards delirium and we will explore how these could be managed in the next section.

Activity 8.1 — *Decision making*

When you are next on placement in a hospital setting:

- review the patients that you have been allocated for risk factors associated with developing delirium;
- if you identify a patient who is at risk, collaborate with the healthcare team and discuss possible options for prevention as shown in Table 8.3;
- continue to observe your patients to monitor any change in their condition that may increase the risk of them developing delirium.

As this activity is based on your own observation, there is no outline answer at the end of the chapter.

How is delirium risk assessed and prevented?

When a patient is admitted to the ward, or unit, part of their assessment on admission should include an assessment of the predisposing and precipitating risk factors for developing delirium.

As with all other elements of assessment, patients should be assessed using the 'Look: Listen: Feel: Measure' and ABCDE criteria. In this case it is very important to include information from the patient's friends and relatives in order to develop a picture of the patient as a person before they were admitted to hospital. Plan and organise the patient's care so that they see familiar faces

Predisposing (vulnerability) factors	Clinical examples
• Increasing old age >65 years. • Existing cognitive impairment/dementia. • Evidence of increasing severity of illness. • Existing physical impairment. • Pre-existing alcohol/substance abuse.	• Any person, male or female who is 65 years or older, has an increased risk of developing delirium. • Patients with existing dementia or depression have an increased risk of developing delirium. • A patient with bronchitis who develops an acute chest infection has an increased risk of developing delirium. • Patients with visual and/or hearing impairments, or with limited mobility, can experience sensory deprivation in hospital, and this predisposes them to developing delirium. • A person who may have abused drugs in the past, but has not taken them for several years, is still at risk of developing delirium as addiction can affect permanent changes on brain cells.
Precipitating (modifiable) factors	**Clinical examples**
Disease • Respiratory disease and associated hypoxia (Chapters 2 and 3). • Cardiovascular disease. • Hypotension. • Severe infection. • Sepsis. • Head injury. • Acute admission for fractures and hip surgery. Physiological imbalance • Imbalance of electrolytes particularly sodium and potassium. • Increased levels of creatinine, urea. • Anaemia. • Metabolic acidosis. • Dehydration. • Vitamin deficiency. • Blood glucose.	• Hanna Mera (67 years) developed hyperactive delirium after her oxygen saturations fell to 87% as the result of an acute exacerbation of her chronic respiratory disease. • Harold Jones (70 years) developed delirium following a delayed diagnosis of myocardial infarction and hypotension. • Sarah Moon (65 years) developed delirium after developing sepsis from a wound infection. • Fred Holloway (78 years) fell and fractured his hip. He had to wait 48 hours after admission before he had surgery to stabilise the fracture. • Fred Holloway developed delirium post-operatively and he was found to have an imbalance in sodium and potassium, dehydration and an increase in his creatinine levels. • Maryam Abdul (57 years) was admitted to hospital with cellulitis and sepsis. She was suffering from hypoxia and metabolic acidosis. She was disorientated and distressed.

(Continued)

Table 8.2   (Continued)

Precipitating (modifiable) factors	Clinical examples
Pharmacology • Polymedication. • Drug withdrawal. • Drug side effects that cause an altered balance of the neurotransmitters, acetylcholine and dopamine. • Failure to provide adequate pain relief. Use of physical and invasive therapy • Physical restraint caused by clinical equipment. • Indwelling catheters. • Immobilisation. • Lack of sleep. • Alien environment such as ICU.	• Ryan Sheppard (20 years) was involved in a road traffic collision. He sustained multiple fractures. He was intubated and ventilated for 24 hours in the post-operative period, after which attempts were made to reduce his respiratory support. As he awoke he appeared to be hyper alert and tried to get out of bed. He was unable to respond to requests to stay in bed and became very agitated. Ryan was a regular user of illegal substances and that, together with his critical illness, had triggered delirium. • Barry Jones (54 years) had been a patient in ITU for 14 days, during which time he had been both physically restrained by catheters and tubes as well as chemically restrained by sedation to support respiratory function. He slept all day and was awake all night. At night he became very agitated and would regularly disconnect his ventilator tubing and attempt to get out of bed.

Table 8.2: Predisposing (vulnerability) and precipitating (modifiable) factors for the development of delirium based on Vasilevskis et al. (2012) with clinical examples

among the carers, as this will provide continuity of care and continuity of assessment and monitoring. Assess for the core features of delirium (Table 8.1), and if any of these are present, your findings need to be validated by a more comprehensive clinical assessment such as the Confusion Assessment Method for ICU (CAM-ICU) (Ely, 2014; Ely et al., 2001; NICE, 2010b). According to Mistraletti et al. (2012), the correct way to approach delirium is to suspect its presence whenever a change in health status occurs and according to NICE (2010a) patients should be assessed for delirium at least once a day. If a diagnosis of delirium is confirmed, the next step is to adopt a multidisciplinary approach to prevent further deterioration and treat any underlying precipitating factors. This process may be summarised as follows.

• Assess the patient and family using a holistic approach to care.
• Risk assess for predisposing factors for developing delirium.
• Promote continuity of care.
• Assess for features of delirium daily and/or if the patient's condition deteriorates.
• If present, validate with the use of an assessment tool (CAM-ICU).
• Risk assess daily for evidence of any changes in risk factors.
• Develop a multidisciplinary plan to risk assess and adopt preventative interventions.

Factors on assessment	Preventative interventions	Preventative interventions for Jack Porter

Cognitive impairment disorientation	• Reorientate the person by explaining:
	    o where they are
	    o who they are
	    o what your role is.
	 • Provide:
	    o a clock
	    o a calendar
	    o appropriate signage.
	 • Provide cognitive stimulation:
	    o reminiscence.
	 • Encourage regular family visits.
		• When Jack awoke the next morning we reminded him where he was and why.
		 • We found his watch in the locker and put it on his wrist, checking it was the right time.
		 • We explained what day it was and encouraged him to talk about his wife and family.
		 • We contacted Jack's family to explain that he had become confused in the night and encouraged them to visit.

Hypoxia	• Assess for hypoxia and treat as necessary with oxygen, other medication, positioning and physiotherapy.	• Jack's oxygen saturations were 94% and we encouraged him to sit up and take regular deep breaths to help his breathing and circulation, while continuing to encourage him to keep his oxygen mask on.
Dehydration Constipation	• Assess fluid balance and bowel activity daily. • Encourage the person to take oral fluids; however, if necessary, supplement with subcutaneous or intravenous fluids.	• Because of Jack's reduced urine output and elevated blood levels of sodium, potassium and creatinine, he was given an infusion of fluids to improve his fluid and electrolyte balance. • Jack had a history of cardiovascular disease so his respirations, pulse and fluid balance were monitored closely in case of fluid overload. • Jack's blood results were checked the next day to review the situation.

(Continued)

Table 8.3 (Continued)

Factors on assessment	Preventative interventions	Preventative interventions for Jack Porter
Imbalance in electrolytes and creatinine Metabolic acidosis	• Monitor blood levels of electrolytes, liver and renal function. • Assess for signs of metabolic acidosis (Chapter 3).	
Infection	• Undertake daily infection and sepsis screening and escalate care as necessary (Chapter 7). • Implement infection control procedures. • Avoid invasive catheterisation unless necessary.	• The results from Jack's catheter specimen of urine directed a change in antibiotic therapy. • The presence of the urinary catheter was reviewed daily. • The catheter was removed three days later. • All infection control procedures were followed.
Multiple medications	• Review the person's medications and assess the risks of side effects and continued requirement for the drugs.	• Jack remained on a reduced dose of antihypertensive medication and metformin for his diabetes.
Medications that alter the balance of neurotransmitters • Anticholinergics: atropine, ipratropium bromide. • Analgesics: opioids such as morphine. • Corticosteroids: hydrocortisone. • Antihistamines: chlorphenamine. • Cardiovascular agents: digoxin. • Hypnotic drugs: benzodiazepines such as **midazolam.**	• Many of the drugs on this list will be vital for the patient's safety and well-being. • It is important that the drugs are only given when necessary and reviewed daily.	• These were reviewed daily by checking blood glucose levels and vital signs.

Pain	• Assess for pain using a holistic approach and manage effectively.	• We continued to assess Jack for evidence of pain and discomfort.
Poor nutrition	• Undertake a nutritional assessment and assess factors that may be affecting adequate nutrition such as ill-fitting teeth.	• Jack's appetite had reduced since being diagnosed with a urinary tract infection. However, over the next few days he gradually improved.
Limited mobility	• Encourage patients who have had surgery to mobilise as soon as possible after surgery. • Encourage people to walk, with support if necessary, as often as possible during the day. • Encourage all patients to carry out active range of movement exercises every day.	• Jack was encouraged to walk around his bed and do a range of motion exercises during the day.
Sensory impairment	• Ensure hearing impairments are assessed and managed. • Ensure people have the appropriate glasses for reading and long-distance vision. • Provide regular stimulation for those patients who are physically isolated.	• We encouraged the family to bring in Jack's reading glasses as well as his regular spectacles so that he could read the paper.
Sleep disturbances	• Avoid undertaking medical and nursing procedures during sleep periods. • Reduce noise to a minimum.	• We kept Jack in the same section of the ward that he was used to and provided an environment to promote restful sleep.

Table 8.3: Clinical assessment factors and interventions to prevent delirium

Table 8.3 provides an example of a multidisciplinary plan for assessing and preventing delirium, using Jack Porter as an example. Jack Porter remained in hospital for three weeks, and he remained in a state of delirium for a week before a gradual improvement was seen. After his discharge Jack was able to go home to his wife with support from community and social services. For patients in acute care, and particularly those patients who have undergone surgery, identifying the risk of delirium and preventing long-term problems for patients has become a priority (NICE, 2010a, 2010b). Your role as a nurse is to be vigilant in the holistic assessment of the patient and family in order to identify the potential for delirium and, if possible, prevent it.

Delirium in ICU

The incidence of delirium among patients in ICU is up to 30% higher than found in acute medical and surgical wards (Vasilevskis et al., 2012; Alce et al., 2014). In the UK, Page (2008) identified that a diagnosis of delirium can occur in up to 69% of patients receiving MIV. Delirium can also be an independent predictor of morbidity, in the form of post ICU cognitive impairment, and mortality in ventilated patients (Ely et al., 2003). In the next section we will explore the relationship between the ICU environment and the development of delirium by exploring Paul Chapman's story.

Case study: Paul Chapman

Paul Chapman (28 years) was walking home from a night out when he was hit from behind by a hit-and-run driver. He was found by a passer-by who called the emergency services. Paul was taken to A&E where he was stabilised and transferred to the operating theatre. Paul's injuries included:

- *facial fractures;*
- *fractured ribs (3 and 4) on the left side and contusion on the right side of his chest;*
- *fractured pelvis;*
- *fractured right shaft of femur, tibia and fibula.*

In theatre Paul received the following.

- *External fixation of a fractured pelvis.*
- *Internal fixation and pinning of his right shaft of femur, tibia and fibula.*

Paul was transferred to ICU from theatre in an unconscious state, intubated and ventilated.

When Paul was admitted to the ED, as well as his fractures, he was suffering from hypoxia, hypovolaemic shock and a metabolic acidosis. When assessed against predisposing and precipitating modifiable factors (Table 8.2), Paul was already considered to be at risk of developing delirium on the basis of hypoxia, hypotension and traumatic fractures. He was resuscitated with oxygen, respiratory support and fluid replacement, including a blood transfusion. Paul had been conscious at the scene, but his level of consciousness had deteriorated by the time he was admitted to hospital and this again is a predisposing factor for delirium (European Delirium Association and American Delirium Society, 2014).

In ICU Paul received a tracheostomy tube to prevent destabilisation of his facial fractures and was supported by MIV. Intravenous medication for the purposes of pain relief and sedation included: fentanyl, which is a potent synthetic opioid used for analgesia and anaesthesia (Marik, 2015), and midazolam for the purpose of sedation. According to Marik (2015) and Vasilevskis et al. (2012) the use of benzodiazepines such as midazolam have been shown to increase the risk and severity of delirium in patients at risk and recommend that early mobilisation and reduction of sedation can reduce this risk. An alternative sedative is dexmedetomidine (Marik, 2015). Paul had a number of invasive and restricting devices inserted in order to monitor his haemodynamic state including central and peripheral infusion lines, arterial line, urinary catheter, a chest drain to drain a pneumothorax on his left side and ECG monitoring. All of these interventions and devices can be described as physically restrictive and invasive forms of therapy and are precipitating factors for delirium (Table 8.2). In summary, the risk of precipitating factors for the development of delirium for Paul were high and it was imperative that he was risk assessed and managed to limit the onset of delirium on a shift-by-shift basis (Ely, 2014).

When Paul was assessed for predisposing factors for the development of delirium, the nurse's initial assessment revealed that the only predisposing factor was that of his increasing severity of illness. This was reviewed, however, when Paul's mother confided in the nurse at the bedside that Paul had experimented with drugs as a teenager but had told his mother that he had given them up eight years ago when he met his wife. This highlights the requirement to continually review your assessments – often not all the relevant information is available from the outset. This finding became significant when 48 hours later Paul was stable enough for the team to reduce his sedation and respiratory support.

Case study: Paul Chapman's sedation is reduced

As Paul started to wake up he became very agitated, and in spite of the use of reorientation and reassurance from Jennie, his nurse, Paul tried to pull out his peripheral and arterial line and ECG leads. Jennie continued to reassure him, explaining where he was and what had happened. She asked him if he had any pain, and Paul responded by beckoning to her to come closer. As Jennie leant forward Paul grabbed her round the waist and wouldn't let go. Jennie instinctively leant back and as she did so Paul came forward in the bed and was in danger of falling out. Jennie shouted for help, and with gentle reassurance from several members of staff Paul eventually let go and appeared to relax. A few minutes later, however, Paul was again trying to pull off anything that appeared to be attaching him to the bed. Jennie decided to invite Paul's wife to the bedside in the hope that this would reassure him. She explained to his relatives why he was more awake and that he was quite agitated at times, but if he was able to settle, they would be able to continue to reduce the sedation and respiratory support as the next step in his recovery. When Paul saw his wife he held out his arms and she leant forward to hold his hands. Paul, seeing her come

(Continued)

continued . . . •

closer, made a grab for her and pulled her onto the bed. We advised her to stay still and tried to persuade Paul to let her go. Paul resisted, and a team decision was made to recommence sedation and review the plan for weaning Paul from respiratory support. Paul's wife was tearful and upset by what had happened, and Jennie tried to reassure her that this situation can occur in critically ill patients and that as Paul began to improve he would become less confused about what had happened.

Treating delirium

For some patients risk assessment and preventative interventions are not enough to prevent severe cases of hyperactive delirium. In the case study, Paul Chapman was suffering from severe symptoms of hyperactive delirium triggered by multiple predisposing and precipitating factors. In cases such as Paul's, a plan of management would begin by dealing with the immediate problem of his distress. Paul was placing himself and others in danger by his actions, and the only option available was to recommence sedation in order to stabilise his condition and protect the safety of others. This can be described as a form of chemical restraint, which in Paul's case was justified in order to protect his safety in the short term (Bray et al., 2004).

When patients develop delirium a treatment plan should always begin with an assessment of the underlying causes and the provision of open and reassuring communication to both the patient and family (Borthwick et al., 2006; NICE, 2010b). The causes of Paul's delirium were related to a history of drug abuse and factors related to his condition, such as fear and anxiety, physical restraint from his multiple therapeutic interventions such as the tracheostomy tube, ECG, infusions and urinary catheter, and the risk of physiological imbalance associated with his critical illness. The most effective method for managing Paul's delirium was to promote recovery and rehabilitation and the subsequent removal of trigger factors.

According to Borthwick et al. (2006), patients with a history of drug abuse and who undergo sedation with benzodiazepines such as midazolam for seven days or more are very likely to experience delirium when the drug is withdrawn. For Paul, a plan for recovery included a gradual reduction of sedation over several days and a daily review of his risk factors for developing delirium. Five days later Paul was awake and no longer requiring respiratory support. He was transferred to the orthopaedic ward where his rehabilitation continued. Paul continued to experience episodes of confusion for several months following his accident and, according to Arend and Christensen (2009), Paul may experience prolonged neuropsychological side effects that can extend beyond his physical recovery.

Key steps in treating delirium include:

- assess patient safety immediately;
- risk assess underlying causes and avoid where possible medication that increases the severity of delirium;
- communicate with, reorientate and reassure the patient;
- involve family and friends;

- encourage early mobility;

- ensure stability and continuity of care using a team approach;

- if the patient is distressed, try verbal and non-verbal reassurance to calm the patient;

- if the patient's distress continues, consider the use of short-term medication such as haloperidol. This drug works by helping to correct the balance of dopamine and acetylcholine activity in the brain (Borthwick et al., 2006).

A systematic toolkit to operationalise interventions to promote prevention of delirium and safety of patients in ICU is accessible through the American Association of Critical Care Nurses (2015) and is based on work by Vasilevskis et al. (2010) and Balas et al. (2012) on their development and evaluation of the ABCDEF bundle for delirium prevention and safety. The bundle of care addresses six key areas and includes the following.

- A: Assess, prevent and manage pain.

- B: Both spontaneous awakening trials and spontaneous breathing trials (this involves daily cessation of sedation in order to assess the patient's suitability for weaning from respiratory support and sedation).

- C: Choice of analgesia and sedation should be patient orientated and goal directed.

- D: Delirium assess, prevent and manage using validated assessment tools such as CAM-ICU.

- E: Early mobility and exercise.

- F: Family engagement and empowerment.

Activity 8.2   *Evidence-based practice and research*

This activity encourages you to think about how you might update and improve practice. Go to the website **www.icudelirium.org/medicalprofessionals.html** or alternatively search for 'CAM-ICU' and the 'ABCDEF' bundle for delirium and explore the toolkits and guides that are available. When you are on your next placement ask the clinical staff how they assess for delirium. The importance of asking questions like this is that it opens up avenues of inquiry that the clinical staff may not have considered and has the potential to improve practice.

The answer is reflective and as such there is no model answer at the end of this chapter.

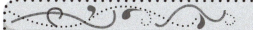

Chapter summary

Within this chapter we have considered the common causes of delirium in patients placed in acute and critical care areas. We have explored ways in which patients can be risk assessed for developing delirium and how it may be prevented and treated. The key messages from this chapter to apply to your practice are the following.

(Continued)

continued . . .

- Patients who develop delirium have increased risk of morbidity and mortality.
- Daily risk assessment of patients for developing delirium can prevent its onset and should be considered a priority of care.
- Promoting good communication and continuity of care is an important factor in preventing delirium.
- If delirium cannot be prevented, then strategies and interventions used must be patient centred and enhance the safety of the patient and others.

Further reading

Bray, K, Hill, K, Robson, W et al. (2004) British Association of Critical Care Nurses' position statement on the use of restraint in adult critical care units. *Nursing in Critical Care*, 9(5): 199–212.

This paper provides advice by the BACCN on the use of physical and chemical restraint for patients who become agitated and combative.

Useful websites

www.icudelirium.co.uk

This website offers general information about the assessment, prevention and management of delirium and, in particular, a list of commonly used medications that can trigger delirium.

www.icudelirium.org/medicalprofessionals.html

This website has educational resources on how to assess patients using the Confusion Assessment Method, CAM-ICU, and the ABCDEF bundle for delirium prevention and safety. The site also provides links to videos that demonstrate the assessment in practice.

www.nice.org.uk/cg103

This website provides you with all NICE guidance documentation of assessing and treating delirium, including a guideline for patients and carers.

Chapter 9
The patient with acute kidney injury

Desiree Tait with Susan Hanson

NMC Standards for Pre-registration Nursing Education

This chapter will address the following draft competencies:

Domain: Nursing practice and decision-making

Generic competencies:

7. All nurses must be able to recognise and interpret signs of normal and deteriorating mental and physical health and respond promptly to maintain or improve the health and comfort of the service user, acting to keep them and others safe.

8. All nurses must provide educational support, facilitation skills and therapeutic nursing interventions to optimise health and wellbeing. They must promote self-care and management whenever possible, helping people to make choices about their healthcare needs, involving families and carers where appropriate, to maximise their ability to care for themselves.

Field-specific competencies:

7.1 Adult nurses must recognise the early signs of illness in people of all ages. They must make accurate assessments and start appropriate and timely management of those who are acutely ill, at risk of clinical deterioration, or require emergency care.

8.1 Adult nurses must work in partnership with people who have long-term conditions that require medical or surgical nursing, and their families and carers, to provide therapeutic nursing interventions, optimise health and wellbeing, facilitate choice and maximise self-care and self-management.

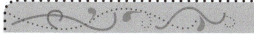

NMC Essential Skills Clusters

This chapter will address the following ESCs:

Cluster: Organisational aspects of care

18. People can trust a newly registered graduate nurse to enhance the safety of service users and identify and actively manage risk and uncertainty in relation to people, the environment, self and others.

(Continued)

continued . . . •••

By entry to the register:

xi. Assesses and implements measures to manage, reduce or remove risk that could be detrimental to people, self and others

Cluster: Nutrition and fluid management

29. People can trust a newly registered graduate nurse to assess and monitor their fluid status and in partnership with them, formulate an effective plan of care.

By the second progression point:

iii. Recognises and reports reasons for poor fluid intake and output.

iv. Reports to other members of the team when intake and output falls below requirements.

By entry to the register:

vi. Identifies signs of dehydration and acts to correct these.

Chapter aims

By the end of this chapter, you should be able to:

- identify and describe risk factors that lead to acute kidney injury;
- differentiate between acute kidney injury and chronic renal disease;
- demonstrate an awareness of how to risk assess patients for acute kidney injury;
- recognise and interpret the clinical signs and symptoms of a person suffering from acute kidney injury and identify appropriate nursing interventions;
- reflect on the clinical examples referred to in this chapter and relate to your own clinical practice.

What is acute kidney injury?

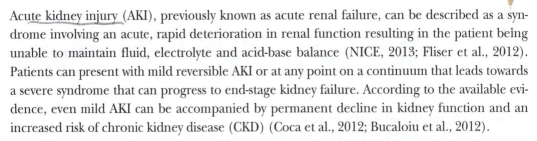

Acute kidney injury (AKI), previously known as acute renal failure, can be described as a syndrome involving an acute, rapid deterioration in renal function resulting in the patient being unable to maintain fluid, electrolyte and acid-base balance (NICE, 2013; Fliser et al., 2012). Patients can present with mild reversible AKI or at any point on a continuum that leads towards a severe syndrome that can progress to end-stage kidney failure. According to the available evidence, even mild AKI can be accompanied by permanent decline in kidney function and an increased risk of chronic kidney disease (CKD) (Coca et al., 2012; Bucaloiu et al., 2012).

The best treatment for AKI is therefore prevention; this is reflected in the clinical guidance offered by NICE (2013) and supported by the European Renal Best Practice (ERBP) group (Fliser et al., 2012).

The medical definition of AKI is based on the following three key physiological factors.

- Urine output.

- Serum creatinine (SCr) level.

- The severity of urine output decline and increase in SCr level from the patient's baseline level at the onset of their current condition.

Degree of severity of AKI	Criteria	Useful points to consider
Stage 1	**One of the following**	
	• Serum creatinine (SCr) increased to 1.5–1.9 times the baseline.	Use the first documented SCr taken from the patient during this current episode of illness.
	• SCr increase >26.5 µmol/L.	
	• Urine output <0.5 ml/kg/hr during a 6 hour block.	Use the patient's ideal weight rather than their actual weight for this calculation.
Stage 2	**One of the following**	
	• SCr increase 2.0–2.9 times baseline.	Use the first documented SCr taken from the patient during this current episode of illness.
	• Urine output <0.5 ml/kg/hr during 2 × 6 hour blocks.	Use the patient's ideal weight rather than their actual weight for this calculation.
Stage 3	**One of the following**	
	• SCr increase >3 times baseline.	Use the first documented SCr taken from the patient during this current episode of illness.
	• SCr increase >353 µmol/L.	
	• Initiation of renal replacement therapy to substitute kidney function.	
	• Urine output <0.3 ml/kg/hr during more than 24 hours.	Use the patient's ideal weight rather than their actual weight for this calculation.
	• Anuria (no urine output) for more than 12 hours.	

Table 9.1: Criteria for determining the severity of AKI in a patient at risk (based on ERBP and KDIGO guidance, Fliser et al., 2012; KDIGO AKI Work Group, 2012)

The ERBP workgroup recommend that each patient should be assessed according to the severity of the AKI rather than an absolute definition of whether AKI exists or not. Table 9.1 provides a summary of the ERBP recommendations and kidney disease improving global outcomes (KDIGO) severity score (Fliser et al., 2012).

Within this chapter we will explore how to assess and interpret situations where people may be at risk of AKI, how to prevent patients from developing AKI and finally how to manage patients who develop AKI.

Why does acute kidney injury occur?

Acute kidney injury occurs as a result of extra cellular volume depletion, decreased renal blood flow and/or toxic inflammatory injury to kidney cells. The most frequent cause of the syndrome is transient hypoperfusion leading to decreased renal blood flow and is referred to as pre-renal AKI. For example, if a patient goes into shock, the body's natural regulatory mechanisms will activate the autonomic nervous system and the renin-angiotensin-aldosterone mechanism (described in Chapter 6). As a consequence, renal blood flow and **glomerular filtration rate** (GFR) are reduced in an attempt to preserve circulating volume and maintain tissue perfusion. At this stage AKI is preventable and/or reversible by treating the cause of the shock.

However, if the underlying cause of the patient's shock is not diagnosed and corrected in a timely manner renal blood flow will continue to be reduced and the kidney will become ischaemic, cells will become damaged due to reduced availability of oxygen and the inflammatory response will be triggered, leading to cell death. This more severe form of the syndrome is referred to as intra-renal AKI. Other causes of intra-renal AKI include toxic damage caused by nephrotoxic drugs and iodinated contrast agents.

Who is most at risk?

Acute kidney injury is common in hospitalised patients and for those patients who are diagnosed with uncomplicated AKI there is a 10% mortality rate. However, in patients where AKI is complicated by multiple failure of their body organs the mortality rate is likely to be more than 50% (Lewington and Kanagasundaram, 2011). The risks associated with AKI are high and the severity of the problem for people at risk has been compounded by a report published by NCEPOD (2009) where they identified serious deficiencies in the care of patients who developed AKI, reporting that only 50% of the patients reviewed received good care. Deficiencies reported include poor attention to detail and inadequate risk assessment of factors for AKI. The recommendations from this report have informed NICE guidance (2013).

Some patients have a higher degree of risk for developing AKI and according to NICE (2013) include people:

- with acute illness;

- with evidence of deteriorating vital signs, particularly hypotension;

- with urine output of less than 0.5 ml/kg/hour (oliguria);

- with sepsis;

- receiving iodinated contrast agents in the previous week;

- having surgery and at risk of hypovolaemia and/or infection;

- with co-morbidities including heart failure, diabetes and liver disease;

- who have a history of previous episodes of AKI;

- with CKD;

- aged ≥65 years;

- who are regularly prescribed nephrotoxic drugs such as non-steroidal anti-inflammatory drugs (NSAIDs), aminoglycosides such as gentamycin, angiotensin converting enzyme (ACE) inhibitors, angiotensin II receptor antagonists (ARBs) and diuretics;

- with a history of or a condition that may lead to urinary obstruction.

Table 9.2 illustrates clinical examples of patients at risk of developing AKI.

What are the nursing responsibilities when assessing patients at risk?

The role of the nurse in risk assessing the patient for the potential, existence and severity of AKI is to:

- know your patients, including their past and recent medical history, recent investigations, prescribed medication and when they last had renal function tests;

- identify if your patient is at risk of AKI (see Table 9.2);

- risk assess and monitor your patients for evidence of deteriorating respiratory function;

- risk assess and monitor your patients for evidence of deteriorating circulation using the ABCDE approach, paying particular attention to:

  o deterioration in fluid balance;

  o deterioration in urine output;

  o deterioration in BP;

  o evidence of sepsis (see Chapter 6);

- communicate your concerns to the relevant medical practitioner using an SBAR approach (see Chapter 1).

People at risk	Why	Clinical example
With acute illness	People with an acute episode of illness are more likely to present with fluid volume depletion due to haemorrhage, diarrhoea and vomiting, burns, acute cardiac failure and failure of other body systems. They are also more likely to need emergency surgery and have a higher associated risk of infection than people receiving elective surgery.	Jenny Brown (19 years old) is admitted following a four day history of acute diarrhoea and vomiting. She refused help from her university friends, initially because she was too embarrassed. On admission Jenny was pale, weak and lethargic: R: 24; P: 102; BP: 80/55. She hadn't passed urine that day and didn't want to.
With evidence of deteriorating vital signs, particularly hypotension	If the early signs of clinical deterioration are missed the patient is likely to experience transient reduced perfusion of the kidneys as a result of hypotension. 55% of people who develop AKI have a transient period of hypotension (Patschan and Müller, 2015).	Terry Jones (35 years old) – a coach driver – had collapsed in a local hotel with haematemesis and melaena. Vital signs on admission were R: 23/min; P: 100/min; BP: 85/58. He received fluid resuscitation as was assessed as having a low risk of a further bleed. Four hours later he became restless: R: 28/min; P: 120/min; BP: 70/40. He received further fluid resuscitation and blood transfusions before his BP stabilised at 110/65. Following a review of Terry Jones's fluid balance since admission the nurse estimated that his urine output had been less than 0.5 ml/kg/hour for the last three hours, increasing his risk of AKI.
With urine output of (less than) <0.5 ml/kg/hour (oliguria)	Possible reasons include: • hypovolaemia and should be assessed with evidence of deteriorating vital signs • obstruction to the flow of urine (see below).	
With sepsis	Sepsis can cause AKI because of: • hypotension • the triggering of a systemic inflammatory response – discussed in Chapter 7.	William Butler (73 years old) had a past medical history of ischaemic heart disease and hypertension. Several days ago he cut and bruised his upper arm on a kitchen door and was admitted with cellulitis. Twenty-four hours later he was risk assessed and diagnosed with

Risk factor	Rationale	Case study
		sepsis and SIRS (Chapter 7). His BP fell to 70/30 and he had passed <0.5 ml/hr for three hours.
Receiving iodinated contrast agents in the previous week	Potential toxicity of these agents increases if patients have any other risk factors listed in the table. Therefore, careful assessment of the risk benefit of undertaking the investigation, e.g. percutaneous intervention (PCI), and effective management of other risk factors should be undertaken before the procedure is undertaken (Fliser et al., 2012).	Harry Smith (58 years old) has a medical history of diabetes, hypertension and hyperlipidaemia. He is prescribed ACE inhibiters, statins and aspirin. This afternoon he was found by his wife in a state of collapse at home. On admission he was diagnosed with ST elevation myocardial infarction (STEMI) and cardiogenic shock. On assessment: R: 24/min; SpO$_2$: 85%; P: 120/min; BP: 83/55.
With chronic kidney disease (CKD)	AKI can occur in patients with existing CKD making the risk of morbidity and mortality higher in this group (Carville et al., 2014).	His estimated glomerular filtration rate was 20 ml/min/1.73m^2 indicating he had stage 4 CKD. He was risk assessed by the cardiac and renal specialist to determine the risks/benefit of PCI and it was decided that without percutaneous intervention and insertion of vascular stents he had a high risk of mortality and they proceeded with the PCI. His co-morbidities, including CKD, PCI and cardiogenic shock, all increased his risk of developing AKI.
Having surgery and at risk of hypovolaemia and/or infection	These patients have a higher risk of hypotension, surgical complications and infection (Aitken et al., 2013; Borthwick and Ferguson, 2010).	Martha Brown (75 years old) lived alone and suffered with congestive heart failure, hypertension, thyroid disorder and rheumatoid arthritis. Her medication included: amiodarone, furosemide, levothyroxine and

(Continued)

Table 9.2 (*Continued*)

People at risk	Why	Clinical example
With co-morbidities including heart failure, hypertension, diabetes and liver disease	Progressive disease increases the risk of chronic inflammatory damage to the nephrons and stimulation of the renin angiotensin system (McCance and Huether, 2014) .	NSAIDs. She was admitted following a fall at home and sustained a fractured neck of femur. During the surgery she sustained moderate to severe blood loss and an episode of hypovolaemia. She was admitted to ITU for post-operative care because the following factors put her at risk of further clinical deterioration and AKI. • Her age. • Co-morbidities. • Medication of NSAIDs and diuretics. • Episode of hypovolaemia.
Age ≥65 years	Increased risk of CKD and co-morbidities as indicated above.	
Who are regularly prescribed nephrotoxic drugs such as: • non-steroidal anti-inflammatory drugs (NSAIDs) • aminoglycosides such as gentamycin • angiotensin converting enzyme (ACE) inhibitors • angiotensin II receptor antagonists (ARBs) • diuretics	Nephrotoxic drugs increase the risk of inflammatory and vascular damage to the functioning nephrons, particularly in patients with existing co-morbidities and with increasing age.	

Who have a history of previous episodes of AKI	This indicates the kidney will have some existing damage from previous episodes thus making the patient more susceptible to further injury.	Barry Taylor (65 years old) has been admitted for a second time in five years to the ITU with acute pancreatitis. On the first occasion he developed AKI secondary to SIRS. On this occasion he was admitted following a period of depression and an increased intake of alcohol. He was diagnosed with acute necrotising pancreatitis, severe sepsis and AKI.
With a history of or a condition that may lead to urinary obstruction	This is a rare cause of AKI unless the patient has only one functioning kidney left or if obstruction affects both kidneys at the same time. For example, a kidney stone can lead to inflammatory damage in the nephrons. A tumour may cause an obstruction to the one ureter or the urethra.	Matthew Richardson (42 years old) presented himself in the emergency unit with a 12-hour history of blood stained urine and severe lower abdominal and loin pain. He was diagnosed with renal colic and advised to increase his fluid intake and was prescribed strong analgesics to manage the pain. He then said: 'Oh by the way I only have one kidney'. He was then admitted and risk assessed for AKI.

Table 9.2: Clinical examples of people at risk of developing AKI

Activity 9.1	*Reflection*

With reference to Table 9.2, think back to your experiences in the clinical setting: can you identify a patient that you have nursed who was at risk of AKI?

If so, now consider the following questions.

- Did your patient fit into one or more of the high risk groups?
- Did you consider them to be at risk of AKI?
- Was your patient identified as being at risk by the clinical team?
- If so, how was the patient managed?
- What was the outcome for the patient?

Hint: These reflective questions will help you to link the chapter content to patients you have nursed.

There is no outline answer at the end of the chapter as this activity is based on your own reflections.

What are the functions of the kidney and what happens when they fail?

The main function of the kidney is the formation of urine, which is produced at a rate of approximately 1.5 L/day. This process occurs within the functional units of the kidney, the nephrons, and involves the processes of filtration, reabsorption and secretion.

The formation of urine begins in the glomerulus. The afferent arteriole subdivides into many smaller capillaries as it enters the Bowman's capsule and arterial pressure within the capillary bed forces water and low molecular weight substances from the blood into the Bowman's capsule. The GFR is a measure of the volume of fluid that is filtrated by all the functioning nephrons in the kidneys. In a healthy person this is 180 L/day. However, in order to maintain homeostasis, 80% of this volume is reabsorbed as it flows through the proximal and distal tubules and collecting duct (McCance and Huether, 2014).

The concentration of urine occurs in the loop of Henle and involves the diffusion and reabsorption of sodium and reabsorption of water. The secretion of ions, including hydrogen and potassium from tubular capillaries, occurs in the proximal and distal tubules. A summary of this process is illustrated in Figure 9.1.

Other functions of the kidney include the following (McCance and Huether, 2014).

- The production of hormones such as:
  - renin: produced by the juxtaglomerular cells in the Bowman's capsule close to the afferent capillary, triggers the renin-angiotensin-aldosterone system (RAAS) if there is a reduction in blood flow to the kidney;

- erythropoietin: produced by interstitial cells in the kidney, controls red cell production;
- calcitriol: produced in the proximal tubules of the nephron, promotes the absorption of dietary calcium.
- Excretion of the by-products of metabolism including:
  - creatinine (produced as a by-product of energy production from muscle contraction);
  - urea (produced as a by-product of protein metabolism);
  - sodium (Na);
  - potassium (K);
  - bicarbonate (HCO_3).
- Maintenance of acid-base balance (see Chapter 3).

The signs and symptoms of impaired kidney function depend on a number of factors, including the progression of the damage (50% of nephrons can be destroyed before signs and symptoms begin to occur), and whether the person is suffering from AKI or CKD (McCance and Huether, 2014). Table 9.3 provides a general summary of physiological signs of malfunction.

How is acute kidney injury different from chronic kidney disease?

For patients experiencing AKI, the syndrome can progress very rapidly, occurring within a few hours or days, depending on the severity of the underlying trigger. AKI is potentially reversible; however, if it is left undiagnosed and unsupported, patients can progress to end-stage renal failure. Patients will experience signs and symptoms based on the acuteness of their clinical condition and recent medical history as well as deterioration in urine output. Serum creatinine levels will increase correspondingly as the urine output deteriorates (see Table 9.1). The extent of changes in creatinine level and urine output determine the severity of, and stage of, AKI (Fliser et al., 2012). When a patient develops AKI they progress through three clinical phases: the initiation phase, the maintenance phase and the recovery phase. Later in the chapter we will introduce you to Tim Hunter and discuss how the syndrome impacted on him and his family as he progressed through the stages of AKI.

For patients experiencing CKD the disease is progressive, developing over months or years. According to the National Kidney Foundation (2006) and KDIGO (2012) there is progressive loss of renal function associated with systemic diseases such as:

- hypertension;
- diabetes mellitus;
- systemic lupus erythematosus;
- existing kidney disease or injury;
- cardiovascular disease.

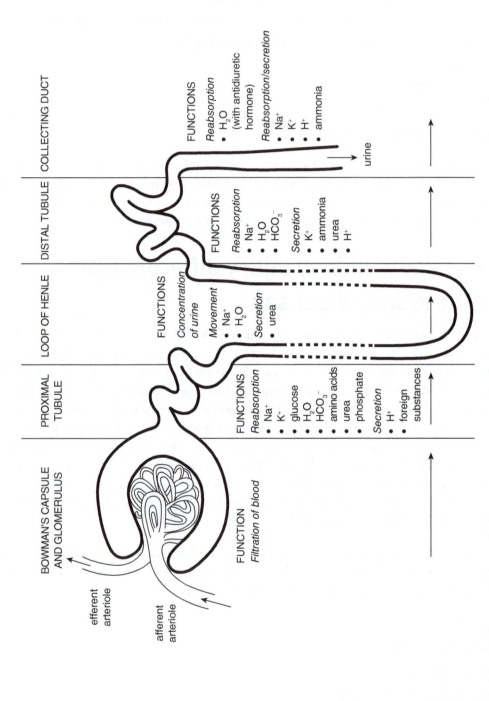

Figure 9.1: Major functions of the nephron

Normal renal function	Signs and symptoms of renal malfunction
Formation of urine	• Reduction in urine production and output. • Fluid overload. • Hypertension. • Heart failure. • Increased risk of pulmonary and interstitial oedema. • Reduction in estimated glomerular filtration rate.

Production of renin	• Inability to control the RAAS leading to loss of control over:
	  ○ blood pressure
	  ○ fluid balance
	  ○ sodium balance.

Excretion of the by-products of metabolism	• Inability to excrete ammonia in the form of urea leading to uraemia and encephalopathy (eventually coma). • Inability to excrete creatinine leading to increased creatinine levels. • Inability to excrete potassium leading to hyperkalaemia. • Anorexia, nausea and vomiting. • Muscle weakness. • Sexual dysfunction.
Maintenance of acid-base balance (see Chapter 3)	• Metabolic acidosis (see Chapter 3).
The production of erythropoietin	• Anaemia, tiredness and lethargy. • Prolonged bleeding time.
The production of calcitriol	• Increased risk of calcium loss and osteoporosis. • Bone pain.

Table 9.3: Kidney functions and the physiological impact of failing renal function

In the early stages of the disease, patients will experience no specific symptoms apart from those of the related disease. The progression of the disease is instead measured by the patient's estimated GFR and urine albumin creatinine ratio (Carville et al., 2014). As the disease progresses from mild to moderate CKD, the patient will begin to show more signs and symptoms of renal malfunction, these becoming more severe as CKD progresses to stage 5 (end-stage kidney disease). CKD is not reversible but early screening and management of underlying co-morbidities, nutrition, vitamin D, fluid and electrolyte balance and erythropoietin, as necessary, can delay its progression.

Table 9.4 provides a summary of the key differences in diagnosis and disease progression.

The initiation phase of acute kidney injury

The initiation phase of AKI occurs when the cause of, or trigger for, evolving renal injury becomes established. The initiation phase can therefore occur in all people who can be identified at risk

Criteria	AKI	CKD
Onset of the condition	Acute onset over hours/days.	Progressive onset over months/years.
Prognosis	Potentially reversible.	Progressive/not reversible.
Classification of severity measurement	>SCr <urine output (see Table 9.1).	<GFR >urine albumin: creatinine ratio.
Risk assessment	<ul><li>Identify people at risk (see Table 9.2).</li><li>Monitor and prevent the development of AKI where possible.</li><li>Recognise early signs and provide physiological support.</li></ul>	<ul><li>Identify people at risk with:<ul><li>hypertension</li><li>diabetes mellitus</li><li>systemic lupus erythematosus</li><li>existing kidney disease or injury</li><li>cardiovascular disease.</li></ul></li><li>Monitor GFR and urine albumin: creatinine ratio.</li><li>**Stages of CKD based on GFR (ml/min) include:**<ul><li>Stage 1: ≥90 *Normal kidney function*</li><li>Stage 2: 60–89 *Mildly reduced kidney function*</li><li>Stage 3: 30–59 *Moderately reduced kidney function*</li><li>Stage 4: 15–29 *Severely reduced kidney function*</li><li>Stage 5: <15 *End-stage kidney failure*</li></ul></li></ul> (Renal Association 2013) <ul><li>Refer patients in stage 4 for specialist assessment (Carville et al., 2014).</li></ul>

Table 9.4: A summary of key differences in the diagnosis and risk assessment of AKI and CKD

of AKI (see Table 9.2). According to McCance and Huether (2014), the general triggers for the initiation of AKI can be summarised as any trigger that has led to reduced tissue perfusion (hypotension) and/or toxic renal damage. The initiation phase of AKI usually lasts for 24–36 hours and if patients at risk are identified during this period, and managed effectively, the maintenance and recovery phases of AKI can be prevented.

How can we prevent progression to established acute kidney injury?

The first priorities of the nurse when preventing patients from progressing to established AKI are the same as the nursing responsibilities for assessing patients at risk of AKI (see page 195) and include:

- knowledge of the patient's past and recent medical history;
- assessment and management of a patient's deteriorating vital signs using the ABCDE approach (in particular hypotension and reduced renal output);
- knowledge of nephrotoxic drugs and interventions that may apply to your patient;
- recognising patients at risk in a timely manner and communicating that information to the patient's medical team using an SBAR approach.

The medical responsibilities for preventing a patient's progression to established AKI include:

- fluid resuscitation and maintenance of intravascular volume in order to restore blood pressure and cardiac output;
- discontinuing and removing nephrotoxic substances from the circulation;
- identifying and treating any related trigger factors such as dysoxia, infection, anaemia (Bellomo, 2014).

Swift action within the first 24–26 hours of the patient being identified at risk is critical to preventing AKI. Prescott et al. (2012) identify ten top tips that describe points along the patient's pathway where we can make a difference.

1. Empower patients to take charge of their healthcare in primary care if they become acutely ill by advising them to increase their fluid intake and avoid nephrotoxic medication while ill.
2. The use of regular updates for healthcare staff on risk assessing for AKI.
3. The effective use and interpretation of the national early warning score (NEWS).
4. All patients should have a consultant review their care within 12 hours of admission (NCEPOD, 2009).
5. The use of an electronic alert system to identify when abnormal serum creatinine levels increase.
6. Follow NICE (2013) guidance for the management of AKI.
7. The use of the AKI care pathway (Map of Medicine, 2014) and timely referral of patients from primary and secondary care for a renal review.
8. Effective communication and handover of care between practice areas and disciplines.
9. Effective clinical coding and audit of the incidence of AKI.
10. The medical follow-up of patients who have been diagnosed with AKI to manage their risk of developing CKD.

In Tim's story we shall see what happens when he enters the initiation phase of AKI.

Scenario: Tim Hunter in the initiation phase of AKI

Tim is a 78-year-old gentleman who lives with his wife Daphne (aged 76) in a small bungalow in the suburbs of the local town. They used to have a good social life but this has dwindled in the last few years and Daphne has recently taken over the driving because of Tim's cataracts.

Situation
Tim has been feeling generally unwell for a few weeks and Daphne has been concerned that he has not been eating properly and seemed tired and lethargic. Tim had been reluctant to go to his GP but was eventually persuaded to go after he became increasingly lethargic with a history of passing small infrequent amounts of red stained urine and complaining of abdominal discomfort.

Background
Tim has a past medical history of:

- *type 2 diabetes for 20 years (prescribed metformin and glipizide);*
- *atrial fibrillation (prescribed digoxin and aspirin);*
- *hypertension for which he is prescribed an ACE inhibitor (ramipril);*
- *awaiting surgery for bilateral cataracts;*
- *he used to smoke but gave up several years ago.*

Assessment
- *The GP assessed Tim and was concerned that he had developed an ascending urinary tract infection as a result of a neurogenic bladder. Tim's blood glucose level in the surgery was 18 mmol/L. In light of his co-morbidities, the GP decided to admit Tim to hospital.*
- *On admission to hospital the following assessment data was collected.*

  - *Airway and breathing:*

    - *R: 22/min, regular rate;*
    - *SpO_2: 97%.*

  - *Circulation:*

    - *HR: 87/min;*
    - *pulse appeared regular with premature beats occurring occasionally;*
    - *BP: 100/65 mmHg;*
    - *urine output: passed 100 ml of urine on admission, tested positive to blood and protein;*
    - *complaining of nausea.*

  - *Disability and exposure:*

    - *blood glucose 18.2 mmol/L;*
    - *lethargic but alert;*

---

o *skin and mucous membranes dry and cracked;*

o *T: 38.2°C.*

Recommendations and ongoing care

- *Commence antibiotic therapy for a suspected urinary tract infection.*
- *Encourage Tim to drink and commence intravenous fluids to correct dehydration.*
- *Insert a urethral catheter and send a catheter specimen of urine (CSU) for culture and sensitivity to antibiotic intervention.*
- *Monitor fluid balance.*
- *Assess serum creatinine and urea and electrolytes.*

Tim's blood results confirmed a high blood glucose of 18.7 mmol/L and an elevated potassium (K) of 6.4 mmol/L. His sodium level was within the normal range (137 mmol/L). Tim's creatinine level was 128 µmol/L, slightly elevated but not indicative of AKI at this stage (see Table 9.1). However, according to NICE (2013), Tim continued to be at high risk of developing AKI due to the following reasons.

- Acute illness.

- Co-morbidities of hypertension and diabetes.

- Nephrotoxic drug prescription (ACE inhibitor) (see Table 9.2).

Tim's immediate problem was hyperkalaemia and he was prescribed an insulin/dextrose regime (GAIN, 2014). The insulin works by moving potassium from the circulation back into the cells thus lowering serum potassium levels. The 50% dextrose is given in order to prevent hypoglycaemia. Once this treatment is complete, the patient's potassium should drop by 0.6–1 mmol/L within 15 minutes (GAIN, 2014). Later that day Tim's serum potassium had reduced to 4.7 mmol/L and his blood glucose level was reduced to 8.9 mmol/L. According to GAIN (2014), hyperkalaemia is commonly associated with AKI and/or CKD and with patients prescribed ACE inhibitors. Based on this finding Tim continued to be at high risk of developing AKI and could be considered to be in the initiation phase of the syndrome.

The following morning Tim was beginning to feel much better, his vital signs were within the normal range and he was in an equal fluid balance. His urethral catheter was removed and he was encouraged to continue to drink a glass of water every hour. He was referred to the dietitian for advice on how to reduce his dietary intake of potassium and the diabetic specialist nurse to monitor his management of the diabetes. He was advised to stay for a further 24 hours to monitor his renal function (because of his risk of developing AKI) but Tim insisted he felt better, he had had enough and decided to discharge himself without further treatment. Daphne became very distressed by the idea of self-discharge and argued that this just wasn't like Tim! However, in the end a taxi was called and Tim and Daphne left the hospital. What Tim and Daphne didn't receive before discharge was information and advice on how to prevent further deterioration in his kidney function and following discharge Tim continued to take his ACE inhibitors, anti-diabetic medication and NSAIDS that he had been prescribed several months before for arthritic pain.

Once at home he became reluctant to drink in spite of being encouraged to do so in the hospital, arguing that he was better now and it was too much effort to keep going to the bathroom so often.

During the last few weeks, according to Jin et al. (2008), certain aspects of Tim's behaviour could be described as non-compliant or non-concordant with his long-term therapy. For example, his hesitance to seek healthcare and after discharge, his hesitance to follow advice from the medical team and his insistence on early self-discharge. Psychological factors that could have influenced this include Tim's feelings of distress around the emotional burden of his disease and possible depression (Walker et al., 2015). In this instance it has led to a further deterioration in his condition and his progression to the maintenance phase of AKI.

Activity 9.2	Communication

Identify three communication strategies you could use to diffuse a situation such as when Tim Hunter insisted he was going home.

A sample answer is found at the end of this chapter.

The maintenance phase of AKI

The maintenance, or oliguric, phase of AKI is synonymous with established renal injury and dysfunction. This period may last weeks or months and its severity is measured by the degree of elevated serum creatinine and evidence of reduced urine output (see Table 9.1). The impact on the patient is severe and the risk of mortality increases correspondingly with rising creatinine levels and reduction in renal function (Fliser et al., 2012). Let us return to Tim's story as he experiences a deterioration in his condition.

Scenario: Tim Hunter in the maintenance phase of AKI

Situation
Tim was discharged from hospital 48 hours ago after being admitted with a urinary tract infection and hyperkalaemia. He took his own discharge against medical advice and has been readmitted with abdominal pain, headache and nausea. He has not passed urine since late yesterday evening (14 hours ago). His wife Daphne said that since returning home he has taken to his bed and been reluctant to eat and drink.

Background

Past medical history remains unchanged.

- *Has been taking NSAIDS for pain.*
- *Neurogenic bladder and urinary tract infection.*

Assessment

- *Airway and breathing:*

  - *R: 25/min, regular rate;*
  - *SpO$_2$: 95%.*

- *Circulation:*

  - *HR: 92/min;*
  - *pulse appeared regular with premature beats occurring occasionally;*
  - *BP: 98/63 mmHg;*
  - *urine output: urethral catheter inserted, drained 80 ml of cloudy urine;*
  - *CSU sent for culture and sensitivity;*
  - *complaining of nausea.*

- *Disability and exposure:*

  - *blood glucose 17.4 mmol/L;*
  - *lethargic but alert;*
  - *skin and mucous membranes dry and cracked;*
  - *T: 38.5°C.*

- *NEWS: 8.*

- *Blood biochemistry and haematology:*

  - *Na: 132 mmol/L;*
  - *K: 5.3 mmol/L;*
  - *creatinine: 630 µmol/L;*
  - *white cell count: 25×10^9/L;*
  - *lactate: 2.9 mmol/L.*

Recommendations

- *Risk assess for AKI and sepsis.*
- *Take blood for culture and commence intravenous antibiotic therapy.*
- *Commence fluid resuscitation.*
- *Monitor urine output hourly.*
- *Contact the critical care outreach team for transfer to ITU.*

When Tim was risk assessed for sepsis and AKI he was found to meet the criteria for both; for sepsis by meeting the recognised criteria for systemic inflammatory response and a likely diagnosis of a urinary tract infection – dysuria (see Chapter 7).

These included:

- R >20/min;

- HR >90/min;

- T >38.3°C;

- WCC >12 × 10^9/L;

- Tim was commenced on the Sepsis Six Care Pathway (see Chapter 7) to achieve goal-directed therapy for managing sepsis.

Tim's diagnosis of stage 3 AKI was confirmed by (see Table 9.1):

- serum creatinine (SCr) increase >353 μmol/L (630 μmol/L);

- anuria (no urine output) for more than 12 hours (immediately prior to admission).

Tim was transferred to intensive care for monitoring and treatment of his condition.

What is the clinical impact of established AKI?

When a patient moves into the maintenance phase of AKI they present with evidence of intra-renal damage and while the precise pathophysiological mechanisms can only be theorised there does appear to be some consensus over the following three events (Patschan and Muller, 2015; Hammer and McPhee, 2014).

1. Initially renal ischaemia leads to renal tubular dysfunction and damage. This triggers apoptosis (programed cell death) and in severe cases necrosis (un-programmed cell death) and an increase in oxidative damage from the release of free radicals. A direct consequence of this damage is that the endothelial lining of the tubules are unable to maintain their functions of secretion and reabsorption and this triggers the functioning tubules to further reduce GFR through a tubule-glomerular feedback mechanism. There is also evidence of backflow of fluid into the interstitial space of the kidney increasing the risk of more generalised damage.

2. Secondly the ischaemic damage causes an interstitial inflammatory response and the release of pro-inflammatory chemicals, such as cytokines, and activation of the immune response, which leads to both pro- and anti-inflammatory effects. The triggering of the pro-inflammatory response can aggravate interstitial tissue damage in AKI but the anti-inflammatory effects are essential for facilitating tissue repair (Patschan and Muller, 2015).

3. Finally ischaemic damage can also lead to renal interstitial microvasculopathy. This occurs when swelling of the endothelial cells in the peritubular capillaries leads to prolonged ischaemia as a result of microvascular occlusion, even when the primary cause of the renal ischaemia has been resolved (Patschan et al., 2012).

Overall the combined impact of these mechanisms leads to acute loss of renal function and the signs and symptoms illustrated in Table 9.3. When we return to Tim's story, the clinical impact of his renal damage becomes evident as his story unfolds.

Scenario: Tim arrives in ITU

Situation
Tim Hunter has been diagnosed with sepsis and AKI. He commenced the Sepsis Six Care Pathway (Survive Sepsis, 2012) 30 minutes ago and was in the process of being transferred to ITU when his condition deteriorated.

Assessment
- *Airway and breathing:*

  - *R: 28/min, rapid shallow breathing;*
  - *central cyanosis;*
  - *producing pink frothy sputum;*
  - *inspiratory crackles heard;*
  - *SpO$_2$: 80% on high-flow oxygen (100%);*
  - *chest X-ray: pulmonary oedema.*

- *Circulation:*

  - *HR: 98/min;*
  - *BP: 70/50 mmHg (mean arterial pressure (MAP) 56.7 mmHg);*
  - *urethral catheter – 10 ml in 30 minutes.*

- *Disability and exposure:*

  - *blood glucose 18.4 mmol/L;*
  - *anxious, disorientated and sweaty;*
  - *T: 38.5°C.*

- *Blood biochemistry and haematology:*

  - *Na: 138 mmol/L;*
  - *K: 5.4 mmol/L;*
  - *creatinine: 630 µmol/L;*
  - *urea: 36.8 mmol/L;*
  - *WCC: 28×10^9/L;*
  - *lactate: 2.9 mmol/L.*

- *Arterial blood gases:*

  - *pH: 7.166;*
  - *PaO$_2$: 7.9 kPa;*

(Continued)

continued . . . . ●

    o *PaCO$_2$: 5.8 kPa;*

    o *HCO$_3$: 17.2 mmol/L;*

    o *BE: −9.9.*

Recommendations

- *Commence mechanical invasive respiratory support to relieve pulmonary oedema and support respiratory function.*
- *Assess Tim's clinical condition against the criteria for continuous renal replacement therapy (CRRT).*
- *Monitor for drug toxicities.*
- *Maintain nutrition.*

By the time Tim arrived in ITU his condition had become critical. The combination of reduced urine production and fluid resuscitation had led to fluid overload, culminating in an increase in pulmonary capillary hydrostatic pressure and pulmonary oedema. Hammer and McPhee (2014) describe the signs and symptoms of pulmonary oedema as: rapid shallow respirations, hypoxaemia and the presence of pink frothy sputum; a pulmonary chest X-ray usually reveals evidence of interstitial and alveolar oedema and inspiratory crackles may be heard on auscultation. These signs and symptoms were consistent with the clinical findings identified on Tim's assessment. He was also demonstrating evidence of an increased cardiac and respiratory workload and a metabolic acidosis triggered by both sepsis and AKI. As a result Tim's cardiovascular and respiratory systems were struggling to cope with his body's increased demand for oxygen and nutrients and his capillary oxygen saturation fell to 80% in spite of high-flow oxygen; he was becoming anxious and disorientated.

An arterial blood sample confirmed that Tim was suffering from type I respiratory failure with a PaO$_2$ of 7.9 kPa and PaCO$_2$ of 5.8 kPa (see Chapter 2). The arterial sample also revealed that Tim had a severe metabolic acidosis with a pH of 7.166 and HCO$_3$ of 17.2 mmol/L. If his respiratory deterioration was allowed to continue he was also progressing towards a combined respiratory and metabolic acidosis caused by a combination of exhaustion, inadequate systemic tissue perfusion and AKI (see Chapters 2 and 3).

It was imperative that as a priority Tim received interventions to support his respiratory and cardiovascular system. He now met the criteria for endotracheal intubation and mechanical invasive ventilation (MIV) for a number of reasons, including:

- type I respiratory failure;
- confusion;
- exhaustion.

(For more information about MIV, see Table 3.6, Indications for mechanical invasive ventilation in the critically ill patient, on pages 73–4.)

Tim was intubated and commenced on bilevel positive airways pressure ventilation with an inspiratory pressure of 20 cm H_2O, an expiratory pressure of 5 cm H_2O and an assisted rate of 18 breath/minute with 80% oxygen. The use of bilevel positive airways pressure, or continuous positive airways pressure support, via a non-invasive route is usually recommended for a patient experiencing pulmonary oedema as it provides a constant flow of positive pulmonary airways pressure in the alveoli to a level higher than the capillary hydrostatic pressure, thus pushing the leaking fluid back into the capillaries (Hammer and McPhee, 2014; Marik, 2015). However, in Tim's case he was unable to cope with non-invasive ventilation due to confusion and exhaustion and thus invasive mechanical ventilation was prescribed. Tim also met the criteria for continuing with resuscitation and maintenance therapy for severe sepsis (Dellinger et al., 2013), however, in his current condition with fluid overload and AKI, the medical team were unable to provide effective support and assessed Tim for treatment with renal replacement therapy.

Assessing Tim for readiness to commence continuous renal replacement therapy

AKI in critically ill patients like Tim frequently develops in situations where there is another critical underlying pathology such as shock, sepsis, major surgery and/or trauma and where there is an increased risk of multiple organ dysfunction. In Tim's case the underlying pathology was sepsis and the AKI has occurred simultaneously with evidence of an ascending renal infection and circulatory failure. The criteria for initiation of continuous renal replacement therapy (CRRT) are listed in Table 9.5 (Bellomo, 2014). An assessment of these criteria in relation to Tim indicated that he met four of the criteria listed and CRRT was deemed essential in order to provide a balanced and controlled removal of fluid and waste products from Tim's circulation.

CRRT in the form of continuous haemodiafiltration can remove plasma water in a controlled process to achieve a desired fluid balance, correct electrolyte abnormalities, remove waste products and correct metabolic acidosis (Richardson and Whatmore, 2014). The two main processes through which this is achieved are:

- haemofiltration: the movement of water across a semipermeable membrane from an area of high pressure (the patient's blood) to an area of low pressure (the filter) at a measured rate of flow. Replacement fluids are titrated in order to maintain the desired fluid balance;

- haemodialysis: the selected diffusion of waste molecules (solutes) from an area of high concentration to an area of low concentration across a semipermeable membrane. For example, dialysis fluid usually contains haemodynamically normal levels of sodium and potassium to ensure the levels in the patient's blood remain within the normal range but may have higher than normal levels of bicarbonate in order to increase bicarbonate levels in the patient's blood and so resolve a metabolic acidosis. Dialysis fluid will contain no creatinine and urea thus increasing the flow of both solutes out of the body and into the dialysis fluid.

The nursing management of a patient who requires CRRT is complex and highly specialised and includes the following principles (Richardson and Whatmore, 2014).

- To assess for indications for CRRT (see Table 9.5).
- To assess, monitor and ensure effective venous access:
  - check patency and flow of the central venous catheter;
  - ensure the catheter is secured with a suture and dressing;
  - monitor the outgoing and return pressures of the blood flow.
- To avoid unnecessary interruptions to CRRT:
  - make sure the pump speed to direct the flow from the patient to the circuit is adequate as prescribed;
  - monitor the use of anticoagulants to maintain blood flow and check for blood clots;
  - ensure the alarm limits have been set.
- To reduce the risk of complications associated with CRRT:
  - reduce the risk of air embolism by flushing the circuit before its use;
  - monitor for fluid and electrolyte imbalance;
  - monitor for haemodynamic stability/instability;
  - reduce the risk of hypothermia;
  - reduce the risk of infection.

If one of the criterion below is present consider the use of renal replacement therapy (RRT)	If two or more criteria are present RRT is essential	Tom's assessment for readiness to commence RRT
Oliguria (<200 ml in 12 hours)		Yes
Anuria (0–50 ml in 12 hours)		
Creatinine >400 µmol/L		Yes
Urea >35 mmol/L		Yes
Potassium >6.5 mmol/L		
Pulmonary oedema		Yes
Uncompensated metabolic acidosis pH <7.1		
Sodium <110 or >160 mmol/L		
Temperature >40°C		
Uraemic complications (encephalopathy, myopathy, neuropathy, pericarditis)		
Overdose with a toxin that can be removed by dialysis (e.g. lithium)		

Table 9.5: Modern criteria for the initiation of renal replacement therapy in ITU (based on Bellomo, 2014) and a column indicating the results of Tom's assessment for readiness to commence CRRT

Tim continued on CRRT together with full respiratory and cardiovascular support and intravenous antibiotic therapy for five days in ITU. The team were able to reduce his respiratory support and sedation after 24 hours and he became more involved in his recovery. Daphne had thought Tim was going to die and seeing him winking at her and holding her hand made her cry and gave her hope. Tim's renal function was slower to return and it was another five days before his renal function improved enough to further reduce his respiratory and renal support. He was progressing towards the recovery phase of AKI.

The recovery phase of AKI

The recovery phase of AKI is the period when renal injury is repaired and normal renal function becomes re-established. As renal function begins to improve there is a progressive increase in urine volume and GFR, and there is a gradual decline in blood urea and creatinine levels. In this early recovery phase, however, the renal tubules are unable to concentrate the filtrate and this leads to increased losses of sodium, potassium and fluid in the urine. The patient becomes at risk of:

- fluid volume depletion due to polyuria (passing large volumes of urine);
- hypokalaemia.

The nursing responsibilities when caring for patients during the recovery phase include the following.

- Assessment of vital signs for dehydration (Thomas et al., 2008):
  o thirst;
  o dry skin and mucous membranes;
  o > pulse;
  o < BP;
  o confusion;
  o negative fluid balance.
- Assessment of vital signs for hypokalaemia (McCance and Huether, 2014):
  o slow or irregular pulse;
  o muscle weakness.
- Risk assess for signs of infection and deterioration in renal function by checking:
  o serum urea;
  o creatinine;
  o electrolyte balance;
  o white cell count;
  o temperature.
- Inform the medical team if there are any signs of deterioration.

- Patient and family education:

  o the process of renal recovery can take from three to 12 months and continue after the patient has been discharged;

  o encourage the patient and their family to understand and work in partnership with the medical team to support recovery and reduce the risk of a decline in renal function and chronic kidney disease.

Activity 9.3   *Decision making*

1. Assess the patients below and based on what you have learnt from this chapter, discuss your recommendations for care.

(a) **Situation:** Mr McDonald (aged 65 years) presented in the emergency department with a history of three days of shortness of breath and wheezing.

Background: known hypertensive, prescribed atenolol.

Assessment:

- R: 26/min, SpO$_2$: 92%.
- Respiratory wheeze.
- Chest X-ray: pulmonary oedema.
- HR: 98/min, BP: 140/95.
- Urine output: 100 ml on admission.
- T: 37.5°C.
- Patient very agitated and confused.
- Creatinine: 1504 µmol/L.
- Urea: 14.2 mmol/L.
- K: 9.2 mmol/L.
- Na: 132 mmol/L.
- Weight estimated at 70 kg.

(b) **Situation:** Mrs Kumar (aged 75 years) has been admitted to the high dependency unit post-operatively following a surgical repair for a fractured hip sustained after a fall. During the surgical procedure Mrs Kumar required a transfusion and fluid resuscitation following severe blood loss. She was breathing spontaneously on 60% oxygen.

Background: history of chronic heart failure, hypertension, rheumatoid arthritis and hypothyroid dysfunction. Medication includes: amiodarone, levothyroxine, furosemide and NSAID.

Assessment:

- R: 40/min, SpO$_2$: 89%.
- HR: 120/min, BP: 190/110.

- Urine output: 25 ml/hr.
- Chest X-ray: pulmonary oedema.
- T: 37.5°C.
- Patient very agitated and confused.
- Creatinine: 216 μmol/L.
- Urea: 16.9 mmol/L.
- K: 4.9 mmol/L.
- Na: 151 mmol/L.
- Weight estimated at 60 kg.

Sample answers can be found at the end of the chapter.

Finally, returning to Tim's story, he continued to make a good recovery and six days after being admitted to ITU he was transferred to the high dependency unit for 48 hours before he was fit enough to return to the ward. He was discharged from hospital a week later. Tim and his wife were informed that because of his critical illness and AKI, diabetes and hypertension he had a high risk of developing chronic kidney disease and would need careful monitoring of his kidney function by the GP as part of his annual diabetes check. Tim admitted that he now realised that he should have sought help sooner and he would be more aware of what to do should he feel unwell again.

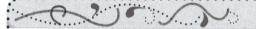

Chapter summary

In this chapter you have been introduced to patients who are at risk of developing AKI and what happens if AKI becomes established: acute and severe deterioration in the patient's condition with an increased risk of developing chronic kidney disease should they survive. The important messages to gain from this chapter are:

- risk assessing patients for AKI, particularly when they are in the initial stage of the syndrome, can prevent established AKI and improve patient morbidity and mortality;
- assessing and knowing your patient's situation and background in order to prioritise assessment of patients who have a high risk of developing AKI;
- working in partnership with patients, particularly those with chronic conditions, encourages patients to feel empowered and more in control of their care.

Activities: brief outline answers

Activity 9.2: Communication (page 208)

Communications strategies you can use when diffusing a situation include the following.

- Be open and questioning: ask Tim what the problem is and whether you can help.
- Use an assertive but democratic approach to the conversation.

- Stay professional.
- Encourage Tim to sit down in a quiet and more private area so that his concerns can be discussed.
- Listen and value what Tim has to say.
- Offer possible solutions.
- Discuss each solution with Tim.
- Encourage Tim to make his decision in a calm environment.

Activity 9.3: Decision making (pages 216–17)

(a) Recommendations – Mr McDonald.

- There is evidence of acute respiratory failure associated with pulmonary oedema: commence bilevel positive pressure ventilation.
- AKI severity is stage 3.
- Meets the criteria for CRRT: creatinine: 1504 µmol/L, presence of pulmonary oedema, K: 9.2 mmol/L. Commence CRRT.
- Assess history for evidence of the use of nephrotoxic drugs or X-ray contrast media.

(b) Recommendations – Mrs Kumar.

- Evidence of acute respiratory failure due to fluid overload and existing heart failure: commence invasive respiratory support.
- Urine output is currently below the required 0.5 ml/kg/hr. Monitor urine output following commencement of MIV and diuretic therapy over the next five hours and review.
- Monitor creatinine levels in an hour for increasing severity of AKI.

Further reading

Peate, I and Dutton, H (2012) *Acute Nursing Care: Recognising and Responding to Medical Emergencies.* Harlow: Pearson.

This book offers more examples of patients with AKI and can be used to support this chapter.

Woodrow, P (2011) *Intensive Care Nursing.* Third edition. London: Routledge.

This book offers an insight into the care of patients with acute renal failure in a critical care setting.

Useful websites

www.renal.org/guidelines/clinical-practice-guidelinescommittee#sthash.6dTGmyRX.dpbs

The Renal Association website offers links to clinical guidance for managing patients with both acute injury and chronic kidney disease.

www.youtube.com/watch?v=bwwQd7xkHNc

This recording describes the pathophysiology of acute renal failure and can be used to support the content of this chapter.

www.youtube.com/watch?v=88ajR62XEcg

Please watch this recording if you are interested in exploring the process of CRRT in more detail.

Chapter 10
The patient with physiological trauma

Catherine Williams

NMC Standards for Pre-registration Nursing Education

This chapter will address the following competencies:

Domain 3: Nursing practice and decision-making

3.1. Adult nurses must safely use a range of diagnostic skills, employing appropriate technology, to assess the needs of service users.

Domain 4: Leadership, management and team working

3. All nurses must be able to identify priorities, and manage time and resources effectively to ensure the quality of care is maintained or enhanced.

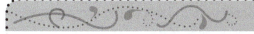

NMC Essential Skills Clusters

This chapter will address the following ESCs:

Cluster: Care, compassion and communication

1. As partners in the care process, people can trust a newly registered graduate nurse to provide collaborative care based on the highest standards, knowledge and competence.

Cluster: Organisational aspects of care

9. People can trust the newly registered graduate nurse to treat them as partners and work with them to make a holistic and systematic assessment of their needs; to develop a personalised plan that is based on mutual understanding and respect for their individual situation promoting health and well-being, minimising risk of harm and promoting their safety at all times.

16. People can trust the newly registered graduate nurse to safely lead, co-ordinate and manage care.

17. People can trust the newly registered graduate nurse to work safely under pressure and maintain the safety of service users at all times.

18. People can trust a newly registered graduate nurse to enhance the safety of service users and identify and actively manage risk and uncertainty in relation to people, the environment, self and others.

Chapter aims

By the end of this chapter, you should be able to:

- interpret the mechanisms of injury to form individualised patient care;
- demonstrate the systematic approach to physiological trauma care;
- describe the primary and secondary survey;
- list the indications for intravenous fluid replacement therapy;
- reflect on clinical examples illustrated in the chapter and apply this to your own clinical situation.

This chapter introduces you to the physical and psychological impact of trauma and how to help patients and their families in their own processes of healing, recovery and restoration.

Case study

Doris, aged 74, is admitted to A&E after tripping over a raised paving slab while running for a bus. Sophia, a student nurse, is working with her mentor, who is triaging patients in A&E. It is the first day of Sophia's placement. On admission Doris is carefully holding her left wrist and is able to give her own account of the accident, although she speaks slowly and deliberately as though she is trying to speak with loose dentures. She has an abrasive graze to her swollen nose and chin and a runny nose. Doris appears embarrassed by her facial injuries and focuses on her wrist injury.

*Sophia did not carry out an accurate primary assessment, GCS and history but focused on secondary survey assessment. Sophia assumes that Doris's wrist probably has a **Colles fracture** because of the classic dinner fork deformity presentation. An X-ray will be needed to confirm this with subsequent reduction of the fracture.*

*However, Sophia's mentor is a very experienced A&E nurse and she prioritises Doris more urgently. After completing an accurate primary and secondary survey she believes that Doris may have sustained max- illofacial injuries based on the abnormal facial mobility and may have a leak of **cerebrospinal fluid** (CSF) from her nose. CSF is clear and has a high sugar (clinistix) and low protein content (electropho- resis) compared to nasal or lacrimal fluid. If CSF is leaking due to a facial injury, the patient may complain of a persistent salty taste in the mouth. Neurological observations are commenced on Doris and she is admitted to the resuscitation bay for urgent medical attention. If left untreated, the type of injuries that cause CSF leaks can represent a life-threatening situation and could lead to meningitis, brain infection, stroke and death. Maxillofacial trauma must be given the same priority as other head injuries.*

There are important messages to learn from Sophia's story.

- Always be alert to changes in your patient's clinical condition, no matter how small. Any patient who has sustained an injury to the face or jaws should be suspected of having an actual head injury.

- The ABCDE order of treatment reflects the importance of the different things that can go wrong, and the primary survey must be completed before moving on to address the obvious injuries. Poor tongue support in **mandibular** fractures can cause airway obstruction.

- Errors are often made in the early management of the trauma patient so a systematic approach is required in order to identify and treat the immediately life-threatening and potentially life-threatening conditions before the limb-threatening ones.

- Timing is of the essence: your patient will continue to deteriorate if prompt action is not taken.

What do we mean by physiological trauma?

This chapter provides an overview of the general causes and treatments of physiological trauma. It examines in detail the care of a patient with physiological trauma and the metabolic response to trauma. The chapter proceeds with an overview of the knowledge and skills required to assess, differentiate and manage the care of a patient who sustains any form of physiological trauma. The underlying physiology and implications of the patient's care will be discussed in the context of diagnostic tests, treatments and collaborative management of care and highlighted through the chapter. The assessment and management of patients with shock is touched upon in this chapter; for a detailed assessment of cardiogenic and **distributive shock** (including sepsis and septic shock), please refer to Chapters 4, 6 and 7.

Trauma care starts at the point of injury and continues through to the end of rehabilitation to ensure the best possible outcome; in any trauma an organisational approach is essential.

What is trauma?

Edwards and Griffiths (2011) define trauma as a blunt or penetrating force to the body resulting in actual injury. Irrespective of the cause of trauma, the medical team must make a systematic assessment in order to ensure that the most important injuries are prioritised. Courses such as the **advanced trauma life support** (ATLS) provide a means of assessing patients that is widely accepted worldwide as a framework of rapid assessment for trauma. Broadly speaking, this comprises a **primary survey** and a **secondary survey** of the patient to ensure that less obvious serious injuries are not missed while healthcare staff deal with more visually apparent patient problems. It is easy to become distracted by obvious injuries when there may be more immediately life-threatening injuries.

Types of trauma to the body can be classified as blunt or penetrating.

- Blunt trauma – can be caused by falls or seat belt injuries but leaves the body surface intact.

- Penetrating trauma – can be caused by stab injuries and the body surface is damaged.

- Perforating trauma – can be caused when an object passes through the body leaving an entry and exit wound (Bersten and Soni, 2003).

A systematic approach to trauma management is not a relatively new concept and has been around since the 1970s, although trauma care has been much improved with systematic approaches that enable effective treatment. Prior to this, survival of major trauma was less likely than it is today.

The **Manchester triage system** (created in 1994, see **www.triagenet.net/en/Overview**) is a formalised standard of triage and is widely used in UK emergency departments. The purpose of a triage system is to detect the critically ill patient by categorising patients into degrees of urgency. Patients are identified by the categories of immediate (zero wait time) to non-urgent (to be seen within four hours).

Case study

Danny, a seven-year-old boy, was a front seat passenger in his uncle's car. He was not in a car seat, and he was not wearing a seat belt. As they drove along the road at around 30 mph, Danny stood up and turned around to wave to the people in the car behind. At that point, his uncle braked heavily and swerved to avoid a car that had pulled out from a junction without looking. While the impact was not particularly serious, Danny was catapulted into the dashboard and had an obvious ankle deformity requiring a visit to hospital for X-rays. An ambulance was called and arrived promptly. On arrival at the hospital, Danny was in a great deal of pain, assumed to be from his ankle injury, and the nurses tried to make him comfortable while the doctor dealt with some other patients. After about 20 minutes the doctor arrived and sent Danny for an X-ray of his ankle. While in the X-ray department, Danny became unresponsive and died within half an hour. Danny's post-mortem report showed massive abdominal bleeding from a ruptured spleen. He also had a fracture to his ankle.

There are important messages to learn from Danny's story.

- All injuries have the potential to be life- or limb-threatening.
- It is essential that problems are anticipated, rather than reacted to once they develop.

Activity 10.1   *Critical thinking*

- What assessment should have been carried out in Danny's case?
- What are you looking for in such an assessment, and why?

There is an outline answer to this activity at the end of the chapter.

The primary survey

The objective of this phase is to identify and correct any immediately life-threatening conditions, including the airway, breathing, circulation, disability and exposure (ABCDE). To do this, the activities in Table 10.1 need to be carried out. The survey follows a simple mnemonic of A, B, C, D, E. These should be worked through in sequence and any issues resolved before proceeding to the next stage of the survey.

On admission to the emergency department the advanced trauma life support/Manchester triage assessment will primarily be the doctor's responsibility. However, all members of the team should be able to contribute to patient safety by having their own awareness of the framework in use. When the primary survey has been completed it should be repeated before proceeding to the secondary survey in order to ensure that new problems have not arisen and nothing important has been missed. This is a rapid assessment to identify time critical emergences that must be treated before assessment continues.

The secondary survey

Once life-threatening conditions have been treated, or excluded, then you can carry out the secondary survey. This is a comprehensive head-to-toe examination of the patient, which provides the basis of the admission documentation. You need to pay close attention to the history of this accident, and of previous medical history, so that important details that may suggest other injuries or complicating factors are not overlooked. You will take a detailed history of the accident from the patient, witnesses, relatives, GP or medical alert jewellery, if worn. If attending paramedics are present, it is essential to gain information from them before they leave (Cole, 2009).

In an emergency situation you may not have the time to obtain certain details such as patient history; therefore, you must focus on the essential information.

Airway and control of cervical spine	Must be considered in conjunction with each other as interventions performed on the airway will impact on the c-spine and vice versa. For example, if you need to perform an emergency intubation for the patient and utilise the usual head tilt, then you may lose control of the c-spine with catastrophic results (jaw thrust should be used until c-spine is cleared). Similarly, intubating the already triply immobilised patient presents its own challenges for the anaesthetist and assisting staff. Intubation would be indicated where respiration is absent, where GCS* <8 or electively where smoke inhalation, oral burns or facial trauma present risks to the airway from gross oedema that may narrow and distort the airway. (*The Glasgow Coma Scale provides a practical method for assessment of impairment of conscious level in response to defined stimuli. The goal of the new updated GCS (2014) is to emphasise on reporting of the three components rather than the total sum, accessed at **http://www.glasgowcomascale.org**)
Breathing	Normal oxygenation and respiration is the aim. Note rate and depth of respirations and listen for normal breath sounds. How is the gas exchange? You may be able to make a quick assumption of this initially from signs of cyanosed skin or laboured breathing although urgent arterial blood gas confirmation will be required. Remember, carbon monoxide poisoning may give the patient a cherry red complexion, and saturations may appear normal

(Continued)

Table 10.1   (Continued)

	as carbon monoxide binds to haemoglobin. Full-thickness circumferential burns to the chest may cause restriction of breathing mechanically.
Circulation	Establishing reliable venous access is a priority at this point in order to carry out any subsequent treatment as you continue with your primary survey. Delays in gaining venous access may make obtaining access more problematic as the patient progresses into shock. Diagnostic blood tests should be taken for full blood count, coagulation, cross match, electrolytes. Arterial blood gas analysis and, where appropriate, carboxyhaemoglobin levels would provide interim information until formal blood results are available. Haemorrhage control should be established and treatment for shock initiated with fluid resuscitation. Examination of chest, abdomen and pelvis should be carried out at this stage.
Disability	Patient responsiveness should be assessed using the GCS and examination of pupil reaction. Blood sugar measurements should be taken at this time.
Exposure	The patient should be undressed for a full body examination, but hypothermia must also be prevented. If possible, thoracic and lumbar spine should be cleared at this stage. Any wounds should be assessed for further management.

Table 10.1: The primary survey

The mnemonic AMPLE helps you to remember what information you need to obtain during the assessment.

- **A**llergies.
- **M**edication.
- **P**ast medical history.
- **L**ast meal/fluid.
- **E**vents relevant to injury.

The secondary survey should revisit all elements of the primary survey in ABCDE priority order, and you should pay attention to important information that may have had to be deferred while the primary survey was establishing the basis of patient survival.

The secondary survey is one of time and detail as an in-depth assessment of each body region is warranted. You must monitor vital signs and examine your patient's head/skull for irregularity or scalp wound, check the ears for blood or CSF leaks, and check eyes for pupil size and reaction (PEARL – Pupils Equal and Reactive to Light). Observe the thorax for bruising and possible fracture. All four limbs need to be checked for irregularity, deformity and fractures; compare limbs with each other and look for shortening and rotation. Finally, the patient's back needs to be checked for fracture and any spinal irregularities. Logrolling should be adopted until the c-spine is cleared by the physicians and documented in the medical notes. Once the primary and secondary surveys have been completed by the medical team, unconscious or confused patients, in particular, are generally reliant on the nurse to anticipate and identify any deterioration in their condition. Thus the principles of the primary survey ABCDE can be utilised in every day practice to provide structure to your own assessment of the patient.

Activity 10.2   *Critical thinking*

Think back to your experiences in the clinical setting and identify examples of situations of when you had to complete a primary survey and a secondary survey.

- In the primary survey, what were the main priorities for the patient and why?
- In the secondary survey, what clinical signs and features were present and did this affect your prioritisation of care?

Hint: These questions will help you to practise linking the importance of treating problems as they are found. The ABCDE order of treatment reflects the importance of treatment priority.

There is no outline answer at the end of the chapter as this activity is based on your own reflections.

Before moving on to each section of the secondary survey, remember to go back and keep checking the patient's ABCs. Avoid the common error of being distracted before the whole body has been inspected, as potentially serious injuries can be missed, especially in the unconscious patient. If the patient deteriorates during the secondary survey, the primary survey needs to start again. For example, the clinical staff may have noted that the patient was wearing rings that were compromising the circulation to the digits during the primary survey, but this would be of little consequence if the patient was not breathing at that time.

In the next section we will consider the clinical features of the metabolic response to trauma and we will explore how you can assess and manage the patient in order to provide clinically effective care.

Metabolic response to trauma

When the body sustains a traumatic injury, an inflammatory response starts from the site of tissue damage as chemical mediators are released (mediators are signalling chemical molecules involved in transmitting information between cells).

The **inflammatory mediators** involved are:

- histamine (organic nitrogenous compound);
- **kinins** (polypeptides);
- **prostaglandins** (fatty acids);
- **leukotrienes** (inflammatory mediators).

All of these mediators in turn cause vasodilation and subsequently increased blood flow, which brings phagocytes and leukocytes to the original injury to deal with infections or foreign agents and to begin repairing the injury. **Vascular permeability** is enhanced by the mediators, which in turn permit clotting proteins, such as fibrin, the enzymatic serum protein complement, kinins and white blood cells, to reach the tissue.

Once the clotting proteins have moved from the blood into the tissues, an osmotic change occurs and oedema forms in the tissue at the site of injury. The clotting proteins then isolate any abnormal agents, such as particles or bacteria, at the source of the injury by forming an encasing clot to isolate it from the surrounding normal tissue.

Now let us consider some minor trauma, which will make it easier for you to understand how the body responds to major trauma.

Case study

Afia, a hard-working student nurse, has decided to attend a ward night out. She has been saving for some lovely shoes, which don't really fit properly but look fantastic. As the evening progresses, the shoes start to rub her heels and they begin to look red. Afia realises that the trauma she is experiencing is **abrasive trauma***.*

Afia is not in a position to change her shoes so they continue to rub until a blister starts to form as fluid leaks into the tissues from the vasodilation that the inflammatory mediators cause as they rush to the injured area. The pain she experiences is caused by localised swelling from the inflammatory response and by mechanical means as the shoes continue to rub. Eventually, the blister breaks, leaving an open wound and a portal for bacterial entry. Nerve endings are now exposed as the top of the blister bursts, causing further pain.

Monitoring the critically ill patient

The critical care setting can be a daunting environment to those unfamiliar with caring for such sick patients. Many pieces of previously unseen equipment are in use for monitoring and treating the patient: for example, blood pressure may be recorded continuously on-screen via an arterial line, giving a blood pressure that varies from beat to beat rather than via a cuff measurement that gives a random, one-off blood pressure reading. Many patients will be assisted with bodily functions that are normally autonomic such as breathing or renal filtration by machinery. Multiple intravenous infusions may be in progress at the same time.

However, as with the patient's initial assessment after injury, the primary survey can be adapted and should be continuously revisited by the nurse caring for the patient in order to ensure the safety of the patient. Once the primary and secondary survey has been completed by the medical team, unconscious or confused patients, in particular, are generally reliant on the nurse to anticipate and identify any deterioration in their condition.

Activity 10.3	Critical thinking

Think back to your experiences in a critical care clinical setting.

- How did you deal with major trauma in a critical care setting and what were your nursing priorities with regard to care delivery and best practice?

These questions will help you prioritise your patient care through examining the means of clinically monitoring and continuously assessing the major trauma patient.

There is no outline answer at the end of the chapter as this activity is based on your own reflections.

Case study

Sharron, aged 25, sustained a 60% flame burn to her upper body from a witnessed suicide attempt in her parked car after suffering from post-natal depression. She was intubated by the paramedics, and 100% oxygen was administered prior to arrival at A&E. Smoke contains dangerous gases such as carbon monoxide that need to be addressed by administering high concentrations of oxygen even before confirmation from blood results (Herndon, 2007).

The c-spine had not been immobilised as Sharron's accident did not involve any impact and the witnesses to the accident were able to state the mechanism of the injury.

Lily, a student nurse, is on duty when Sharron arrives. Lily observes the primary survey being undertaken by the medical and nursing staff.

Airway *is deemed to be patent following intubation.*

Breathing *is occurring with assistance, but bagging the patient is difficult and the chest is not rising much with each breath delivered. Arterial blood gas analysis reveals significant respiratory and metabolic acidosis. Lily notes that Sharron's trunk is burned circumferentially, and the anaesthetist explains that this is why it is difficult to ventilate the patient. An emergency* **escharotomy** *is performed on the spot by the doctors to release the taut burned skin that is restricting chest movement. This involves making an incision with a sterile blade through the depth of the burned tissue and extending into unburned skin. This results in an immediate improvement in chest expansion as the patient is easier to bag, with better oxygenation and gas exchange evident on the next arterial blood gas. From this, Lily realises that a secured airway does not automatically mean that the patient will be able to breathe: steps need to be taken to ensure that breathing can take place, such as bagging to manually inflate the chest or addressing other complicating factors, in this case the deep burns to the chest, making bagging difficult and requiring emergency intervention. Escharotomies are performed under general anaesthetic except in an emergency situation such as this where time delays could mean that the patient will not survive.*

(Continued)

continued . . . •

Sharron's arterial blood gases were as follows.

Prior to escharotomy	1 hour post escharotomy
pH 7.05	pH 7.30
PCO_2 9.0 kPa	PCO_2 7.0 kPa
PO_2 10.5 kPa	PO_2 14 kPa

Note the rapid improvement in Sharron's arterial blood gases following escharotomy once she is able to fully expand her chest and exhale carbon dioxide more efficiently. While the blood gases have not yet reached normality, you will recognise a significant improvement from the earlier blood gas analysis.

Blood gas analysis may be measured in millimetres of mercury or kilopascals depending on the blood gas analyser (see Table 10.2).

Kilopascal measurements	Millimetres of mercury measurement
pH 7.35–7.45	pH 7.35–7.45
PO_2 11.5–13.5 kPa	PO_2 80–100 mmHg
PCO_2 4.5–6 kPa	PCO_2 35–45 mmHg
HCO_3 25–30 mmol/L	HCO_3 25–30 mmol/L
Base excess –2 to +2	Base excess –2 to +2

Table 10.2: Normal values for arterial blood gases

Only once the airway, breathing and cervical spine elements of the primary survey have been addressed, should consideration be given to the other elements of the primary survey such as circulation, disability and exposure. Initially, the circulation component of the survey will be concerned with checking that the pulse is present and noting whether it is strong and bounding or weak and thready. Then capillary refill can be checked by applying pressure to an area of skin (unburned area in this patient). The skin should blanch and return to normal within two seconds. If it does not, then you may have a hypovolaemic patient.

However, other limbs should be tested in order to exclude a localised problem with the circulation. For example, if the limb has a circumferential burn, circulation may be sluggish locally but fine generally. Excluding the possibility of major haemorrhage is the immediate priority. Establishing venous access, while important, should not come before first aid for bleeding. Direct pressure should be applied where serious bleeding occurs. Commencing intravenous fluid resuscitation can be dealt with during the secondary survey, provided access has already been established. If access cannot be gained intravenously, then intraosseous access may have to be considered. When these have been addressed, other factors such as disability can be considered. As Sharron has already been intubated, this could prove to be difficult as the normal AVPU measures of Alertness, Vocal Stimulus, Response to Painful Stimuli and Unresponsiveness may be affected by sedatives. However, the aim is to exclude signs of head injury and maxillofacial trauma, and in this situation pupil reaction to light would need to be assessed before proceeding to complete exposure of the patient in order to ensure that no other life-threatening injuries have been missed. Care must be taken to keep the patient warm during this part of the assessment. If a warm environment cannot be provided, then the patient may have to be exposed in stages to prevent hypothermia. Jewellery should be removed and kept safe at this stage.

With all forms of major trauma, regardless of cause, the risk of hypovolaemic shock is present, along with sepsis either from the original injury or the invasive devices used to monitor the patient's condition. These risk factors may perpetuate the inflammatory response in a negative way, so that it moves from being beneficial to becoming detrimental to the patient.

Activity 10.4   *Decision making*

Read the case study below and list the potential problems that might be easy to overlook. Ask a colleague to do the same then compare and discuss your lists before looking at the answer.

There is an outline answer to this question at the end of the chapter.

Case study

Tayvin is a 31-year-old man who sustained a crush injury to his abdomen from heavy machinery at work. Primary and secondary surveys are conducted in A&E and he is taken straight to theatre to explore an open abdominal wound.

A student nurse, John, is working under supervision with Christine, his mentor, who is allocated as Tayvin's nurse when he arrives from theatre. Tayvin has multiple injuries including pelvic fractures. His peritoneum has been found to be intact but a vacuum-assisted closure (VAC) drain is in situ due to a large surface of skin loss over the abdomen with a small but steady drainage of **haemoserous fluid**. *On arrival from theatre, Tayvin's vital signs are remarkably stable. He appears pale, but he is pre-scribed a further two units of red blood cells post-operatively that were not completed in theatre, and these are in the process of being ordered. He has intravenous fluid running and a patient-controlled analgesia (PCA) pump for analgesia but is not dependent on inotropic support. Tayvin's family have been spoken to by the surgeon as he remains on a ventilator in ITU. John's mentor Christine starts the admission paperwork after setting up the first unit of blood. As John begins to document the patient's observations, the VAC begins to alarm.*

(Continued)

continued . . .

John checks the cause of the alarm and notices that the 1 litre VAC chamber has completely filled with frank blood. Tayvin remains pale but otherwise does not appear to have deteriorated drastically. His heart rate has increased a little and he is now mildly tachycardic. Blood pressure is not yet affected. John draws Christine's attention to the situation. Another nurse is asked to contact the medical staff as John and Christine reassess the patient.

Using the primary survey as a framework, John realises that airway and breathing are secure and stable as Tayvin remains on the ventilator but is able to initiate his own breaths. There is a slight rise in respiratory rate from 16 previously to 24 breaths per minute. Circulation has become a concern due to the blood loss into the VAC, and closer inspection of the patient reveals a significant amount of blood into the bed underneath the patient, although the abdominal dressing does not appear unduly saturated with blood as the fluid has leaked downwards under the dressing as the patient has been lying in a semi-recumbent position. John realises the importance of exposure of the patient as one of the components of the primary survey, as some issues may not be initially obvious.

As the medical staff arrive, Tayvin becomes hypotensive with a blood pressure of 83/50. After checking an arterial blood gas measurement, which reveals a haemoglobin level of 6.8 and slight metabolic acidosis, the medical staff request that the unit of blood in progress is given at a faster rate and the next unit is ordered immediately. Arrangements are made for Tayvin to return to theatre for exploration of the source of the bleeding. Tayvin returns from theatre before the end of the shift. The second surgery identifies that a small artery in the existing abdominal wound was bleeding. This was repaired and Tayvin made good progress, culminating in his discharge from the critical care unit several days later.

Activity 10.5   *Critical thinking*

- With reference to the case study, what clinical signs would indicate that Tayvin's condition was getting worse?
- What could be the possible causes for his metabolic acidosis?

There is an outline answer to this activity at the end of the chapter

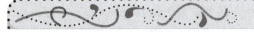

Chapter summary

The aim of this chapter was to help you to assess, recognise and respond to patients who sustain physiological trauma. In this chapter we have focused on the assessment and management of primary and secondary surveys and the metabolic response to trauma. In all of the clinical examples illustrated the key responsibilities of the nurse are the same.

- The ABCDE order of treatment reflects the different things that can go wrong for trauma patients.
- Problems are treated as they are found – if a problem is found and treated and the patient deteriorates, you start again and work through ABCDE.
- Knowledge about a pattern of injury is helpful as a discovery of one injury should prompt you to search for a related injury.

Activities: brief outline answers

Activity 10.1: Critical thinking (page 222)

Missed intra-abdominal injuries and concealed haemorrhage are frequent causes of increased morbidity and mortality, especially in patients who survive the initial phase after an injury. Danny's abdomen should have been exposed and examined during the primary/secondary survey, which was not completed as Danny did not appear to have life-threatening injuries. Inspection of the abdomen would have revealed distension associated with bleeding and may have saved his life.

Activity 10.4: Decision making (page 229)

Things that can be overlooked in this situation are airway burns, major trauma and inhalation exposure to carbon dioxide. Tayvin's scenario represents a textbook situation in which the principles of the ATLS have been utilised to their full potential. Tayvin will remain very ill for many more weeks, but giving the patient the best possible start on their road to recovery begins at the scene of the accident and continues through the emergency unit and onto specialist services such as the burns centre.

Activity 10.5: Critical thinking (page 230)

Tayvin would have an increased respiratory rate, increased heart rate and decreasing blood pressure as the body attempts to compensate for the sudden blood loss.

The main cause of his metabolic acidosis would be hypovolaemia due to the excessive hydrogen ions produced in shock.

Tayvin's story demonstrated to John the importance of checking a patient thoroughly (exposure), and he also learned how quickly a seemingly stable patient can deteriorate after major trauma and major surgery. It is essential to keep utilising the principles of the primary and secondary surveys even when a patient may seem to be on the road to recovery.

Further reading

Bosworth, C (2003) *Burns Trauma: Management and Nursing Care.* Second edition. London: Bailliere Tindall.

This book considers the treatment needs of patients of all ages with different types of burn injury, in a variety of clinical environments, and it is a valuable resource for all grades of staff within the multidisciplinary team caring for patients with burn injuries.

Edwards, M and Griffiths, P (2011) *Emergency Nursing Made Incredibly Easy.* Philadelphia, PA: Lippincott, Williams and Wilkins.

This book covers emergency care basics including patient assessment and triage, trauma, disease crises, and patient and family communication, as well as legal issues such as handling evidence and documentation and holistic issues such as pain and end-of-life care. It offers essential information on emergency, trauma and critical care in an easy-to-follow format.

Mackway-Jones, K, Marsden, J and Windle, J (2006) *Manchester Triage Group: Emergency Triage.* Second edition. Oxford: Blackwell Publishing.

This practical handbook will be an essential purchase for all health service staff who deal with emergencies. It guides the user through the basic methodology of triage, and then demonstrates how to apply the principles of all the major emergency presentation using easy-to-follow flow charts.

Useful websites

www.nice.org.uk

This website allows you to access a series of national clinical guidelines to secure consistent, high quality, evidence-based care for patients using the NHS.

www.who.int/publications/en

This is an easy, user-friendly website that provides summaries of the best available evidence relating to best practice and supporting policy.

www.glasgowcomascale.org

This website explains the rationale for the Glasgow Coma Scale. It explains how to conduct an assessment and how to chart responses. There are video links to narrated demonstrations.

Chapter 11
The patient with altered consciousness

Jane James

NMC Standards for Pre-registration Nursing Education

This chapter will address the following competencies:

Domain 3: Nursing practice and decision-making

Generic competencies:

7. All nurses must be able to recognise and interpret signs of normal and deteriorating mental and physical health and respond promptly to maintain or improve the health and comfort of the service user, acting to keep them and others safe.

Field-specific competencies:

7.1. Adult nurses must recognise the early signs of illness in people of all ages. They must make accurate assessments and start appropriate and timely management of those who are acutely ill, at risk of clinical deterioration, or require emergency care.

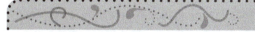

NMC Essential Skills Clusters

This chapter will address the following ESCs:

Cluster: Care, compassion and communication

1. As partners in the care process, people can trust a newly registered graduate nurse to provide collaborative care based on the highest standards, knowledge and competence.

By entry to the register:

viii. Demonstrates clinical confidence through sound knowledge, skills and understanding relevant to field.

ix. Is self-aware and self-confident, knows own limitations and is able to take appropriate action.

Cluster: Organisational aspects of care

9. People can trust the newly registered graduate nurse to treat them as partners and work with them to make a holistic and systematic assessment of their needs; to develop a personalised plan that is based on mutual understanding and respect for their individual situation promoting health and well-being, minimising risk of harm and promoting their safety at all times.

(Continued)

continued . . . •

By entry to the register:

xx.   Acts autonomously and appropriately when faced with sudden deterioration in people's physical or psychological condition or emergency situations, abnormal vital signs, collapse, cardiac arrest, self-harm, extremely challenging behaviour, attempted suicide.

xxi. Measures documents and interprets vital signs and acts autonomously and appropriately on findings.

Chapter aims

By the end of this chapter, you should be able to:

- identify causes of altered consciousness;
- describe the clinical features of altered consciousness in relation to trauma, toxicity, cerebrovascular and neurological problems, and the clinical implications for the patient;
- undertake a neurological assessment;
- diagnose and differentiate between possible causes of patient deterioration and identify most appropriate nursing interventions;
- relate the clinical examples in the chapter to your own practice.

Introduction

Consciousness is not fully understood, however, we use the term generally in relation to awareness and control of ourselves and our environment. Different areas of the cerebral cortex on the surface of the brain are responsible for interpreting awareness of different sensations, such as sight, sound, smell, touch and taste. We also have awareness of self and our own thoughts. This is cognition and is represented by mental activity. Awareness of self, thoughts and sensations enables us to respond through controlled activities such as thinking, talking, looking and moving.

Other parts of the brain (the brain stem, diencephalon and cerebellum) work subconsciously, meaning that we are not aware of them and we cannot control them (Tortora and Derrickson, 2014).

In order to process information accurately and to elicit appropriate controlled responses, the cerebral cortex relies upon information being sent from, or received by, the subconscious parts. This means that full consciousness is only possible when the brain stem, diencephalon, cerebellum and cerebrum are working properly. Altered levels of consciousness show themselves in different ways depending upon the area of the brain affected, but loss of awareness and control are always evident to some extent. It is the nurse's responsibility to recognise these signs and to assess, report and act appropriately.

This chapter gives an overview of the possible causes of unconsciousness. It examines in detail the care of three patients suffering with altered consciousness resulting from head injury, stroke and seizure. It looks at the underlying physiology, social psychology and ethical implications of all three patients in the context of risk assessment and collaborative management and care.

The chapter begins with a case study followed by an explanation of unconsciousness. An overview of the knowledge and skills required to recognise, assess, prioritise and manage care for patients with altered consciousness is given. Neurological assessment skills are explored based upon the requirements of the Glasgow Coma Scale (GCS). Confusion is seen in this chapter as an indication of altered consciousness, but is discussed in detail in Chapter 8.

Case study: Unconsciousness

Julia, a student nurse, was walking through the park with her friend on a cold wintry morning when they found a young man lying on the path. Julia approached with caution while calling to him. As she got closer, she could see that his eyes were closed and he was clearly breathing. He was snoring loudly and his breath smelled of alcohol. Julia assessed his responsiveness using AVPU (alert, responsive to voice or pain, or unresponsive) and was unable to rouse him by speaking loudly to him, by shaking him gently or by pinching his trapezius muscle. While Julia continued her assessment, her friend used her mobile phone to call for an ambulance. In order to open his airway, Julia lifted the young man's chin and tilted his head back until he stopped snoring. She watched and listened to his breathing and counted his pulse rate before looking in his eyes and using sound and pressure to stimulate him to respond. Starting at his head, Julia quickly looked and felt for visible injury on the parts of his body that were accessible. She found bruises and swelling on his head, face and abdomen, and his skin was cold to touch. Her friend found a wallet nearby that contained photographic identification of the young man and the name Mark Spencer on it.

There are many possible reasons why Mark was lying on the ground, and it was most important for Julia and her friend not to put themselves at risk. After excluding any danger, Julia recognised her professional obligation to help, knowing it was important to assess Mark's condition quickly using AVPU followed by ABCDE (see Chapter 1) and to get help. She knew of several reasons for unresponsiveness, and that more detailed assessment would yield clues as to what had happened to Mark.

Julia's experience highlights the fact that patients with altered consciousness may not be able to give information to help with their assessment. Patients with altered conscious states are vulnerable and at risk of deterioration, and even death, from untreated causes as well as being unable to protect themselves from other harm. Mark's unconsciousness might not have been due to alcohol. Any additional findings that Julia noted on her assessment could be significant, and it was most important for Julia to keep Mark safe from further harm. She could do this by getting expert help, by ensuring his airway, breathing and circulation are protected (ABC) and by looking for any additional disabilities (D) and any other environmental factors (E).

Julia found a young man unconscious in the park. She had no way of knowing the circumstances of the situation. She knew that she must keep him safe, get help and assess the degree of unconsciousness as well as look for signs of the cause. What can we learn from this? There are several important messages in Julia's story.

- In emergency situations, always ensure that you do not put yourself or others in danger.

- Use a systematic approach to assess the situation and look for clues as to the causes.

- Be non-judgemental and continue your assessment to the end as there may be more than one problem.

- Organise the people around you and get professional help.

- You may not be able to do anything other than keep the patient safe in the short term, but this can reduce risk of long-term complications.

What are the causes of unconsciousness?

Unconsciousness is a state of unrousable unresponsiveness where the victim is unaware of their surroundings and no purposeful response can be obtained (Martin, 2010). The brain requires a constant supply of oxygenated blood and glucose to function. Interruption of this supply can be sudden, causing unconsciousness within a few seconds. If the interruption is prolonged to ten minutes or more, permanent brain damage occurs as the brain tissue becomes ischaemic and dies. Other causes of unconsciousness can manifest more slowly as the severity of the problem progresses. Even with a gradual decline in consciousness, if the cause is left unattended, unconsciousness will eventually result and the likelihood of permanent disability increases with the period of unconsciousness (Woodward and Waterhouse, 2009). Causes can be classified into four broad groups as detailed in Table 11.1.

General cause	Possible root cause	Clinical examples
Problems with oxygenation causing hypoxia	• Asphyxiation/drowning/ asthmatic attack/smoke inhalation/anaphylaxis.	1. Liz had a severe asthma attack and the bronchospasm restricted the flow of air through her airways – she was irritable and restless.
	• Carbon monoxide poisoning – inhalation of noxious gases.	2. Bob's gas fire was faulty and he suffered carbon monoxide poisoning – he was unresponsive when found.
	• Trauma/injury to lungs/ pneumothorax.	3. Peter sustained broken ribs when a tree fell on him, causing pneumothorax and precluding him from taking deep breaths – he couldn't remember his phone number.
	• Chest infection – sputum retention. Infection – increases oxygen consumption.	4. Sally has pneumonia and secretions have consolidated the bases of both lungs – she was confused and disorientated.

Problems with cerebral circulation	• Occlusion of carotid artery by plaque, clot or compression.	1. Audrey suffered a transient ischaemic attack – she was incoherent and her face was drooping on the left, but she is better now.
	• Occlusion of vertebral arteries due to hyperextension of the head.	2. Bill collapsed in the library when he was looking up to get a book from the top shelf. He recovered almost immediately.
	• Rupture of cerebral vessels as in subarachnoid haemorrhage.	3. Katherine felt an explosion in her head like an elastic band snapping. She had a massive headache and is now responding only to sound.
	• Hypotension/low cardiac output or slow heart rate.	4. Jennifer feels dizzy every time she stands up. Yesterday she fainted at work when she was rushing.
	• Increased intracranial pressure caused by cerebral oedema, tumour, bleed, hydrocephalus causing reduced cerebral perfusion.	5. Andrew has a shunt for drainage of hydrocephalus. He is becoming increasingly drowsy, his eyes are half closed and he doesn't seem to be able to concentrate – the doctor thinks his shunt is blocked.
Metabolic problems	• Overdose of drugs/alcohol.	1. Ian drank a bottle of whisky and now his friends can't wake him up.
	• Hypoglycaemia.	2. Shanta is a diabetic. She is shopping with her friend and is being uncharacteristically aggressive to everyone and cannot be consoled.
	• Electrolyte imbalance.	3. Sheilagh has had copious diarrhoea. She complained of thirst and headaches, became restless and agitated and has just had a fit – her blood results show high sodium levels.
	• Sepsis.	4. Hugh was admitted with confusion and a urine infection. He is now hypotensive, tachycardic and responding only to sound.

(Continued)

Table 11.1   (Continued)

General cause	Possible root cause	Clinical examples
Central nervous system problems	• Epilepsy – convulsions (post-ictal).	1. Robin had his medication changed and has had violent fits. He is now very sleepy and responding only to pressure stimuli.
	• Injury or insult to brain tissue.	2. Diane was hit by a car some weeks ago and sustained brain stem injury. She is now breathing spontaneously, yawns a lot and makes moaning sounds. She opens her eyes but doesn't look at you and she goes rigid when stimulated.
	• Meningitis or encephalitis.	3. Ruby's lumbar puncture shows meningitis. She is photosensitive, has a terrible headache and is confused, irritable and just wants to sleep.

Table 11.1: Causes of diminished consciousness

Julia had no way of knowing whether Mark's unconsciousness was sudden or gradual, but to assess Mark effectively, she had to consider all possible causes of unconsciousness. She must also be mindful that combinations of different causes may be present – for example, a head injury as well as the influence of alcohol or drugs.

Activity 11.1   *Critical thinking*

Look again at the case study with Mark Spencer. What possible causes of Mark's unconsciousness can you identify from those shown in Table 11.1?

A brief outline answer is given at the end of the chapter.

Quickly recognising signs of deteriorating consciousness, and understanding the possible underlying causes, allows early detection of physiological problems and early instigation of correct treatment and care. This can prevent the development of unconsciousness and further risk. Mark's most immediate risk was obstruction of his airway and respiratory arrest leading to cardiac arrest. Julia recognised this and acted immediately by performing the head-tilt, chin-lift manoeuvre. She then continued with a more detailed neurological assessment.

Assessing consciousness level

The two aspects of consciousness generally considered in nursing neurological assessment are arousal, which indicates function of the reticular activating system (RAS) in the brain stem, and awareness or cognition, which indicates function of the cerebral hemispheres. Varying degrees of unconsciousness can occur depending upon the cause and extent of brain dysfunction. Julia used AVPU as a rapid initial assessment to determine any reduced responsiveness, followed by the more detailed GCS (Teasdale et al., 2014). The GCS helped to establish Mark's degree of unconsciousness and which neurological responses were affected. The AVPU assessment findings can be loosely equated to ranges of the GCS score (see Table 11.2) indicating the urgency for more detailed neurological assessment.

The GCS is a widely used neurological assessment tool recommended by Teasdale et al. (2014) to assess patients with altered consciousness and for use in adults and children over five years of age. It measures three indicators of neurological function.

- Eye opening (E).
- Verbal response (V).
- Motor response (M).

Scores are attributed to each indicator (Table 11.3) and should be considered separately, but may also be combined to give the overall coma score. The highest possible score is 15 and the lowest is three. Woodward and Waterhouse (2009) define coma as a GCS of eight or less. Because Mark did not respond to painful stimulus when Julia did the AVPU score, it suggested his GCS was dangerously low, indicating a state of coma.

In addition to noting GCS, it is important to assess pupil size, shape and reaction to light, and limb movements, as well as respiratory rate, oxygen saturations, pulse, blood pressure and temperature. Together these will give more accurate indications of your patient's neurological deficits and degree of risk.

AVPU score	Approximate GCS score
Alert	14–15
Responds to voice	9–13
Responds to pain	4–8
Unresponsive	3

Table 11.2: AVPU and equivalent GCS scores

Source: Cook, 2006

Activity 11.2   *Evidence-based practice and research*

Visit the web link to see information and guidance on how to conduct a GCS assessment and to rate your findings. Follow the links to the video for a demonstration.

www.glasgowcomascale.org/whats-new

Try to check, observe, stimulate and rate your patients in this way when you next need to conduct a neurological assessment.

As this is your own research, there is no answer to this activity at the end of the chapter.

Activity 11.3   *Evidence-based practice and research*

Take some time to read the anatomy and physiology of the central nervous system. Make a note of the main structures of the brain and identify the parts that contribute to the neurological functions tested by the three indicators used in the Glasgow Coma Scale assessment in Table 11.3.

Because you will find this in your anatomy and physiology textbooks, there will be no answer provided for this activity. However, you may find Table 11.3 useful in linking the pathophysiology to your practice.

Case study

When Julia assessed the three indicators of Mark's GCS, he did not open his eyes to central pressure stimulus, nor did he make any vocal sounds. Julia noticed some flexion in response to trapezius pinch when Mark seemed to move his left arm upwards towards her hand. Checking a second time, she could also see that his left knee rose slightly. She considered his best motor response to be normal flexion because his hand did not reach above his clavicle, but he moved one side of his body, thus scoring E1, V1, M4 (see Table 11.3). This gave a total score of 6 out of 15, confirming that Mark's conscious level was dangerously low and he was at risk of stopping breathing.

Julia had noted bruising and swelling of Mark's face, but was still able to lift his eyelids to look at the size and shape of his pupils. She opened both Mark's eyes simultaneously in order to compare the pupil size and shape. Both were round, although the left pupil looked slightly larger than the right. Julia used her friend's mobile phone to shine a light directly at each pupil in turn. She moved the light across Mark's left eye, from the outer aspect to rest over the pupil, then back again and repeated this on the right side to check the right pupil. Noting each pupil response, Julia could see that the left pupil was slower to constrict than the right pupil, which moved so quickly that she could only really see it dilating when she took the light away. Julia made a point of repeating the observation, looking at the non-stimulated pupil, and noted that the right pupil still constricted quickly when light was shone into the left eye, but the left pupil remained sluggish in response when light was shone into the right eye.

Indicator	Score	If the patient …	When you …	Because …
Eye opening	4	Opens eyes spontaneously, without stimulation.	Approach your patient or gently touch them if there is a known hearing impairment.	This demonstrates arousal or wakefulness which is dependent upon the reticular activating system (RAS: a dense network of neurons) within the brain stem being fully functional. Spontaneous eye opening should **not** be equated to alertness or awareness.
	3	Opens eyes to sound.	Make a noise or say something loud enough to elicit a response (e.g. his/her name). Or touch your patient's hand, arm or shoulder and shake gently.	Trauma or increased intracranial pressure could impair neurone pathways within the RAS requiring increased sensory stimulation to evoke eye opening. Speech is used, then touch and lastly pain.
	2	Opens eyes in response to pressure.	Exert graded painful peripheral stimuli by first using the side of a pen or pencil to apply pressure to the fingertip for a short time, then exerting painful central stimulus by pinching the trapezius muscle, and finally applying supraorbital notch pressure. Only if there is no response to the previous, lesser stimulus, and there are no fractures in this region.	A central painful stimulus may result in the patient grimacing, thus closing their eyes. An initial peripheral stimulus could avoid misleading results if there is no response to sound or touch. Alternate the finger tested in order to minimise damage. It is important to elicit the best response, so central stimuli may be applied.
	1	Does not open eyes to stimuli.	Apply painful central stimulus (supraorbital pressure). If eye opening is not possible due to orbital swelling, you need to note this and write 'C' against 'none' on the neurological observation chart.	Intracranial pressure or neural damage due to trauma could be severely impairing the function of the RAS.
	NT	Eyes are closed by a local factor such as eye swelling or surgery.	Find that eye opening is not testable.	In this instance the combined score of all three components of the GCS will be invalid and scores in the sub-scales must be considered separately.

(Continued)

Table 11.3 (Continued)

Indicator	Score	If the patient …	When you …	Because …
Verbal response	5	Is orientated.	Ask questions about the time, place and person, e.g. what the month or year is, where they are and who they are. Avoid questions requiring only yes/no answers. If the patient is expressively dysphasic, write 'D' instead. It is not essential to know the exact day, date or location due to the disorientating effect of prolonged hospital stays and hospital transfers.	The highest level of consciousness requires a person to be totally aware of their surroundings, being orientated to time, place and person. Questions requiring only yes/no answers are not conclusive as answers can be predicted. It is important to be able to recognise and distinguish between receptive and expressive dysphasia as these can detract from accurate assessment for orientation. More detailed observation may be required.
	4	Is confused.	Ask the questions above and the patient cannot answer correctly but is able to converse through coherent phrases or sentences.	Deterioration of consciousness begins with impaired ability to think clearly, repetition, impaired perception and responsiveness with reduced memory of current stimuli relating to time, place and person in that order.
	3	Uses words.	Ask the questions above. Single-worded answers or the inability to make a sentence of words is classed as 'words'.	The cerebral hemispheres of the brain are most susceptible to damage and are responsible for verbal and analytical abilities, perception of language and performance of speech. Poor comprehension and impaired ability to express thoughts into words could indicate reduced cerebral function.

2	Makes sounds.	Apply graded stimuli (noise to supraorbital pressure). Noises such as moans or grunting sounds are classed as 'sounds'.	This is a sign of further deterioration of cerebral function extending to deeper structures of the brain. There is usually associated psychomotor impairment at this stage.
1	Makes no attempt at verbal response to stimuli.	Apply graded stimuli (noise to supraorbital pressure).	Stupor and coma are indicated by little or no spontaneous activity and by being unrousable and unresponsive to external stimuli. These are signs of advanced brain failure.
NT	Has local factors that interfere with communication.	Find that no verbal response is possible due to an endotracheal tube or tracheostomy (without a speaking valve), write 'T' against 'none'.	Intubated patients cannot speak although they may be conscious. They may attempt to mouth words, which are often very difficult to determine, so alternative scores may be misleading, unless by written test of orientation.
Best motor response	6	Obeys commands.	Give the patient a two-part command to squeeze and release your hand, raise and lower their arm or leg or put out and pull back their tongue. If there are varying responses from the different limbs you must note the best limb response and record the appropriate score for the response. Deficits in individual limbs will be recorded separately under 'limb movement'.	This indicates how well the brain is functioning as a whole by testing the areas of brain that precipitate motor responses to sensory stimuli. Following commands indicates the ability to process instructions. Grasping is a primitive reflex that may happen spontaneously, thus giving misleading scores if a one-part only command is used. One limb responding worse than the other gives indication of the site of focal brain damage, so is worth noting.

(Continued)

Table 11.3 (*Continued*)

Indicator	Score	If the patient …	When you …	Because …
	5	Is localising.	Apply a graded pressure stimulus on the head or neck (trapezius pinch to supraorbital notch pressure) if there is no motor response to speech or touch.	Central stimulus used as peripheral pain may evoke a spinal reflex action. Purposeful or semi-purposeful movements are known as localising and the hand must be brought above the clavicle towards the stimulus. Localising may be asymmetrical and when associated with clouding of consciousness as a result of the RAS being squeezed, can indicate increased intracranial pressure. This causes downward displacement of the cerebral hemispheres and structures of the upper brain to the level of the tentorium cerebelli, a transverse fold in the meninges that separates the structures of the upper and lower brain. The oculomotor nerve emerges to control pupillary constriction around the mid brain and can become trapped if the pressure continues to increase. It is at this point when changes in pupil reactions to light might begin.
	4	Displays normal limb flexion.	Apply a graded pressure stimulus on the head or neck (trapezius pinch to supraorbital notch pressure) if there is no motor response to speech or touch.	Flexion of limbs in response to pain is less well targeted to the stimulus than localisation, and indicates advancing brain dysfunction. Fluctuating respiratory function may be noticed at this point, identified by yawning or irregular breathing patterns.

3	Displays abnormal limb flexion.	Apply a graded pressure stimulus on the head or neck (trapezius pinch to supraorbital notch pressure) if there is no motor response to speech or touch.	Abnormal flexion or decorticate rigidity (see Figure 11.1, page 246) may indicate a lesion in the cerebral hemisphere or internal capsule where motor neurones originate.
2	Displays limb extension.	Apply a graded pressure stimulus on the head or neck (trapezius pinch to supraorbital notch pressure) if there is no motor response to speech or touch.	Extension or decerebrate rigidity (see Figure 11.1) can be an indication of a lesion in the diencephalon, mid brain or pons. It can also result from severe metabolic disorders, hypoxia or hypoglycaemia.
1	Does not respond.		
NT	Is paralysed or has other limiting factors.	Find that limb response is not testable.	In this instance the combined score of all three components of the GCS will be invalid and scores in the sub-scales must be considered separately.

Table 11.3: Glasgow Coma Scale: how to score

Source: based on information from Grossman and Porth, 2014 and Teasedale et al., 2014.

Take a torch with a bright white light and narrow beam, and ask a friend to allow you to shine it in their eyes, using the same technique as Julia.

1. Note what happens.
2. What are the difficulties in this technique of pupil assessment?
3. Look at Table 11.3. What might be happening to Mark to elicit the pupil response Julia noted? What might happen next?

An explanation of what you might notice and the answers to the questions can be found at the end of this chapter.

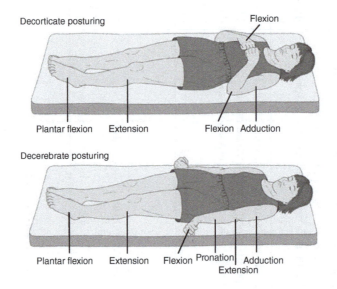

Figure 11.1: Decorticate and decerebrate posturing are examples of 'abnormal posturing'. They are involuntary flexion or extension of the arms and legs, indicating severe brain injury. They occur when one set of muscles becomes incapacitated while the opposing set is not, and an external stimulus such as pain causes the working set of muscles to contract. These types of posturing are indicators of the amount of damage that has occurred to the brain, and are used to measure the severity of a coma with the Glasgow Coma Scale.

Julia informed the paramedics of her findings on assessing Mark. They quickly undertook a further ABCDE assessment including GCS and secured Mark's airway with an endotracheal tube (see Chapter 3). This would allow them to administer oxygen and assist with his respirations should his consciousness deteriorate further, affecting the central areas of the brain that control the vital functions. Julia had kept Mark safe until professional help arrived.

In the A&E department Mark's GCS was reassessed within fifteen minutes according to the guidelines (NICE, 2014b). Blood tests and radiological investigations enabled the medical and nursing team to eliminate many of the causes of unconsciousness that you may have identified earlier. For patients with GCS less than 13 on initial assessment in the A&E department, a computerised tomography (CT) scan should be performed within one hour and provisional results available within a further hour (NICE, 2014b). It later emerged that Mark had been assaulted and kicked repeatedly in the head after leaving the pub where he had been for a drink with his friend the previous evening to celebrate his twenty-third birthday.

Even though there was no evidence of intracranial haematoma or skull fracture on the CT scan, Mark had suffered head trauma causing obvious external bruising and swelling. His neurological assessment suggested changes to the cerebral hemispheres and oculomotor nerve that could be due to intracranial bruising and cerebral oedema (swelling of his brain tissue).

What are the nursing priorities of the unconscious patient?

Case study: Head injury

David is a third-year student nurse on critical care placement in the intensive care unit. Penny, his mentor, agreed that he should look after a newly admitted patient in order to focus on priorities of care. They prepare a bed area for Mark, who was in A&E, having suffered a closed head injury following assault. He was to be sedated, ventilated and closely monitored for 24 hours. While Mark is being prepared for transfer, Penny asks David what would be the nursing priorities in caring for Mark.

David was aware that he and Penny would need to work collaboratively with the medical team to reduce the risk of death or long-term brain damage for Mark. Any initial damage to Mark's brain (primary damage) was irreversible, but the main objective was to prevent further (secondary) damage resulting mainly from a rising intracranial pressure (ICP), which was Mark's biggest threat.

A quick ABCDE assessment and response (see Chapter 1) would address any immediate dangers, but David really needed to know which aspects of care could affect Mark's ICP. He was unsure how to prevent further increase and how best to aid reduction of ICP. Penny points out some important specific nursing considerations to help with reducing the risk of secondary damage. These are identified in Table 11.4.

How can secondary brain injury be prevented?

Preventing secondary brain damage depends upon the quality and quantity of circulation to the brain. For Mark, this means having adequate oxygenation and blood pressure, and maintenance of normal ABGs and blood glucose levels. Increases in ICP result from cerebral oedema, infection, haematoma, tumour or hydrocephalus taking up space within the skull (Grossman and Porth, 2014). Because the skull is rigid, the increase in contents causes them to become squeezed and the intracranial pressure rises. Mark's raised ICP was due to cerebral oedema, which can subside naturally as healing processes take place. Sometimes intravenous infusion of hypertonic sodium chloride solution may be prescribed (Mortazavi et al., 2012). This uses osmosis to draw fluid from the swollen brain tissue into the cerebral circulation, which contains the high concentration salt solution. The extra fluid from the brain tissue is returned to the central circulation and excreted by the kidneys. Whether natural process or medical interventions are employed, the injured tissue requires a good blood supply for the swelling to reduce.

Intracranial pressure and arterial blood pressure work in opposition, so cerebral perfusion depends on the blood pressure being higher than ICP. Thus, if Mark's ICP rises, his mean arterial blood pressure (MAP) must also rise by the same amount as his ICP. If Mark's MAP dropped too low, cerebral circulation would be compromised and his brain tissue would be poorly perfused. Poor perfusion can lead to further swelling, thus compounding the problem.

Problem	Intervention	Rationale
Cerebral oedema may increase during first 24–48 hours, causing ICP to rise further.	• Keep sedated and minimise stimulation. • Nurse in a 15–30° head-up tilt. • Keep head in neutral alignment with body. Ensure ET tube ties are not tight around neck. • Avoid hip flexion.	• Prevents coughing, sneezing and straining, which temporarily increase ICP. • To optimise cerebral venous drainage. • Avoids obstructing jugular veins, which would prevent cerebral venous drainage. • Prevents raised intra-abdominal pressure leading to raised intra-thoracic pressure, which in turn impedes cerebral venous drainage.
Inadequate oxygen delivery to the brain tissues will cause further cerebral damage and exacerbate oedema.	• Care of ET tube. Perform endotracheal suction to remove secretions if needed. • Titrate inspired oxygen and ventilator settings against ABG and SpO_2 results to keep PaO_2 normal. • Keep sedated – monitor sedation score.	• Ensures airway remains patent and optimises gaseous exchange. • Optimises ventilation and avoids increased blood flow to the brain which takes up space and increases ICP. • Reduces cerebral oxygen demand.

	• Avoid infection – use aseptic techniques, monitor body temperature, and aim to keep it normal.	• Raised body temperature increases O_2 demand and CO_2 production, thus increasing cerebral oxygen use. Patients with head injury are susceptible to chest infection, which can lead to sepsis. High ICP can squeeze the hypothalamus, causing temperature regulation to be lost.
Inadequate cerebral perfusion pressure (CPP) will compromise oxygen delivery to the brain, exacerbating cerebral oedema. Good perfusion is needed to help to reduce the cerebral oedema.	• Monitor heart rate. • Monitor fluid input and output – replace fluids to prevent hypotension. • Keep MAP <70 mmHg and CPP <60 mmHg. • Titrate prescribed inotropic drugs to correct hypotension. • Keep $PaCO_2$ on low side of normal. • Use correct patient positioning and care of ET tube ties.	• Changes in heart rate can indicate early BP compensating mechanisms, increasing ICP or inadequate sedation, which may need to be acted upon. Cardiac dysrhythmias need correcting. They reduce efficiency of the heart causing hypotension. • Ensures adequate circulating volume. Gives early identification of excessive diuresis (diabetes insipidus) resulting from pituitary gland being squeezed. Gives indication of renal function. • MAP counteracts rise in ICP to allow adequate cerebral perfusion pressure (CPP = MAP–ICP). • Higher CO_2 levels cause vasodilation. This takes up space and increases ICP. Increased ICP reduces CPP. • Aids cerebral venous drainage, thus reducing cerebral vascular congestion.
Head injury can cause hyperglycaemia and increase metabolism.	• Monitor and correct glucose levels as per policy. • Commence enteral feeding as soon as possible.	• Reduces mortality. • Prevents catabolism (breakdown of complex substances to produce energy), which creates more CO_2.

Table 11.4: Priorities of care to prevent secondary damage in head injury

Activity 11.5 — *Communication*

Imagine you are Mark's nurse in the A&E department. Using the SBAR communication tool (see pages 23–4), make a note of the content and sequence of your handover to David and Penny in ICU.

A plan of Mark's handover can be found at the end of this chapter.

Case study

David and Penny prioritised Mark's care for the next 24 hours. Mark remained stable but his repeat CT scan showed evidence of cerebral oedema. It was agreed that he should be kept sedated and ventilated for a further 24 hours to allow this to settle down. When Mark's sedation was reduced, he was restless and agitated, requiring re-sedating. One day later, Mark developed sepsis, secondary to pneumonia. On day seven Mark's sedation was stopped and he was extubated successfully. He was not agitated, but his GCS remained low at 9/15 (E3, V2, M4) indicating residual brain damage. Mark's recovery from this point was very uncertain, and it was impossible to know whether the brain damage resulted from primary or secondary injury.

Being alert to subtle changes in patient behaviour

Scenario: Stroke

Imagine you are working on the rehabilitation ward and looking after Mrs Pam Green, who suffered a haemorrhagic stroke ten days ago. This morning when you woke her she resisted getting out of bed and did not appear to be making her usual effort with her exercises. Communication can be difficult because of her expressive dysphasia, but today she did not appear to be concordant and she was yawning, so you left her in bed. You return two hours later to find Pam slumped in her bed. On assessment of her GCS, she scores 5 (E1, V1, M3) and her pupils are fixed and dilated. There is no response to light.

Activity 11.6 — *Critical thinking*

Consider Pam's scenario and answer the following questions.

- What signs of altered consciousness were missed?
- What could these signs have indicated?

- What could have been done?
- Why do you think Pam did not get the required attention?

Answers to these questions can be found at the end of this chapter.

Pam's deterioration appeared to be a sudden event, but clues were evident some time before she became unresponsive. You should make objective assessments despite communication difficulties and avoid any preconceptions. You will experience situations similar to Pam's in all spheres of nursing. It is important to be aware of the subtle changes in patient behaviour as these are the earliest indicators of altered consciousness. If you are alert to these changes then, in many cases, early intervention can prevent deterioration.

Because Pam had previously suffered a stroke and had some residual neurological deficits, continued assessment using the GCS would not only identify any deterioration but could also be used to measure progress. Limb assessment may be specifically useful in this instance.

Limb assessment

Limb assessment usually forms part of the overall neurological assessment with the GCS, pupil responses and vital signs. Changes in limb movements can help to pinpoint more specifically the area and degree of brain injury, although it is important to eliminate any pre-existing conditions that may affect limb movement, such as previous stroke or injury (Woodward and Waterhouse, 2009). Ideally, the patient should be able to obey commands, so despite expressive dysphasia, Pam should have been able to respond. Some patients with receptive dysphasia may benefit from a demonstration of what is expected of them.

It is important to compare left side with right side of arms and then legs, rather than assess each limb independently, although results for each limb should be recorded separately. Pam could have been asked to lift her limbs against gravity or slight resistance. This is more useful than asking her to squeeze your hands as grasping is a primitive reflex and may give misleading results. Deviation from previous recorded findings is most significant and this may well have been revealing in Pam's scenario.

Spontaneous or involuntary movement should be recorded, as well as limb strength, which is classified as:

- normal – usual power and strength;
- mild weakness – inability to fully lift limbs or difficulty in moving against resistance;
- severe weakness – unable to lift limbs but can move them laterally.

Patients who are unable to obey commands can be assessed for limb movement in response to pressure as in the motor response section of the GCS. Any difference between responses in left and right must be noted in the limb movement assessment.

When Pam seemed to be resisting care, her condition was deteriorating. A thorough GCS, including limb assessment, would have revealed that she opened her eyes to voice (E1), made sounds or words (V2 or 3) and localised to pressure (M5), but that her best motor response was weaker than her last limb assessment had shown. With this information, medical attention could have been summoned much earlier. Unfortunately, it is likely that Pam suffered another intracerebral bleed, and prognosis in this instance is extremely poor.

Seizure: what action is needed?

Seizures are transient episodes of neurological deficit and take many different forms depending upon their origin and cause. They are often associated with epilepsy, but can be triggered by drugs, alcohol, metabolic disorders, pre-eclampsia, head injury or cerebral hypoxia and pyrexia in children (Woodward and Waterhouse, 2009). Abnormal electrical activity can start in one part of the brain and spread, sometimes involving localised areas and sometimes affecting the whole cerebral cortex. Various symptoms result, depending upon the area and location of brain involvement.

Case study: Seizure

Student nurse, Claire, was returning to the ward from an errand when she met a young lady in the ward entrance. She seemed to be walking aimlessly, but on approach Claire established that she was Josie Watkins who was visiting her mother, Maureen, a patient on the ward. Claire directed Josie to the correct bed, but saw her stop. She was fiddling with her hands, then collapsed on to the floor. Her arms were jerking and she was making choking sounds. Claire shouted for help and cleared the area of obstacles. She was unsure of what to do next and was relieved when Satya, the ward sister, appeared.

Josie was showing early signs of onset of seizure when Claire met her. The subtle behaviour that Claire noticed is significant and will be useful for Josie and her family members to recognise in future. The most important and immediate concern was to keep her safe for the duration of the seizure, using the ABCDE approach, and to protect her from injury.

It is not recommended, or safe, to open the mouth of someone having a seizure to insert an oropharyngeal airway because of jaw clenching, and stimulation may further exacerbate the seizure. It is usual to allow short seizures to run their course, observing closely, and to intervene once the seizure stops (Woodward and Waterhouse, 2009). It is not advisable to restrain the victim. If seizures are continuous, prescribed emergency medication such as diazepam should be administered through an accessible route with quick absorption.

Activity 11.7   *Evidence-based practice and research*

Visit the International League Against Epilepsy website at **www.ilae.org** to find out more about the classification of seizures, current research and recommendations.

As this is your own research, there is no answer to this activity at the end of the chapter.

Case study: Seizure (continued)

Satya, the ward sister, removed Josie's neck scarf and cushioned her head with a pillow. She asked Claire to record the duration of the seizure and all the different components, such as noises, movements and progression, skin colour and injuries. Another nurse brought emergency equipment and positioned it at Josie's head ready for Satya to use if needed. Once Josie seemed to relax (after 75 seconds), Satya asked Claire for help to put Josie into the recovery position. Josie's airway was protected using a head tilt and chin lift, and Satya had oxygen and a face mask ready. Claire carried out a full set of observations, including respirations, oxygen saturations, pulse, blood pressure, temperature and neurological assessment. Josie began to respond after a further two minutes and was helped onto a bed to recover.

Satya found out from Maureen that her daughter suffered with epilepsy, and had recently had her medication regime reviewed.

Claire's experience could have happened outside the hospital where no emergency equipment is available. However, despite the help from experienced healthcare professionals, we can see that the initial actions required only common sense. Claire acted appropriately by:

- noting symptoms leading up to the seizure;
- calling for help;
- preparing a safe environment;
- staying with the patient;
- being prepared to intervene with the ABCDE approach afterwards.

The duration of seizures is often surprisingly short, so it is important to note components and timings of all the phases. The patient may not remember events, so information is useful for them and their families for future management and care. It is important to reassure the patient and to be able to provide accurate and reliable information regarding the cause and possible triggers of their seizures and their likely course. The nurse has a role in patient education and health promotion, as well as recognising signs of impending and actual problems.

In patients not known to have epilepsy, alternative causes of seizure should be considered and subsequently treated to avoid further seizures. Repeated, convulsive seizures and those of longer duration pose increased risk of hypoxia to the patient as cerebral oxygen consumption increases and there may be insufficient oxygen supply. This is a life-threatening situation and demonstrates why it was important for the ward sister to have oxygen ready to administer to Josie if she needed it. Seizures lasting longer than 60 minutes can lead to acidosis, dehydration, hypoglycaemia, possible fractures and muscle breakdown, which in turn can cause acute kidney injury. It is important to respond quickly to support airway, breathing and circulation in this instance and to summon urgent expert and medical help in order that appropriate medical treatment can be given (NICE, 2012).

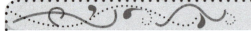

Chapter summary

This chapter highlights the nursing responsibilities of rapid and accurate neurological assessment and subsequent prioritisation of care for patients with altered consciousness and at risk of deterioration. Nurses can come across patients with altered consciousness in all clinical settings, and early intervention and prioritisation of care can reduce complications. Outcomes are not always good, but increased understanding of neurological problems will enable you to make evidence-based clinical judgements.

Activities: brief outline answers

Activity 11.1: Critical thinking (page 238)

Several of the causes identified in Table 11.1 could apply to Mark: alcohol intoxication; drug overdose; head injury; hypoglycaemia; hypotensive episode such as fainting; hypoxia; infection such as meningitis or encephalitis; post-ictal (post-fit); spontaneous intracranial bleed such as subarachnoid haemorrhage.

Activity 11.4: Evidence-based practice and research (page 246)

1. Normally, when a bright narrow beam of light is shone into one eye and held there, the pupil of that eye constricts briskly to a pinpoint size of about 1 mm. The pupil dilates again, usually back to its original size, when the light is removed. To avoid misleading results in pupil size difference, it is important to check equality of pupil sizes prior to subjecting them to light stimulus. Normally, both pupils respond when light is shone in only one of them – this is the consensual response that helps to test the optic nerve.
2. Difficulties with this technique.

   - You may find some healthy people have unequal pupils ordinarily.
   - With brown eyes it is sometimes difficult to determine the margin of the pupil from the iris, so the motor response may need to be noted from the dilation of the pupil on removing the light rather than looking for constriction on applying the light stimulus.
   - The brightness of light in the room, and the width and strength of the light beam, affects starting pupil size and may hinder response.
   - Moving the light stimulus across the bridge of the patient's nose can hinder response, so it is better to introduce the light from the outer aspect of the eye.
   - Patients who are photosensitive will find this very uncomfortable and may resist the assessment.
   - Likewise, orbital oedema that precludes eye opening hinders assessment in the patients who may need to be monitored.

3. Mark's direct pupil responses indicated that his optic and oculomotor cranial nerves were functioning. The fact that his left pupil was slow to constrict suggests that either the left optic nerve had impaired sensitivity to light, or that the conduction pathway of the left oculomotor nerve was impeded. The brisk consensual response of the right pupil when light was shone into the left eye demonstrates that the left optic nerve was sensing the light. These findings give strong clues as to the extent of intracranial pressure increase (see Table 11.3) and suggest that Mark's left oculomotor nerve was getting squeezed, and the intracranial pressure was such that the cerebral hemispheres were being pushed down towards the tentorium cerebelli. If the pressure continued to rise, the next sign would be a change in left pupil shape to oval, then a fixed and dilated left pupil, accompanied by reduced motor responses to painful stimuli and haemodynamic changes as the diencephalon and brain stem start to get squeezed. This is a dangerous situation for Mark.

Activity 11.5: Communication (page 250)

Introduce self and department.

Patient's name: Mark Spencer, 23-year-old male.

Situation

- Unconscious closed head injury.
- Intubated and ventilated.
- Bruising and swelling to head, face and abdomen.
- No other injuries.

Background

- Give home situation if known.
- Went out for a drink last night.
- Assaulted – kicked repeatedly in the head.
- Found unconscious in park this am – give original GCS – and has been unconscious since.
- No significant past medical history.
- Usually fit and well.
- Takes no medication.

Assessment

- Airway – intubated by paramedics at the scene.
- Breathing – spontaneously on admission, now sedated and ventilated. Give breathing rate, % oxygen delivered and oxygen saturations readings.
- Circulation – give heart rate, blood pressure, temperature measured and peripheral temperature to touch. Fluid input and output.
- Disability – give latest GCS score and pupil assessment, blood glucose result, CT scan and X-ray results. Summarise blood results and give any significant deviations from normal. Give information relating to medication and fluid administered and diuretic response to hypertonic saline if given.
- Exposure – if not already mentioned, give urine output and state if catheterised. Indicate other injuries and how they have been treated.

Response

Outline proposed plan

- Keep sedated and ventilated for next 24 hours.
- Repeat CT scan tomorrow to check for reduction in cerebral oedema.
- Repeat ABGs one hour after transfer.
- Keep PaO_2 normal and $PaCO_2$ on low side of normal.
- Give any information regarding family, police and property.
- Agree a time for transfer.

Activity 11.6: Critical thinking (pages 250–1)

First of all, Pam may not have been asleep, but she opened her eyes to sound. Resisting getting out of bed and lack of effort and concordance may not have been stubbornness but due to reduced awareness, cognition and control. Early signs of deterioration in consciousness include decreased concentration, agitation, dullness and lethargy. These fit with Pam's changed behaviour, but because of her usual expressive dysphasia, her falling GCS went unnoticed. Depending upon the degree of Pam's expressive dysphasia, it may be difficult to ascertain confusion and words lacking order from sounds not resembling words. Yawning is an early respiratory indicator of rising intracranial pressure.

Had Pam's GCS been thoroughly assessed, it should have been possible to note that she could not obey commands and that she was losing control of motor function. Assessment of vital signs, limb movement and pupil reactions may have helped to conclude findings.

It is not clear whether the course of Pam's deterioration could have been halted.

It is not safe to assume that recovering patients are safe from deterioration.

Further reading

Edwards, M and Griffiths, P (2011) *Emergency Nursing Made Incredibly Easy!* London: Lippincott Williams & Wilkins.

This book gives easy-to-understand explanations of emergency care and includes a specific chapter dedicated to neurological problems.

Geraghty, M (2005) Nursing the unconscious patient. *Nursing Standard,* 20(1): 54–6.

This article gives comprehensive coverage of the nursing management of unconscious patients, taking into account all activities of living based on life-like scenarios.

Goulden, I (2011) Traumatic brain injury, in Clarke, D and Ketchell, A (eds) *Nursing the Acutely Ill Adult: Priorities in Assessment and Management.* Basingstoke: Palgrave Macmillan.

This chapter deals with traumatic brain injury, considering medical and surgical interventions in a clearly laid out format.

NICE (2014) *Head Injury: Triage, Assessment, Investigation and Early Management of Head Injury in Infants, Children, Young People and Adults.* London: NICE.

This gives comprehensive guidance on care of patients with head injury. Nurses involved in caring for acutely ill patients should have this information.

Useful websites

www.ilae.org

The International League Against Epilepsy website presents a wealth of information about epilepsy. The different classifications and manifestations are explained. There are presentations, research papers and practice guidelines.

www.stroke.org.uk

The Stroke Association website gives information for patients and professionals about the different stages of stroke. There are links to research articles as well as information and advice that you can pass on to your patients.

www.glasgowcomascale.org/whats-new

This website explains the rationale for the Glasgow Coma Scale. It explains how to conduct an assessment and how to chart responses. There are video links to narrated demonstrations.

Chapter 12
The patient with an endocrine disorder

David Blesovsky

Chapter aims

By the end of this chapter, you should be able to:

- demonstrate an understanding of the causes of endocrine problems;
- identify the three main reasons for emergency admission of the person with diabetes mellitus;
- describe the role of the nurse in caring for endocrine emergencies, especially those concerning diabetes mellitus;
- demonstrate how to assess, record and respond to these patients;
- demonstrate knowledge of rapid risk assessment within holistic care;
- reflect on the case studies in the chapter to enhance your own clinical skills.

Case study: Millie's story

Millie is coming to the end of her second year of a degree in adult nursing. She came on duty for an early shift on the acute medical ward and was put with her mentor for the shift. She was keen to show that she had some skills as this was the last placement of her second year and when she was asked to go and do the observations for four patients she was more than happy to carry out this request. All four patients had type 2 diabetes mellitus and three had been admitted for reasons other than their diabetes. The fourth patient, Mr John Evans, was on the ward because he was having trouble stabilising his blood glucose levels. When Millie talked to Mr Evans he appeared not interested in her and was aggressive in his responses. He was not happy about having his blood glucose recorded and Millie explained that she would get her mentor to come and do this as she was not currently allowed to record blood glucose levels. Millie recorded John's pulse, blood pressure, respirations and temperature, which were all within the normal ranges. Millie documented the results and continued with the other observations. She informed her mentor about Mr Evans and her mentor came and recorded John's blood glucose which was 12.8 mmol/L.

Activity 12.1   *Critical thinking*

After reading the case study: Millie's story, answer the following questions.

1. If you were in Millie's position, what else should you have done?
2. Did Millie miss some signs of hyperglycaemia in Mr Evans?
3. What needs to be done now to stabilise Mr Evans's condition?
4. Is this level of blood glucose problematic?

Answers to these questions can be found at the end of the chapter.

Endocrine problem	Hormone(s) involved	Specific disease	Population affected	Treatment
Diabetes mellitus	Insulin	Type 1 diabetes.	Usually children and young people at onset.	Insulin injections.
		Type 2 diabetes.	Until a few years ago, this was a disease of adults aged 40+. However, increasing obesity levels and sedentary lifestyles worldwide have resulted in younger people – even some children – being diagnosed.	Diet and lifestyle changes. Tablets (oral hypoglycaemics). Insulin injections (most people will need these as they get older).
		Gestational diabetes.	Women during pregnancy.	Combination of diet control, oral therapy and sometimes insulin.
Adrenal disorders	Aldosterone Cortisol	Addison's disease. Addisonian crisis.	Can affect people of any age, although most commonly seen between ages 30–50 years and more common in women.	Maintain ABC, monitor ABCDE and GCS closely, rapid fluid replacement (5% dextrose in normal saline), monitor blood glucose and rapidly treat hypoglycaemia, cortisol administration (IV hydrocortisone), identify and treat cause of crisis (infection, surgery, trauma).
	Adrenaline Noradrenaline	Pheochromocytoma (very rare tumour of adrenal gland).	Can occur at any age but, as above, peak incidence is between 30–50 years.	Rapid blood pressure stabilisation and then prepare for surgery for tumour removal.
Thyroid disorders	Thyroid hormone T_3 T_4	Hyperthyroidism. Thyroid crisis.	Can occur at any age, more common in women: 8% compared to 1% of men developing the disease.	Reduction of the effects of raised hormone levels until stable. Close monitoring of ABCDE (see page 14). Treat with drug therapy that includes beta-blockers, sedatives, hydrocortisone and specific anti-thyroid drugs such as carbimazole.

(Continued)

Table 12.1 (Continued)

Endocrine problem	Hormone(s) involved	Specific disease	Population affected	Treatment
		Myxoedema (including Hashimoto's disease). Myxoedema coma.	Can be a rare congenital problem, far more common in women than men and in people over the age of 60. Hashimoto's disease is an autoimmune disease with strong familial links and commonly seen in women after having their first baby.	Management of coma is around organ support and addressing the cause and administration of thyroxine, close monitoring of ABCDE.
Pituitary disorders	Antidiuretic hormone	Diabetes insipidus (DI).	An acquired disorder: 30% **idiopathic**, 25% brain or pituitary tumour, 20% cranial surgery and 16% head trauma. Can be a rare congenital problem. Some people can have kidneys that are insensitive to ADH (nephrogenic DI) although this is very rare.	Rapid administration of desmopressin (DDAVP) and close monitoring of ABCDE.
		Syndrome of inappropriate antidiuretic hormone hypersecretion (SIADH).	Can affect any age group, but more common in the elderly and hospitalised patients. Some evidence that menstruating women are more at risk.	Initial close monitoring of ABCDE with concurrent fluid restriction and monitoring.

Table 12.1: Disorders of the endocrine system: a summary

This chapter will look at how you can gain an understanding of the most common endocrine problems by describing diabetic emergencies of hypoglycaemia and hyperglycaemia, diabetic ketoacidosis (DKA) and hyperosmolar hyperglycaemic syndrome (HHS), and briefly discuss some of the other more rare endocrine emergencies.

Emergency admission of medical problems are many and varied and approximately 2% of these are related to endocrine problems. By far the most common of these are related to diabetes mellitus with the other endocrine conditions accounting for only around a hundred emergency admissions a year (Kearney and Dang, 2007). The nurse needs to be able to rapidly assess this group of patients so that early identification and treatment can occur. To be able to do this you need to have an understanding of glucose metabolism and management otherwise caring for the patient with diabetes mellitus will be problematic. Table 12.1 provides a summary of the main endocrine problems by identifying the hormone and the disease caused by either lack of the hormone or, in some cases, over production.

Millie's story is a common one for student nurses as diabetes mellitus is a complex collection of disorders classed into type 1 and type 2 diabetes. Mr Evans's aggression could easily have been a symptom of his rising blood glucose. There are key differences between type 1 and type 2 diabetes, as can be seen in Table 12.2.

Type 1 diabetes mellitus	Type 2 diabetes mellitus	Gestational diabetes mellitus
<ul><li>Less common at around 10%.</li><li>Sudden onset at any age, but more common in the young (<40 years).</li><li>Usually underweight at diagnosis.</li><li>Caused by cessation of insulin production from the beta cells of the pancreatic islets. Thought to be an immune response frequently following an infection.</li><li>Treatment is insulin injections for life.</li></ul>	<ul><li>Most common form of diabetes mellitus seen with 90% of all cases.</li><li>Gradual onset over weeks or months more commonly in the elderly, or overweight and sedate adult.</li><li>Combination of insulin resistance at cellular level and reduction in insulin production at the beta cells of the pancreatic islets.</li><li>Treatment is lifestyle change, diet, oral agents and in later life insulin therapy.</li></ul>	<ul><li>Diabetes that occurs during pregnancy and with an incidence of 2–5%.</li><li>Closely resembles type 2 diabetes mellitus.</li><li>Frequently self corrects following childbirth.</li><li>Mothers have an increased risk of developing type 2 diabetes mellitus in later life (50%).</li></ul>

Table 12.2: Differences between types of diabetes mellitus

The three emergency problems associated with diabetes mellitus are hypoglycaemia and hyperglycaemia in the form of DKA and HHS. Hyperglycaemia is classified as blood glucose above the normal level (4–7 mmol/L), but it is not uncommon for patients with diabetes mellitus to run their blood glucose levels between 5–10 mmol/L, particularly those with type 1 diabetes who have suffered frequent hypoglycaemic attacks.

Hypoglycaemia

For the person with diabetes mellitus, hypoglycaemia is the most frightening side effect of having the disease. Hypoglycaemia can be characterised by a blood glucose of less than 4 mmol/L. The person will show signs of autonomic (neurogenic) effects caused by elevated levels of adrenaline in the system and neuroglycopenic symptoms (see Table 12.3), which occur because of glucose deprived brain cells. The symptoms in Table 12.3 are not definitive as symptoms vary from patient to patient.

Assessment	Observation	Hypoglycaemia
Airway	• Airway patent.	• Most commonly normal.
Breathing	• Respiratory rate and pattern. • O_2 saturations.	• Normal respiratory rate and pattern.

Circulation	• Blood pressure.
	• Pulse.
	• Capillary refill time (CRT).
	• Skin.
	• CVP.
	• Urine output.
		• Autonomic effects:
		  o sweating
		  o palpitations
		  o dry mouth.
		• CRT normal.
		• Skin clammy.

Disability	• AVPU/GCS.
	• Pain assessment.
	• Blood glucose.
		• Anxiety (autonomic).
		• Neuroglycopenic symptoms:
		  o irritability
		  o difficulty thinking and speaking
		  o tiredness
		  o poor coordination
		  o visual problems
		  o shakiness
		  o drowsiness
		  o confusion
		  o seizures
		  o coma
		  o low GCS.

Exposure	• Other. • Temperature.	• Nausea (autonomic). • Paraesthesia (neuroglycopenic). • Normal temperature.

Table 12.3: ABCDE assessment of hypoglycaemia

As can be seen from Table 12.3 the symptoms of hypoglycaemia are many and varied and patients need to learn the signs so that they can recognise the symptoms and treat themselves before collapse occurs. There are three levels of hypoglycaemia:

- mild: recognised symptoms, these tend to be autonomic in nature, and self-treated (blood glucose of 3–4 mmol/L); no assistance required. Treated with dextrose tablets or refined carbohydrates, the patient will know what works for them, followed by long-acting carbohydrate (unless they are on an insulin pump). Repeat blood glucose 10–15 minutes later;

- moderate: recognition of symptoms, but symptoms are neuroglycopenic in nature (blood glucose of 2.5–3.5 mmol/L). The patient could be confused and irritable and have difficulty concentrating; they may need help. Give dextrose tablets if the patient can swallow or 30% glucose gel (hypostop) applied to the buccal mucosa. Repeat blood glucose 10–15 minutes later and if no increase then give more dextrose and contact doctor;

- severe: assistance is required urgently, could be very drowsy, losing consciousness or in a coma (blood glucose <2.5 mmol/L). A blood glucose of less than 1.5 mmol/L is a medical emergency and if action is not taken rapidly, then there is a great risk of brain damage occurring. One mg of glucagon can be administered intramuscularly or intravenously to an unconscious patient or one who cannot maintain their own airway. They will need rapid and continuous assessment using ABCDE until medical help arrives.

Hypoglycaemia is caused by either too much insulin being administered, too much exercise or not enough food eaten, or a combination of these. The patient needs to learn how their body reacts to exercise and work out how to reduce insulin and/or increase carbohydrate intake. Unfortunately iatrogenic hypoglycaemia is not uncommon; the National Diabetes Inpatient Audit (Health and Social Care Information Centre, 2014) identified that 25% of patients with diabetes made medication errors. This suggests that there is a need for nurses to be able to recognise hypoglycaemia in their patients.

Activity 12.2 — *Evidence-based practice and research*

Go to the InDependent Diabetes Trust website (**www.iddt.org**) and investigate the incidence of medication errors related to diabetes. What do you think can be done to reduce this major problem?

An outline answer to this activity is given at the end of the chapter.

Hyperglycaemia

Acute hyperglycaemia has two presentations: diabetic ketoacidosis (DKA) and hyperosmolar hyperglycaemic syndrome (HHS). Both DKA and HHS are initiated post infection, but can occur through non-compliance with treatment and following other major medical events such as myocardial infarction (see Table 12.4). DKA and HHS are two acute complications of diabetes that can result in increased ill health and death if not competently and effectually treated. Mortality rates are 2–5% for DKA and 15% for HHS, and mortality is usually a consequence of the underlying precipitating cause(s) rather than a result of the metabolic changes of hyperglycaemia. Effective standardised treatment protocols, as well as prompt identification and treatment of the precipitating cause, are important factors affecting outcome and these are frequently initiated by the nurse.

Condition	Presenting features	Signs and symptoms	Demographics
Diabetic ketoacidosis	• Blood glucose >14 mmol/L (rarely above 40 mmol/L). • pH <7.3 • Bicarbonate <18 mmol/L. • Anion gap >11 (sign of metabolic acidosis). • Ketonaemia/ ketonuria.	• Rapid onset. • **Polyuria, polydipsia**, vomiting, weight loss, abdominal pains. • Signs of hypovolaemia: tachycardia, hypotension, low CVP if measured. • Confusion rarely.	• Most commonly younger slimmer patients with type 1 diabetes. • Mortality less than 5% but still the most common cause of death in young people with diabetes.
Hyperosmolar hyperglycaemic syndrome	• Blood glucose >35 mmol/L (frequently much higher). • pH normal 7.35– 7.45. • Bicarbonate >15 mmol/L. • Serum osmolality >320.	• Insidious onset (several days or weeks). • Polyuria, polydipsia, vomiting, occasionally weight loss. • Signs of hypovolaemia: tachycardia, hypotension, low CVP if recorded. • Confusion common.	• Most commonly older, obese patients with type 2 diabetes. • Mortality rate: 15%.

Table 12.4: Presenting features and signs and symptoms of DKA and HHS

Diabetic ketoacidosis

DKA is a life-threatening complication of type 1 diabetes, although it is seen in type 2 diabetes during acute illnesses. Presenting features and signs and symptoms can be found in Table 12.4 above. The underlying cause for most patients – 50% – is an infection and because of this it is more commonly seen during the winter months. Also it is commonly seen as the presenting problem of patients newly diagnosed with type 1 diabetes. Other factors are poor compliance with treatment and psychological stress; a combination of these factors have been identified in young women with type 1 diabetes, who think that it will help them lose weight quickly, which rapidly leads to DKA (Umpierrez et al., 2002).

DKA is caused by an absolute deficiency of circulating insulin with the subsequent increase in glucagon, catecholamines, cortisol and growth hormone, all of which raise the glucose levels in the blood through **glucogenolysis** (splitting up of glycogen) in the liver. The body starts to digest its own fat stores and muscle mass through the digestion of amino acids and glycerol, the waste products of which are ketones. Ketones are an acid and so acidaemia occurs (further information on this can be gained from the *Handbook of Diabetes* (Bilous and Donnelly, 2010).

Once identified then the diabetes specialist team must be involved with the management of every patient admitted (Joint British Diabetes Societies (JBDS), 2013). The team need to be involved as it has been shown that it improves safety and reduces length of patient stay (JBDS, 2013). All care needs to be in line with local and national clinical guidelines and nurses need to be aware of these to provide the high standards of safe care required.

The nurse's role is based around ongoing clinical assessment and observation of vital signs using the ABCDE rapid assessment process (see Table 12.6) and management should be aimed at:

- measurement of blood ketones, venous (not arterial) pH and bicarbonate and their use as treatment markers;
- monitoring of ketones and glucose using bedside meters when available and operating within their quality assurance range;
- replacing 'sliding scale' insulin with weight-based fixed rate intravenous insulin infusion (FRIII), see Table 12.5;
- use of venous blood rather than arterial blood in blood gas analysers;
- monitoring of electrolytes on the blood gas analyser with intermittent laboratory confirmation;
- continuation of long-acting basal insulin analogues as normal;
- involvement of the diabetes specialist team as soon as possible.

The diabetes clinical nurse specialist, once the patient is stable, has to try and identify what the cause of the DKA was; this is not so difficult if the patient is newly diagnosed and presenting with DKA, but it becomes more difficult if other reasons are involved.

Hyperosmolar hyperglycaemic state

Hyperosmolar hyperglycaemic state – commonly referred to as HHS – is classed as a medical emergency and is different to DKA, as is treatment. HHS is far more common in the elderly,

Weight in kg	Insulin dose per hour (units)
60–69	6
70–79	7
80–89	8
90–99	9
100–109	10
110–119	11
120–129	12
130–139	13
140–149	14
>150	15 (any dose higher than this should be on the advice of the diabetes specialist team)

Table 12.5: FRIII rates per weight of patient

Source: JBDS, 2013

Assessment	Observation	DKA	HHS
Airway	• Patent.	• Most commonly normal.	• Most commonly normal.
Breathing	• Respiratory rate and pattern. • O$_2$ saturations.	• Tachypnoea. • **Kussmaul breathing**. • Normal.	• Normal respiratory rate and pattern. • Normal.
Circulation	• Blood pressure. • Pulse. • Capillary refill time (CRT). • Skin. • CVP. • Urine output.	• Signs of hypovolaemia: hypotension, tachycardia, low CVP. • Raised CRT. • Dysrhythmias due to electrolyte imbalance. • Polyuria due to the hyperglycaemia.	• Signs of hypovolaemia: hypotension, tachycardia, low CVP. • Raised CRT. • Dysrhythmias due to electrolyte imbalance. • Polyuria due to hyperglycaemia
Disability	• AVPU/GCS. • Pain assessment. • Blood glucose.	• Confusion, lethargy, reduced level of consciousness. • Blood glucose >13 mmol/L.	• Confusion probably because of increased serum osmolality. • Blood glucose >30 mmol/L.

Exposure	• Other. • Temperature.	• Nausea, vomiting, abdominal pain and acetone smell on breath because of raised ketones. • Tendency to be hypothermic.	• Tendency to be hypothermic.

Table 12.6: ABCDE assessment of DKA and HHS

but as younger people and teenagers develop type 2 diabetes they can present with HHS. Underlying infections are the most common precipitating cause for the development of HHS. It has a higher mortality rate than DKA and is usually accompanied by vascular complications such as myocardial infarction, stroke or peripheral arterial thrombosis. Seizures and cerebral oedema are uncommon but known complications of HHS which take many days to develop, resulting in more severe dehydration and metabolic disturbances. Table 12.4 showed the presenting features and signs and symptoms of HHS and as soon as they are identified the diabetes specialist team should be informed and involved in the management of the patient. The key role of the nurse is the rapid assessment of the patient using the ABCDE approach (see Table 12.6) and recording observations from admission and during treatment to stabilise symptoms. The treatment goals for HHS are to treat the underlying cause and gradually:

- normalise the osmolality;
- replace fluid and electrolyte losses;
- normalise blood glucose.

Other goals include the prevention of:

- arterial or venous thromboses;
- other potential complications, e.g. cerebral oedema;
- foot ulceration.

Activity 12.3   *Evidence-based practice and research*

Using the internet (Diabetes UK: **www.diabetes.org.uk** and UpToDate: **www.uptodate.com**) research the physiology of DKA and HHS and try to identify why it is that HHS is non-ketotic and DKA is ketotic.

An outline answer to this activity is given at the end of the chapter.

Scenario: Sanjit – HHS

Harry is a third-year student nurse on placement in A&E. One Saturday morning, a young man, Ashya Gupta, comes in with his father, Sanjit. The older man seems to have trouble staying awake and doesn't appear to know where he is or why.

Carole, the triage nurse, asks Ashya how long his father has been unwell. Ashya replies that he has been running a temperature for a couple of days. He phoned his GP, who advised him to take a few days rest and drink plenty of fluids as the problem was likely to resolve itself. Sanjit did as advised, but this morning, he was incoherent and drowsy. The family didn't want to phone an out-of-hours GP, but they were sure that Sanjit needed urgent medical attention.

Harry is surprised when Carole asks Ashya what Sanjit has been drinking. Sanjit said his father has a lot of tea (black, with two sugars) as well as plenty of orange juice. It also transpires that Sanjit has been needing to pass urine often. However, when asked if his father suffers from diabetes, Sanjit replies that he doesn't.

To Harry's surprise, Carole tests Sanjit's blood sugar level and finds it to be 42 mmol/L. She explains to Ashya that his father is suffering from severe dehydration, which will need to be treated with intravenous fluids in hospital. He will also need to be treated with insulin to bring his blood glucose level under control.

Later, when Carole and Harry are eventually able to take a break, Carole explains that Sanjit is very likely to have HHS and that he has underlying type 2 diabetes, which will need ongoing treatment once the acute condition has been brought under control.

Activity 12.4	*Evidence-based practice and research*

If you were in Harry's position, where might you go to find out more about HHS and other complications of diabetes?

Go to **www.diabetes.org.uk** and see if you can find the answer to the following question.

What should Ashya look for if he suspects Sanjit is not looking after himself?

An outline answer to this activity is given at the end of the chapter.

Once on the ward, the priorities of care for Sanjit are based around education and developing his self-caring. The ward team are skilled in teaching Sanjit about type 2 diabetes and how to manage his diet and exercise with the medication he will need to control his diabetes.

Harry visits Sanjit on the ward a few days later. He is completely different – alert and aware of what is going on around him. He knows that he has now been diagnosed with type 2 diabetes and shares with Harry his worries about what this is going to mean for him and his family in the future. He is very concerned about becoming ill again after discharge, especially as the doctor has told him that he won't need to carry on having insulin injections.

Speaking to Carole, his mentor, Harry discovers that communication is the key; Sanjit and his family must come to terms with the disease and be fully aware of what to look for so that Sanjit doesn't become this ill again. Learning and understanding his disease is a steep learning curve, but the clinical diabetes teams are trained to deal with this – Carole suggests Harry spends a couple of days with them.

Activity 12.5   *Communication*

Put yourself in Harry's shoes. Imagine you are a nurse on the medical ward with responsibility for Sanjit's care. What advice can you give to Ashya and Sanjit to make sure that this doesn't happen again?

How would you:

(a) reassure him about his treatment, especially the fact that he has been told he won't need to carry on taking insulin?
(b) advise him about any lifestyle changes that will help to ensure he stays as healthy as possible?

An outline answer to this activity is given at the end of the chapter.

Other acute endocrine problems

Addison's disease

Addison's disease is a chronic condition where there is a deficiency of the cortical hormones, cortisol and aldosterone. Deficiency of cortisol will produce:

- muscle weakness;
- fatigue;
- hypoglycaemia;
- ileus;
- reduced immunity;
- low cardiac output.

Deficiency of aldosterone causes:

- polydipsia;
- polyuria;
- dehydration;

- hypovolaemia;
- **hyponatraemia**;
- **hyperkalaemia**;
- postural hypotension;
- arrhythmias.

The patient will be on hormone replacement therapy for life. Your role in caring for a patient with this condition is one of prevention through close monitoring and strict administration of steroid therapy. Omission of just one dose can cause steroid deprivation and push the patient into crisis. It is not uncommon for these patients to suffer more than one endocrine problem and if they have type 1 diabetes mellitus, then the combination of steroid therapy and insulin becomes time specific: they must be administered at the exact time required. Addisonian crisis can occur when demand for cortisol cannot be met; this is frequently triggered by a gastric infection and is the most important predictor of impending Addisonian crisis (White and Arlt, 2010). Eight per cent of patients with Addison's disease will fall into crisis and this is invariably through poor management. You need to use your rapid assessment skills to fully monitor the patient and any changes that may occur, making sure that you provide full holistic care and give medication at correct times. It is advisable to listen to the patient as he or she will often be the expert on their disease.

Scenario: Linda – Addison's disease

Linda is a 42-year-old marketing executive who has Addison's disease. This means her body is unable to produce adequate levels of the hormones, aldosterone and cortisol. She is admitted to hospital following a bad bout of diarrhoea and vomiting accompanied by pain and fever.

On admission, Linda is found to have the following.

- *BP: 95/60 mmHg*
- *Blood glucose level: 4.1 mmol/L*
- *Temperature: 38.6°C*

The immediate management of the patient is rapid assessment, prompt rehydration and correction of the hypoglycaemia. IV hydrocortisone should be administered and then a full history taken to identify the trigger for this crisis event. Antibiotic therapy will have to be considered if the underlying problem is an infection. You will need to assess, record and report findings on a regular basis so as to prevent this problem worsening.

Activity 12.6   *Critical thinking*

Linda's observations gave cause for concern because of her underlying condition.

What action would need to be taken if a patient presented with similar results but also had:

- type 1 diabetes?
- an underactive thyroid?
- no known pre-existing condition, but aged over 70?

An outline answer to this activity is given at the end of the chapter.

Pheochromocytoma

Pheochromocytoma is a very rare tumour of the adrenal medulla that causes extremely high levels of adrenaline and noradrenaline to be secreted into the systemic circulation. It is an emergency that will require the patient to be cared for in intensive care where close monitoring and observation can be carried out continuously. Symptoms of raised catecholamines are:

- tachycardia;
- very severe hypertension;
- hyperglycaemia;
- headaches;
- blurred vision;
- bowel disturbances.

The aim of care is to control and stabilise hypertension with alpha- and beta-blockers followed, once stable, with surgical removal of the tumour. Again, you need to use your sound rapid assessment skills to monitor heart rate and blood pressure and record and report all findings.

Thyroid crisis

Thyroid crisis is a life-threatening condition where sufferers of hyperthyroidism show exaggerated signs and symptoms of hyperthyroidism – fortunately it is very rare. A study by Akamizu et al. (2012) looking at the incidence of thyroid crisis across Japan identified that 0.2 per 100,000 per year were recorded, showing the low numbers of this problem. Thyroid crisis is precipitated by stressors such as:

- infection;
- trauma;
- DKA;
- surgery;
- heart failure;
- stroke.

This oversecretion of thyroid hormones leads to symptoms such as hyperpyrexia, tachycardia, hypertension, agitation and shakes. Management is aimed at reducing the effects of thyroid hormones, T_3 and T_4, until the patient is stable and comfortable. There are some drug therapies that are used and these include sedatives, beta-blockers, hydrocortisone and specific anti-thyroid drugs such as Lugol's iodine and carbimazole. Through good assessment, observation, recording and reporting of findings, the priorities of nursing care for this group of patients include:

- reducing metabolic demands and supporting cardiovascular function;
- providing psychological support;
- preventing complications;
- providing information about disease process/prognosis and therapy needs.

Myxoedema coma

Myxoedema coma is a rare life-threatening form of hypothyroidism, commonly seen in untreated patients. It is a medical emergency and even with early diagnosis and best possible treatment has a high mortality rate of 60% (Vivek et al., 2011). Causes are usually associated with those who have hypothyroidism who are then faced with additional trauma or stress. Most cases appear in winter and hypothermia may play a part, although infections are seen as a predisposing factor. The discontinuation of thyroid supplements needs to be closely managed and sudden discontinuation can be a factor.

Symptoms are those of decreased thyroid hormone secretion and hypometabolic state and are listed in Table 12.7. This hypometabolic state will cause bradycardia and hypotension, which in turn will lead to poor tissue perfusion and metabolic acidosis. Management is aimed at organ support and identifying what has caused the problem, such as administering thyroxin.

The nursing care is rapid assessment using ABCDE approach, with the airway, breathing and circulation as a priority. Patients are usually transferred to ICU for ventilation, CVP monitoring and fluid management.

Cardiovascular	Respiratory	Neurological	Renal	Gastrointestinal	Metabolic
Bradycardia.	Hypoxia.	Confusion.	Fluid retention.	Anorexia.	Hypothermia.
Hypotension.	Hypercarbia.	**Obtundation**.	Hyponatraemia.	Nausea.	Hypoglycaemia.
Low cardiac output.	Pneumonia.	Lethergy. Seizures.	Oedema.	Abdominal pain.	
Cardiogenic shock.		Coma.		Constipation. Paralytic ileus.	

Table 12.7: Symptoms of myxoedema coma

Diabetes insipidus

Diabetes insipidus occurs when the posterior pituitary gland does not produce enough antidiuretic hormone (ADH). There are two forms of diabetes insipidus:

- central diabetes insipidus – inadequate production of ADH caused by neuropathology affecting the pituitary and/or hypothalamus;

- nephrogenic diabetes insipidus – a rare form of the disease where the kidneys become insensitive to ADH.

In both cases it results in polyuria and polydipsia causing intense hypovolaemia and hyponatraemia. Treatment is with replacement ADH in the form of desmopressin (DDAVP).

Syndrome of inappropriate antidiuretic hormone hypersecretion

Syndrome of inappropriate antidiuretic hormone hypersecretion is a problem of persistent abnormally high levels of ADH in the absence of stimuli, with normal renal function. The feedback mechanism is impaired and the posterior pituitary continues to release ADH (Gross, 2012), and the renal tubules continue to absorb free water regardless of serum osmolality. It is caused by neuropathology such as head injury, subarachnoid haemorrhage and surgery on the pituitary gland, and also by some carcinomas, pulmonary infections (pneumonia), nervous system infections (meningitis) and drugs. The disease causes fluid retention with the potential for fluid overload and resulting haemodilution of solutes. It is a common cause of hyponatraemia accounting for almost a third of all cases.

Management involves treating the underlying cause and fluid restriction (500–1000 ml/day). In severe hyponatraemia 3% saline can be given with care and frusemide can be given with close monitoring of potassium levels. Nursing management involves:

- frequent neuro assessment with mental status and assessment of level of consciousness;

- pulmonary assessment and watching for signs and symptoms of fluid overload;

- cardiac assessment watching for dysrhythmias and BP abnormalities;

- monitoring for seizure activity;

- accurate measurement of input/output;

- daily weighing, same time each day, same scale, same clothes;

- oral hygiene;

- reducing stress, pain and discomfort.

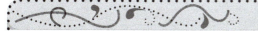

Chapter summary

This chapter has outlined the most common endocrine problems likely to be seen in clinical practice, and explored the skills needed for assessing, recognising and responding to patients presenting with these problems. It has concentrated on the conditions most likely to present as emergencies, primarily complications of diabetes mellitus: hypoglycaemia,

(Continued)

continued . . . . •

DKA and HHS. The nurse's responsibilities are similar in all of these problems, but as the causes are different, health professionals need to be alert to the possible meaning of different clusters of symptoms.

Nurses can come across patients with diabetes mellitus in any clinical speciality but, with good assessment and early recognition, prioritisation and intervention, problems can be minimised.

This chapter has also looked at other endocrine disorders that may be encountered, and has emphasised that often it is patients themselves who are the experts on their own condition.

Activities: brief outline answers

Activity 12.1: Critical thinking (page 258)

1. Mr Evans's aggression could have been a developing problem and Millie should have sought help from her mentor at this point.
2. Aggression is a common sign of raised or rising blood glucose levels.
3. Mr Evans needs to be given insulin, usually as fixed rate intravenous insulin infusion (FRIII) (see Table 12.5) in the first instance.
4. Yes, as it is above the normal limits of 4–7 mmol/L and probably rising if no treatment is given.

Activity 12.2: Evidence-based practice and research (page 263)

This is predominantly a discussion issue, but from the work of the NDIA it is clear that errors in insulin prescribing, medication and administration keep occurring at an alarming level. The key to preventing this is continuous education at all clinical levels from nursing staff through to consultants. By mining into the data that the NDIA provide it can be seen that a lot of the problem is in the prescription, where new doctors have written up the insulin in the incorrect way, but it is clear to see that administration errors still occur and these can only be prevented with good education and awareness of the problem.

Activity 12.3: Evidence-based practice and research (page 267)

Those with type 2 diabetes mellitus are still producing a small level of insulin and this protects against **gluconeogenesis** and the production of ketone bodies.

Activity 12.4: Evidence-based practice and research (page 268)

Look for symptoms such as:

- frequent urination
- thirst
- nausea
- dry skin
- disorientation leading to drowsiness and gradual loss of consciousness.

Activity 12.5: Communication (page 269)

Advice for Ashya and Sanjit should include the following.

- Always take your diabetes medication, even if you feel unwell and can't eat.
- If you monitor your blood glucose, you may need to test more frequently.

- Contact your healthcare team if your blood glucose levels remain high (>15 mmol/L).
- Drink plenty of unsweetened fluids.
- If you can't eat, replace meals with snacks and drinks, containing carbohydrate.

If the above advice is followed, then control of Sanjit's blood glucose will stabilise. This will mean that he will not continue to need insulin although, as he gets older, he may find that taking insulin as part of his type 2 diabetes treatment will become necessary. He will have to balance his dietary habits, eating more complex carbohydrates, non-starchy vegetables, less fat and protein and increase his exercise.

Do be aware that people don't always remember information that is given to them by word of mouth, especially if they are unwell or upset at the time they are told it. So make sure you have leaflets and other written materials to give the family to take away. This will both back up what you have said and ensure that they continue to have access to information.

Leaflets on many aspects of diabetes and its management can be downloaded from the Diabetes UK website: **www.diabetes.org.uk**.

Activity 12.6: Critical thinking (pages 270–1)

Type 1 diabetes mellitus – treatment would be the same as Linda's but with the emphasis also being on getting glucose into the patient to increase their blood glucose levels.

An underactive thyroid – up to 1–5 people with Addison's disease will develop autoimmune thyroid problems with the most common being hypothyroid disease. Bloods would be needed for thyroid levels:

- thyroid-stimulating hormone (TSH) assay result is >4.0 mU/L (normal values: 0.5–1.5 mU/L). Normal value excludes primary hypothyroidism and a markedly elevated value confirms the diagnosis;
- thyroxine (T4) radioimmunoassay decreased (normal values: 5.0–12.0 µg/dL). Reflects underproduction of thyroid hormones; monitors response to therapy;
- tri-iodothyronine (T3) radioimmunoassay decreased (normal values: 80–230 ng/dL). Reflects underproduction of thyroid hormones.

Other tests required:

- electrocardiogram (ECG) reveals low voltage, T wave abnormalities;
- other tests: 24-hour radioactive iodine uptake; thyroid autoantibodies; antithyroglobulin.

Once Addison's disease is stable then the patient could go home with regular appointments for blood levels until thyroid levels are under control.

No known pre-existing condition, but aged over 70 – those with Addison's disease can expect to live a long and normal life as long as they have control and manage the disease properly. Therefore, this group of patients would be treated the same, but with the extra care that the elderly need.

Further reading

Bilous, R and Donnelly, R (2010) *Handbook of Diabetes*. Fourth Edition. London: Wiley-Blackwell.

See especially Chapter 1 (Introduction to diabetes), Chapter 12 (Diabetic ketoacidosis, hyperglycaemic hyperosmolar state and lactic acidosis) and Chapter 13 (Hypoglycaemia).

White, K and Arlt, W (2010) Adrenal crisis in treated Addison's disease: a predictable but undermanaged event. *European Society of Endocrinology*. Jan 1, 162, 115–20.

Useful websites

www.diabetes.org.uk

Diabetes UK has a very informative website, with pages for professionals and pages for patients. There are also a lot of resources and information sheets to download or purchase. As well as exploring the site yourself, you should also make sure any patients with diabetes, and their family members, know about it.

www.Idf.org

International Diabetes Federation.

www.iddt.org

Independent Diabetes Trust.

www.uptodate.com

UpToDate – useful for all endocrine problems.

www.youtube.com/watch?v=yIc2XFNLhm8

Physiology of DKA.

Chapter 13
Conclusion
Lessons learned – an action plan for practice
Desiree Tait

The chapters in this book have provided an opportunity for you to explore the clinical assessment and rapid decision-making skills required to manage acute and critically ill patients. The patient case studies and scenarios used in the book are fictional, but the physiological and psychological data used are based on real situations. Reading the scenarios and working through the activities in each chapter have given you an opportunity to rehearse situations in a safe environment and reflect on their outcome. The key messages that have emerged from this book can be summarised as follows.

- Always use a comprehensive, systematic and holistic approach to nursing assessment.
- Always interpret the findings from your assessment and determine a diagnosis of the current situation.
- Always respond to your findings in a timely manner, ensuring that you communicate your concerns and review the situation.
- Always provide support and protection for vulnerable people in your care.
- Always provide a person-centred approach to care and ensure that you acknowledge and communicate the wishes and concerns of the patient and families when delivering nursing care.
- Always demonstrate a collaborative approach to care.

Within the chapters we have discussed the care of acutely ill patients and those at risk of deterioration in acute and critical care settings in both community and hospital environments. It is important to recognise that the rapid decision-making skills required to manage these patients safely are the same wherever the patient is located, although the access to interventions may vary depending on the facilities available.

Developing an action plan for practice

In your role as a senior student and as a qualified nurse, your priority will be to ensure that you meet the standards and competencies set by the NMC (2010). After you qualify as a registered nurse, these standards will continue to be a basis from which to develop your practice as well as to teach others. According to Benner et al. (2011), rapid assessment and understanding of the patient's condition is based on the nurse's ability to interpret, recognise and respond to patterns and trends in the patient's behaviour and physiological data. This ability comes from knowledge and experience developed over time, the presence of leadership and organisational skills, and the presence of clinical forethought (the ability to anticipate and act on potential problems). The development towards proficient and expert practice involves the refinement of clinical knowledge and evidence-based practice so that an intuitive and automatic understanding of practice is achieved. In order to continue to develop and expand your clinical decision-making skills, we have identified five action points that you can use on your journey.

1. *Never lose your willingness to learn.* Nursing and healthcare practice is a dynamic and innovative environment; use every opportunity you have to learn and develop your practice.

2. *Know your patients and always be receptive to their condition.* The patient, or client, is the person who lives with the experience of their condition. They know and sense when something has changed and it is reasonable to assume that knowing and understanding your patient will help you to interpret their condition quickly and effectively.

3. *Reflect on your nursing experiences and question the issues raised.* When reflecting on your practice, question and challenge your decision making. Can you justify the decisions you made with an evidence base? How strong is that evidence base? Do you need to explore this issue in more detail?

4. *Combine your knowledge from experience with evidence-based practice.* Clinical reasoning and decision making can be guided by an evidence base such as clinical pathways and care bundles, research and theoretical frameworks. It is also important to remember that each patient is an individual, and the clinical value of all evidence-based interventions needs to be judged in the context of individualised patient care.

5. *Continue to work collaboratively with colleagues and demonstrate emotional intelligence when communicating with others.* In order to collaborate effectively with others you need to be aware of your own emotions and their impact on others, know your strengths and limitations, and have a sense of self-worth. You need to have an empathic awareness of others, with political and social awareness, so that you can interpret and manage communication between individuals and groups.

These action points will guide you on the path to professional maturity when involved in direct care and when collaborating with others. Nursing is a dynamic and exciting profession with a continuing demand to question, and learn from, practice and is a journey to be enjoyed.

Glossary

abrasive trauma   a process of wearing away a surface area of the skin/mucous membrane by friction resulting from trauma.

activated partial thromboplastin (APPT)   a measure of the efficiency of activation and duration of clotting time.

acute pain   pain that is temporary, resulting from surgery, an injury or an infection.

acute pancreatitis   a sudden and often severe inflammation and swelling of the pancreas. The pancreas is normally protected from the digestive enzymes that it produces; however, during an acute episode the pancreatic enzymes begin to digest the tissue of the pancreas. In severe cases this is described as acute necrotising pancreatitis. The most common cause is alcohol abuse.

adenosine triphosphate (ATP)   a chemical in cells that is able to release energy during a chemical reaction. It is the major source of energy for all the body's cellular functions.

advanced trauma life support   a safe reliable method for immediate management of the injured trauma patient.

aldosterone   a hormone that increases the reabsorption of sodium ions and water. This increases circulating blood volume and blood pressure.

aminophylline   a drug used to prevent and treat wheezing, breathlessness and dyspnoea associated with asthma and COPD. It works by relaxing and dilating the bronchi in the respiratory system and making it easier for the patient to breathe. Side effects include an increase in heart rate and risk of cardiac arrhythmias, restlessness and irritability.

angiotensin I   an inactive chemical that is triggered by the release of renin and activated by an enzyme to produce angiotensin II.

angiotensin II   once activated by the renin angiotensin system, angiotensin II exerts a vasoconstrictor effect, increases a sensation for thirst and ultimately increases blood pressure.

angiotensin converting enzyme (ACE)   an enzyme secreted by the pulmonary endothelial cells to act as a catalyst in the conversion of angiotensin I to angiotensin II.

antidiuretic hormone (ADH)   a hormone that increases the concentration of urine (osmolarity) and reduces the excretion of water by the kidneys. It also has a powerful vasopressor effect, thus increasing peripheral resistance and blood pressure; also known as vasopressin.

benzodiazepines   a group of drugs that have a number of sedative, muscle relaxant and amnesic effects. They are prescribed to relieve anxiety, induce sleep, as an anticonvulsant in the management of seizures, to relieve muscle spasm and to manage alcohol withdrawal.

beta agonist   a group of drugs that include salbutamol and are effective in causing bronchodilation. They relieve bronchospasm, wheezing and breathlessness. They are most frequently administered by the inhalation route and can have an effect in just a few minutes. Side effects include an increase in heart rate and risk of cardiac arrhythmias, restlessness, anxiety and shaking/tremor in the limbs. The side effects usually last for only a few minutes.

bradykinin   a protein found in the body that when released causes vasodilation during the inflammatory response and when systemic can lead to a reduction in blood pressure.

carbon monoxide poisoning   occurs following enough inhalation of carbon monoxide gas (CO), a colourless, odourless and tasteless toxic gas found in appliances such as gas boilers and in exhaust fumes from older vehicles. CO poisoning is potentially fatal because of the ability of the CO to bind to haemoglobin. As a result the body is unable to carry enough oxygen to the tissues and organs.

cardiogenic shock   occurs when there is an inadequate circulation of blood to the body's organs and tissues due to primary failure of the ventricles of the heart to function effectively.

central venous pressure   the blood pressure in the vena cava, the blood vessel returning to the right atrium of the heart. Measuring the CVP allows you to measure the amount of blood returning to the heart and is an indication of fluid balance in the circulation. When the CVP is low, the patient may be suffering from hypovolaemia; when it is high, the patient may be fluid overloaded or suffering from right-sided cardiac pump failure leading to a backlog of blood in the venous circulation.

cerebrospinal fluid   a bodily fluid that occupies the subarachnoid space and the ventricular system around and inside the brain and spinal cord.

chronic pain   pain that lasts longer than three months. It is different from acute pain in that it is not easy to find the cause, and diagnosis can reveal no injury in the body at all, yet the patient can be experiencing very debilitating pain.

clotting time   the time required for blood to form a clot.

Colles fracture   a fracture of the distal radius in the forearm with dorsal (posterior) displacement of the wrist and hand. The fracture is sometimes referred to as a 'dinner fork' or 'bayonet' deformity due to the shape of the resultant forearm.

compensatory stage of shock   the second stage of shock, which occurs when the body has triggered compensatory mechanisms to improve blood supply to organs and tissues in order to maintain homeostasis.

complement system   a system made up of plasma proteins that react with one another to make pathogens such as a bacterial infection easier to break down and digest. Overall the system induces a series of inflammatory responses that help to fight infection.

CRP   a blood test to measure the levels of C-reactive protein in the blood. This gives information about the presence of infection.

distributive shock   occurs when there is inadequate circulation of the blood to the body's organs and tissues due to the systemic dilation of blood vessels. This is found, for example, in anaphylactic shock and septic shock.

dobutamine   a drug that stimulates the beta receptors of the sympathetic nervous system. It is used to improve cardiac output in patients with cardiogenic shock.

dopamine   a neurotransmitter acting on receptors in the brain. It acts on the sympathetic nervous system to increase heart rate and blood pressure.

dysoxia see   tissue dysoxia.

dyspnoea   a term used to describe difficult or laboured breathing and is often associated with breathlessness.

empirical antibiotic therapy   refers to the commencement of treatment before a firm diagnosis is reached. In the case of infection, patients are prescribed broad spectrum antibiotics until the microorganisms are cultured and diagnosed. The antibiotics may then be changed if the micro-organisms are not sensitive to the prescribed medication.

escharotomy   provides a release of tissue constriction that compromises the underlying structures, whether those are circulatory or respiratory structures. Untreated, the tissue constriction will lead to loss of limbs by compromising the circulation, or death by constricting chest movement and preventing lung expansion.

FBC   full blood count – a test to discover whether the different elements of a person's blood are in the correct proportions.

gate control theory   a theory proposed by Ronald Melzack and Patrick Wall in 1965 to explain the multidimensional nature of pain. The theory explains that an individual's pain experience can be modulated by stimulating neural gates in the spinal cord to open or close. Thus the pain experience can be moderated by, for example, rubbing it better or diversionary therapy.

glomerular filtration rate   the number of millilitres of blood the kidneys are able to filter in one minute. The lower the rate, the less effectively the kidneys are working.

glucogenolysis   the splitting up of glycogen in the liver, yielding glucose.

gluconeogenesis   the synthesis of glucose from non-carbohydrate sources, such as amino acids and glycerol. It occurs primarily in the liver and kidneys whenever the supply of carbohydrates is insufficient to meet the body's energy needs.

Guillain-Barré syndrome   a neurological disorder that occurs when the body's immune system attacks part of the peripheral nervous system. This can lead to symptoms such as muscle weakness, paralysis, breathing difficulties and an unstable heart rate and blood pressure. Most people who get the disease can make a complete recovery although initially the disorder is considered a medical emergency.

haemoserous fluid   blood-stained fluid that is leaking from the wound (haemoserous means 'stained with blood').

histamine   chemical released by the mast cells as part of the inflammatory response. Its action is to dilate blood vessels and increase capillary permeability to white blood cells in order to fight the pathogens in infected tissues.

hyperkalaemia   the medical term that describes a potassium level in the blood that's higher than normal. The blood potassium level is normally 3.6 to 5.2 millimoles per litre (mmol/L).

hyperlipidaemia   refers to raised blood levels of cholesterol. Raised levels of cholesterol, in combination with other risk factors, can increase the risk of stroke and/or heart disease.

hyponatraemia   the medical term for low sodium levels in the blood. The normal range is 135–45 mEq/L. Many medical illnesses, such as congestive heart failure, liver failure, renal failure, diabetes or pneumonia, may be associated with hyponatraemia.

hypovolaemic shock   occurs when there is inadequate circulation of the blood to the body's organs and tissues due to loss of blood or body fluids.

idiopathic   relating to or denoting any disease or condition which arises spontaneously or for which the cause is unknown.

inflammatory mediators   various chemicals that, when released by immune cells, cause vasodilation and bring about an inflammatory response.

initial stage of shock   the first stage of shock, which occurs when the body begins to recognise and respond to a reduction in blood flow to the organs and tissues.

inotropic therapy   includes the use of drugs that improve the force of muscle contraction and are said to have a positive inotropic effect.

interleukins   a family of proteins that control some aspects of the immune response. They do this by conveying signals between white blood cells.

intubated (intubation)   the placement of a flexible, cuffed tube into the trachea in order to maintain an open airway and facilitate processes such as assisted ventilation, administering anaesthesia during surgical procedures and to prevent airway obstruction and/or accidental inhalation of toxic substances; referred to as tracheal intubation.

invasive ventilation   intubation and respiratory support provided either to assist normal breathing or, in some cases, to replace normal breathing. Patients usually require sedation when receiving invasive ventilation.

iron lung   a large cylindrical steel chamber. Patients lay in the chamber with only their head and neck free. The chamber was airtight, and at set intervals the atmospheric pressure inside the chamber was reduced to lower than atmospheric pressure. This change in pressure reduced the work of breathing for the patient and the patient was able to take a deeper breath (increase their tidal volume). When the interchamber pressure returned to normal, the patient exhaled normally.

ischaemia   a restriction in blood supply, and therefore in the supply of oxygen, to tissues.

kinins   any of a group of substances formed in body tissue in response to injury.

Kussmaul breathing   a very deep, repetitive, gasping respiratory pattern associated with profound acidosis (e.g., diabetic ketoacidosis).

laparoscopic cholecystectomy   the surgical removal of the gall bladder using a minimally invasive technique.

leukotrienes   any of a group of physiologically active substances that possibly function as mediators during acute inflammatory responses.

lymphocytes   a family of white blood cells that are responsible for defending the body against infection and damage. They include B lymphocytes that attack bacteria and toxins, and T lymphocytes that attack cells that have been taken over by a damaging organism such as a virus or by cancerous cells.

Manchester triage   a formalised standard of triage relying on a list of presenting complaints, each with its own flow chart to aid determining the priority of the presenting complaint.

mandibular   refers to any tissue or bony structure that makes up the lower jaw.

midazolam   a short-acting drug of the benzodiazepine family. It is used to induce sedation and amnesia before and during medical procedures, to treat acute seizures, and as sedation in the management of ventilated patients.

monocyte   a type of white blood cell that plays a role in the inflammatory and immune response. Monocytes can develop either into dendritic cells that play a role in the antibody antigen response or into macrophages, which are cells that eat other damaged cells.

muscarinic antagonist   a group of drugs, also known as anticholinergic drugs, and include ipratropium bromide (atrovent). They work causing bronchodilation in the lungs and are used to treat asthma and COPD. They are administered by inhalation and patients may complain of a dry mouth when taking these drugs.

nephrotoxic   the poisonous effect of medication on the kidneys.

neutrophil   the most common type of white blood cell that acts as the first line of defence when the inflammatory response is triggered. Neutrophils will recognise anything that should not be present in the body as an invader and destroy it.

nitric oxide   a compound that acts as a vasodilator, helps to regulate the uptake of oxygen in cells and can destroy viruses and cancer cells as part of the immune system.

nitrous oxide   a colourless, non-flammable chemical compound used in medicine for its analgesic, anaesthetic and anxiolytic effects, usually administered by inhalation and distributed through the lungs by diffusion.

nociceptive pain   is caused by stimulation of peripheral nerve fibres that respond only to stimuli approaching or exceeding harmful intensity, the most common categories being thermal, mechanical and chemical.

nociceptors   sensory neurons that are found in any area of the body that can sense pain either externally or internally.

non-steroidal anti-inflammatory drugs (NSAIDs)   a group of drugs that have analgesic, anti-inflammatory and antipyretic effects. These drugs can cause dyspepsia and gastric ulceration.

obstructive shock   occurs when there is inadequate circulation of the blood to the body's organs and tissues due to physical obstruction of blood flow from the heart or aorta, such as in cardiac tamponade when the pericardial sac fills with blood and squashes the ventricles.

obstructive sleep apnoea   a condition characterised by repeated intermittent obstruction or collapse of the upper airways during sleep, often accompanied by loud snoring. The patient experiences periods of apnoea (no breathing), tiredness and lethargy.

obtundation   less than full alertness.

oedema   an excessive accumulation of serous fluid in the intercellular spaces of tissue.

osmolarity   the measure of the concentration of solute particles in a solution.

phagocytosis   the process that cells such as neutrophils use to destroy dead or foreign cells by ingesting or engulfing them.

phlebitis   the inflammation of the walls of the vein.

pneumothorax   a collection of air that has leaked into the space between the layers of the lung sac. The lung is contained in two sacs: the visceral and parietal layers of the pleura. The parietal layer lines the thoracic wall and the visceral layer covers all the surfaces of the lungs. Leakage of air into the pleural space can build up and cause the lung to collapse. When this happens the patient is unable to take a deep breath and becomes breathless and dyspnoeic.

polydipsia   abnormally great thirst as a symptom of disease (such as diabetes) or psychological disturbance.

polyuria   production of abnormally large volumes of dilute urine.

primary survey   a methodical process used to quickly identify immediate life-threatening injuries and conditions that require immediate attention.

progressive stage of shock   the third stage of shock, which occurs when the underlying cause of the shock has not been corrected and the body is no longer able to compensate for the reduction in blood flow. Cell damage becomes more severe over time and can be irreversible.

prostaglandins   a group of substances that influence a number of body functions such as the dilation and constriction of blood vessels, control of blood pressure and the inflammatory response. They are also influential in the promotion of uterine contractions during childbirth.

prothrombin time (PT)   a blood test that measures how long it takes blood to clot. It is also known as an INR test (international normalised ratio) when the results are standardised to facilitate wider standard interpretation.

pulmonary embolism   occurs when a blood vessel supplying blood to the lungs becomes clogged by a blood clot or embolus. This prevents an amount of blood from perfusing the alveoli and as a result the body receives a reduced supply of oxygenated blood.

refractory stage of shock   the fourth and final stage of shock, which occurs when the body's organs begin to fail due to a sustained lack of oxygen and nutrients; eventually the organs completely fail and this leads to death.

renin-angiotensin-aldosterone mechanism   a hormone system that helps to regulate fluid balance and blood pressure. The system forms part of the body's response to shock.

respiratory depression   a respiration that has a rate below 12 breaths per minute or that fails to provide full ventilation and perfusion of the lungs.

revascularisation   restoration of circulation to tissues after this has been compromised by accident or ischaemia.

secondary survey   a complete examination of the patient from top to toe, both front and back.

septic shock   shock caused by decreased tissue perfusion and oxygen delivery as a result of severe infection and sepsis, and it can cause multiple organ dysfunction syndrome (formerly known as multiple organ failure).

somatic pain   pain arising from tissues such as skin, muscle, tendon, joint capsules, fasciae and bone.

ST segment   this is the normally flat line between the s and t segment of the pqrst wave form found in an electrocardiograph (ECG). The ECG records the electrical wave pattern of conduction as the message for the heart muscle to contract spreads through the heart recording the pattern of a person's heartbeat.

STEMI   This is an abbreviation of 'ST elevation myocardial infarction'. The ST segment located over the damaged area of the heart in a 12-lead ECG becomes elevated as part of the inflammatory response and indicates an area of muscle that has been starved of a blood supply.

tachypnoea   rapid breathing or respiration.

tissue dysoxia   a very low concentration of oxygen in the body tissues.

tumor necrosis factor (TNF)   one of the cytokines that is influential in the inflammatory response. TNF induces cell death in cancer cells and is involved in stimulating the inflammatory response.

U&E   a blood test to measure the levels of urea and electrolytes in a person's blood. This can give valuable information about the person's kidney function.

vascular permeability   the degree to which one substance allows another substance to pass through it.

vasodilation   the widening of blood vessels resulting from the relaxation of the muscular wall of the blood vessels.

vasopressin   see antidiuretic hormone (ADH).

ventilation a method used to assist spontaneous breathing. The techniques available include non-invasive ventilation where respiratory support is provided through a tight-fitting mask and the patient continues to breathe with support.

visceral pain pain arising from the internal organs; patients state the pain feels like squeezing, cramping or pressure.

References

Adam, S, Odell, M and Welch, J (2010) *Rapid Assessment of the Acutely Ill Patient*. Oxford: Wiley Blackwell.

Akamizu, T, Satoh, T, Isozaki, O et al. (2012) Diagnostic criteria, clinical features, and incidence of thyroid storm based on nationwide surveys. *Thyroid*, 22(7): 661.

Alce, T, Page, V and Vizcaychipi, M (2014) Delirium, in Bersten, A and Soni, N (eds) *Oh's Intensive Care Manual*. Seventh edition. Oxford: Butterworth Heinemann Elsevier.

Aldemir, M, Ozen, S, Kara, O et al. (2001) Predisposing factors for delirium in the surgical intensive care unit. *Critical Care*, 5: 265–70.

American Association of Critical Care Nurses (2015) *Implementing the ABCDE Bundle at the Bedside*. Accessed at: www.aacn.org/wd/practice/content/actionpak/withlinks-ABCDE-ToolKit.content?menu=practice

American College of Surgeons (2008) *ATLS, Advanced Trauma Life Support Program for Doctors*. Chicago, IL: American College of Surgeons.

American Psychiatric Association (2013) *Diagnostic and Statistical Manual of Mental Disorders (DSM-5)*. Fifth edition. Virginia: The American Psychiatric Association.

Arbour, C, Gélinas, C and Michaud, C (2011) Impact of the implementation of the critical-care pain observational tool (CPOT) on pain management and clinical outcomes in mechanically ventilated trauma intensive care units patients: a pilot study. *Journal of Trauma Nursing*, 18(1): 52–60.

Arend, E and Christensen, M (2009) Delirium in the intensive care unit: a review. *Nursing in Critical Care*, 14(3): 145–54.

Babaev, A, Frederick, P, Pasta, D, Every, N, Sichrovsky, T and Hochman, J for the NRMI Investigators (2005) Trends in management and outcome of patients with acute myocardial infarction complicated by cardiogenic shock. *Journal of the American Medical Association*, 294(4): 448–54.

Balas, M, Vasilevskis, E, Burke, W et al. (2012) Critical care nurses' role in implementing the 'ABCDE bundle' into practice. *Critical Care Nurse*, 32(2): 35–48.

Beel-Bates, C and Rogers, A (1990) An exploratory study of sundown syndrome. *Journal of Neuroscience Nursing*, 22: 51–2.

Bellomo, R (2014) Acute kidney injury, in Bersten, A and Soni, N (eds) *Oh's Intensive Care Manual*. Seventh edition. Oxford: Butterworth Heineman Elsevier.

Benner, P, Hooper-Kyriakidis, P and Stannard, D (2010) *Clinical Wisdom and Interventions in Critical Care*. Second edition. Philadelphia, PA: WB Saunders Company.

Bersten, A (2014) Acute respiratory distress syndrome, in Bersten, A and Soni, N (2014) *Oh's Intensive Care Manual*. Seventh edition. Oxford: Butterworth Heinemann Elsevier.

Bersten, A and Soni, N (eds) (2014) *Oh's Intensive Care Manual*. Seventh edition. Oxford: Butterworth Heinemann Elsevier.

Bilous, R and Donnelly, R (2010) *Handbook of Diabetes*. Fourth edition. London: Wiley-Blackwell.

Blitz, M, Blitz, S, Hughes, R et al. (2005) Aerosolized magnesium sulfate for acute asthma: a systematic review. *Chest*, 128(1): 337–44.

BMA (British Medical Association), Resuscitation Council (UK) and RCN (Royal College of Nursing) (2014) *Decisions Relating to Cardiopulmonary Resuscitation*. London: British Medical Association.

BNF (2013) *BNF 66 September 2013 – March 2014*. London: BMA Royal Pharmaceutical Society.

Borthwick, M, Bourne, R, Craig, M, Egan, A and Oxley, J (2003) *Evolution of Intensive Care in the UK*. Intensive Care Society. Accessed at: www.ics.ac.uk/ics-homepage/guidelines-and-standards

Borthwick, M, Bourne, R, Craig, M et al. (2006) *Detection, Prevention and Treatment of Delirium in Critically Ill Patients*. Leicester: United Kingdom Clinical Pharmacy Association.

Bray, K, Hill, K, Robson, W et al. (2004) British Association of Critical Care Nurses' position statement on the use of restraint in adult critical care units. *Nursing in Critical Care*, 9(5): 199–212.

Brenner, B, Corbridge, T and Kazzi, A (2009) Intubation and mechanical ventilation of the asthmatic patient in respiratory failure. *Proceedings of the American Thoracic Society*, 6: 371–9.

Bridges, E and Dukes, S (2005) Cardiovascular aspects of septic shock: pathophysiology, monitoring and treatment. *Critical Care Nurse*, 25(2): 14–40.

BTS, RCP and ICS (2008) *The Use of Non-Invasive Ventilation in the Management of Patients with Chronic Obstructive Pulmonary Disease Admitted to Hospital with Acute Type II Respiratory Failure*. Accessed at: www.brit-thoracic.org.uk/document-library/clinical-information/niv/niv-guidelines/the-use-of-non-invasive-ventilation-in-the-management-of-patients-with-copd-admitted-to-hospital-with-acute-type-ii-respiratory-failure

BTS (British Thoracic Society) and SIGN (Scottish Intercollegiate Guidelines Network) (2014) *British Guidelines on the Management of Asthma*. Accessed at: www.brit-thoracic.org.uk/guidelines-and-quality-standards/asthma-guideline

Bucaloiu, I, Kirchner, H, Norfolk, E, Hartle, J and Perkins, R (2012) Increased risk of death and de novo chronic kidney disease following reversible acute kidney injury. *Kidney International*, 81(5): 477–85.

Carbery, C (2008) Basic concepts in mechanical ventilation. *Journal of Perioperative Practice*, 18(3): 106–14.

Carville, S, Wonderling, D and Stevens, P (2014) Early identification and management of chronic kidney disease in adults: summary of updated NICE guidance. *British Medical Journal*, 349: g4507.

Cecconi, M, De Backer, D, Antonelli, M et al. (2014) Consensus on circulatory shock and haemodynamic monitoring. Task force of the European Society of Intensive Care Medicine. *Intensive Care Medicine*, 40(12): 1795–815.

Chen, H, Liu, J, Chen, L and Wang, G (2014) Effectiveness of daily interruption of sedation in sedated patients with mechanical ventilation in ICU: a systematic review. *International Journal of Nursing Sciences*, 1(4): 346–51.

Coca, S, Singanamalas, S and Parikh, C (2012) Chronic kidney disease after acute injury: a systematic review and meta-analysis. *Kidney International*, 81: 442–8.

Cole, E (2009) *Trauma Care: Initial Assessment and Management in the Emergency Department*. Oxford: Blackwell Publishing.

Coulter Smith, MA, Smith, P and Crow, R (2014) A critical review: a combined conceptual framework of severity of illness and clinical judgement for analysing diagnostic judgements in critical illness. *Journal of Clinical Nursing*, 23(5–6): 784–98.

References

Creed, F and Spiers, C (eds) (2010) *Care of the Acutely Ill Adult: An Essential Guide for Nurses.* Oxford: Oxford University Press.

Creed, F, Dawson, J and Looker, K (2010) Assessment tools and track and trigger systems, in Creed, F and Spiers, C (eds) *Care of the Acutely Ill Adult: An Essential Guide for Nurses.* Oxford: Oxford University Press.

Daniels, R (2013) *Survive Sepsis.* Third edition. Sutton Coldfield: UK Sepsis Trust.

Daniels, R and Nutbeam, T (eds) (2010) *ABC of Sepsis (ABC Series).* Oxford: Wiley-Blackwell.

Dayton, E and Henriksen, K (2007) Communication failure: basic components, contributing factors and the call for structure. *Joint Commission Journal on Quality and Patient Safety,* 33(1): 34–47.

De Gaudio, A (2014) Severe sepsis, in Bersten, A and Soni, N (eds) *Oh's Intensive Care Manual.* Seventh edition. Oxford: Butterworth Heinemann Elsevier.

Dellinger, R, Levy, M, Rhodes, A et al. (2013) Surviving sepsis campaign: international guidelines for management of severe sepsis and septic shock: 2012. *Critical Care Medicine,* 41(2): 580–637.

Department of Health (2000) *Comprehensive Critical Care: A Review of Adult Critical Care Services.* London: The Stationery Office.

Dougherty, L and Lister, S (2008) *The Royal Marsden Hospital Manual of Clinical Nursing Procedure.* Seventh edition. Oxford: Wiley-Blackwell.

Duffield, C, Roche, M, Diers, D, Catling-Paull, C and Blay, N (2010) Staffing, skill mix and the model of care. *Journal of Clinical Nursing,* 19: 2242–51.

Edwards, M and Griffiths, P (2011) *Emergency Nursing Made Incredibly Easy.* London: Lippincott Williams & Wilkins.

Elliot, M, Worrall-Carter, L and Page, K (2014) Intensive care readmission: a contemporary review of the literature. *Intensive and Critical Care Nursing,* 30: 121–37.

Ely, E (2014) *Confusion Assessment Method for the ICU (CAM-ICU): The Complete Training Manual.* Vanderbilt University Medical Centre. Accessed at: www.icudelirium.org/docs/CAM_ICU_training.pdf

Ely, E, Margolin, R, Francis, J et al. (2001) Evaluation of delirium in critically ill patients: validation of the confusion assessment method for the intensive care unit (CAM-ICU). *Critical Care Medicine,* 29(7): 1370–9.

Ely, E, Truman, B, Shintani, A et al. (2003) Monitoring sedation status over time in ICU patients: reliability and validity of the Richmond Agitation-Sedation Scale (RASS). *Journal of the American Medical Association,* 289(22): 2983–91.

Eom, J, Lee, M, Chun, H et al. (2014) The impact of a ventilator bundle on preventing ventilator-associated pneumonia: a multi-centre study. *American Journal of Infection Control,* 42: 34–7.

European Delirium Association and American Delirium Society (2014) The DSM-5 criteria, level of arousal and delirium diagnosis: inclusiveness is safer. *Biomed Central Medicine,* 12(141): 1–4.

Fairbrother, G, Jones, A and Rivas, K (2010) Changing model of nursing care from individual patient allocation to team nursing in the acute inpatient environment. *Contemporary Nurse,* 35(2): 202–20.

Fleming, S and Todd, N (1998) Cardiorespiratory physiology, in Shuldham, C (ed) *Cardiorespiratory Nursing.* London: Stanley-Thornes.

Fliser, D, Laville, M and Covic, A (2012) A European Renal Best Practice (ERBP) position statement on the Kidney Disease Improving Global Outcomes (KDIGO) clinical practice guidelines on acute kidney injury:

part 1 – definitions, conservative management and contrast-induced nephropathy. *Nephrology Dialysis Transplant*, 27(12): 4263–72.

Franklin, C and Matthew, J (1994) Developing strategies to prevent in hospital cardiac arrest: analysing responses of physicians and nurses in the hours before the event. *Critical Care Medicine*, 22: 244–7.

Frost, P (2015) Intravenous fluid therapy in adult inpatients. *British Medical Journal*, 350: g7620.

Fulbrook, P and Mooney, S (2003) Care bundles in critical care: a practical approach to evidence based practice. *Nursing in Critical Care*, 8: 249–55.

GAIN (2014) *Guidelines for the Treatment of Hyperkalaemia in Adults* GAIN. Accessed at: www.gain-ni.org/images/Uploads/Guidelines/GAIN_Guidelines_Treatment_of_Hyperkalaemia_in_Adults_GAIN_02_12_2014.pdf

Gao, H, McDonnell, A, Harrison, DA et al. (2007) Systematic review and evaluation of physiological track and trigger warning systems for identifying at-risk patients on the ward. *Intensive Care Medicine*, 33: 667–79.

Gowda, R, Fox, J and Khan, I (2008) Cardiogenic shock: basics and clinical considerations. *International Journal of Cardiology*, 123: 221–8.

Green, D, Ervine, E and White, S (2003) *Fundamentals of Perioperative Management.* London: Greenwich Medical Media.

Gross, P (2012) Clinical management of SIADH. *Therapeutic Advances in Endocrinology and Metabolism*, 3(2): 61–73.

Grossbach, I, Chlan, L and Tracy, M (2011) Overview of mechanical ventilator support and management of patient- and ventilator-related responses. *Critical Care Nurse*, 31(3): 30–44.

Grossman, S and Porth, CM (2013) *Porth's Physiology: Concepts of Altered Health States.* Ninth edition. Philadelphia, PA: Wolters Kluwer/Lippincott Williams & Wilkins.

Hall, J (2011) *Guyton and Hall: Textbook of Medical Physiology.* Twelfth edition. Philadelphia, PA: Saunders Elsevier.

Hammer, G and McPhee, S (2014) *Pathophysiology of Disease: An Introduction to Clinical Medicine.* Seventh edition. New York: McGraw Hill Education/Medical.

Hastings, M (2009) *Clinical Skills Made Incredibly Easy.* Philadelphia, PA: Lippincott Williams & Wilkins.

Health and Social Care Information Centre (2014) *National Diabetes Inpatient Audit.* London: HSCIC.

Herndon, DN (2007) *Total Burn Care.* Third edition. London: WB Saunders.

Hockman, J, Sleeper, L, Webb, J et al. (2006) Early revascularization and long term survival in cardiogenic shock complicating acute myocardial infarction. *Journal of the American Medical Association*, 295(21): 2511–15.

ICS (Intensive Care Society) (2009) *Levels of Critical Care for Adult Patients.* London: ICS.

ICSI (Institute for Clinical Systems Improvement) (2009) *Diagnosis and Treatment of Chest Pain and Acute Coronary Syndrome (ACS).* Bloomington, MN: ICSI.

Identifying Sepsis Early Group (2006) *Identifying Sepsis Early.* Edinburgh: University of Edinburgh.

IHI (Institute for Healthcare Improvement) (2009) *Improvement Map: Patient Care Processes – Pressure Ulcer Prevention.* Accessed at: www.ihi.org/offerings/initiatives/improvemaphospitals/Pages/default.aspx

IHI (2011a) *Rapid Response Team Data Collection and SBAR Communication Tool.* Accessed at: www.ihi.org/knowledge/Pages/Tools/SBARToolkit.aspx

References

IHI (2015) *Implement the IHI Central Line Bundle.* Accessed at: http://app.ihi.org/imap/tool/processpdf. aspx?processGUID=e876565d-fd43-42ce-8340-8643b7e675c7

Jarvis, H (2006) Exploring the evidence base for the use of non-invasive ventilation. *British Journal of Nursing,* 15(14): 756–9.

Jeffries, D, Johnson, M and Griffiths, R (2010) A meta-study of the essentials of quality nursing documentation. *International Journal of Nursing Practice,* 16: 112–24.

Jevon, P and Ewens, B (2007) *Monitoring the Critically Ill Patient.* Second edition. Oxford: Blackwell Publishing.

Jin, J, Sclar, G, Oh, V and Li, S (2008) Factors affecting therapeutic compliance: a review from the patient's perspective. *Therapeutics and Clinical Risk Management,* 4(1): 269–86.

Joint British Diabetes Societies (2013) *The Management of Diabetes Ketoacidosis in Adults.* Malmesbury: JBDS.

KDIGO AKI Work Group (2012) KDIGO clinical practice guidelines for acute kidney injury. *Kidney International* 2 (Supplement): 1–138.

Kearney, T and Dang, C (2007) Diabetic and endocrine emergencies. *Postgraduate Medical Journal,* 83, 79–86.

Kelly, C and Lynes, D (2011) Best practice in the provision of nebuliser therapy. *Nursing Standard,* 25(31): 50–6.

Kumar, P and Clark, M (2012) *Clinical Medicine.* Eighth edition. London: Saunders.

Lane, D and Lip, G (2012) Use of the CHA2DS2-VASc and HAS-BLED Scores to aid decision making for thromboprophylaxis in nonvalvular atrial fibrillation. *Circulation,* 126: 860–5.

Lassen, HC, Bjorneboe, M, Ibsen, B and Neukirch, F (1954) Treatment of tetanus with curarisation, general anaesthesia and intratracheal positive pressure ventilation. *Lancet,* ii: 1040–4.

Lawrence, P and Fulbrook, P (2011) The ventilator care bundle and its impact on ventilator-associated pneumonia: a review of the evidence. *Nursing in Critical Care,* 16(5): 222–34.

Leander, M, Lampa, E, Rask-Andersen, A et al. (2014) Impact of anxiety and depression on respiratory symptoms. *Respiratory Medicine,* 108: 1594–600.

Levy, M, Fink, M, Marshall, J et al. (2003) International sepsis definitions conference. *Critical Care Medicine,* 31: 1250–6.

Levy, M, Dellinger, R, Townsend, S et al. (2010) The surviving sepsis campaign: results of an international guideline-based performance improvement programme targeting severe sepsis. *Intensive Care Medicine,* 36: 222–31.

Lewington, A and Kanagasundaram, S (2011) *Clinical Practice Guidelines: Acute Kidney Injury.* Renal Association. Accessed at: www.renal.org/guidelines/modules/acute-kidney-injury#sthash.yn97aOPJ.dpbs

Lim, W, Baudouin, SV, George, RC et al. (2009) Guidelines for the management of community acquired pneumonia in adults: Update 2009. Pneumonia guidelines. Committee of the British Thoracic Society Standards of Care Committee. *Thorax,* 64 (Supplement 3): 1–55.

Lim, W, Mohammed Akram, R, Carson, K et al. (2012) Non-invasive positive pressure ventilation for treatment of respiratory failure due to severe acute exacerbations of asthma (review). *Cochrane Database of Systematic Reviews.* Issue 12.

Ludikhuize, J, Smorenburg, SM, de Rooij, SE and de Jonge, E (2012) Identification of deteriorating patients on general wards: measurement of vital parameters and potential effectiveness of the Modified Early Warning Score. *Journal of Critical Care*, 27(4): e7–13.

McCaffery, M and Pasero, C (1999) *Pain: A Clinical Manual.* St Louis, MO: Mosby.

McCance, V and Huether, S (2014) *Pathophysiology: The Biological Basis of Disease in Adults and Children.* Seventh edition. St Louis, MO: Elsevier Mosby.

McGloin, H, Adam, S and Singer, M (1999) Unexpected deaths and referrals to intensive care of patients on general wards: are some cases potentially avoidable? *Journal of the Royal College of Physicians of London*, 33: 255–9.

McPherson, D, Griffiths, C, Williams, M, Baker, A, Klodawski, E and Jacobson, B (2013) Sepsis-associated mortality in England: an analysis of multiple cause of death data from 2001 to 2010. *British Medical Journal Open*, 3: 1–7.

McQuillan, P, Pilkington, S, Allan, A et al. (1998) Confidential inquiry into quality of care before admission to intensive care. *British Medical Journal*, 316(748): 1853–8.

Mackway-Jones, K, Marsden, J and Windle, J (eds) (2014) *Emergency Triage.* Third edition. Manchester Triage Group. New York: Wiley.

Maiden, M and Peake, S (2014) Overview of shock, in Bersten, A and Soni, N (eds) *Oh's Intensive Care Manual.* Seventh edition. Oxford: Butterworth Heinemann Elsevier.

Map of Medicine (2014) *Acute Kidney Injury.* London: Map of Medicine LTD.

Marik, P (2015) *Evidence-Based Critical Care.* Third edition. Cham (Switzerland): Springer.

Martin, EA (ed) (2010) *Oxford Concise Medical Dictionary.* Oxford: Oxford University Press.

Massey, D, Aitken, LM and Chaboyer, W (2009) What factors influence suboptimal ward care in the acutely ill ward patient? *Intensive and Critical Care Nursing*, 25(4): 169–80.

Mattson Porth, C and Matfin, G (2009) *Pathophysiology: Concepts of Altered Health Status.* Eighth edition. Philadelphia, PA: Lippincott Williams & Wilkins.

Medoff, B (2008) Invasive and non-invasive ventilation in patients with asthma. *Respiratory Care*, 53(6): 740–50.

Mellor, J (2013) *Time to Act: Severe Sepsis – Rapid Diagnosis Saves Lives.* London: Parliamentary and Health Service Ombudsman.

Melzack, R (1996) Gate control theory: on the evolution of pain concepts. *The Journal of Pain*, 5(2): 128–38.

Merritt, S (2009) Chronic obstructive pulmonary disease, in Smith, SA, Price, AM and Challiner, A (eds) *Ward-Based Critical Care: A Guide for Health Professionals.* Keswick: M & K Publishing.

Miller, M, Bosk, E, Iwashyna, T and Krein, S (2012) Implementation challenges in the intensive care unit: the why, who, and how of daily interruption of sedation. *Journal of Critical Care*, 27(2): 218.e1–218.e7.

Mistraletti, G, Pelosi, P, Mantovani, E, Beradino, M and Gregoretti, C (2012) Delirium: clinical approach and prevention. *Best Practice and Research Clinical Anaesthesiology*, 26: 311–26.

Morandi, A, Pandharipande, P, Jackson, J, Bellelli, G, Trabucchi, M and Ely, E (2012) Understanding terminology of delirium and long term cognitive impairment in critically ill patients. *Best Practice and Research Clinical Anaesthesiology*, 26: 267–76.

Mortazavi, MM, Romeo, AK, Deep, A et al. (2012) Hypertonic saline for treating raised intracranial pressure: literature review with meta-analysis. *Journal of Neurosurgery*, 116: 210–21.

Murray, J (2011) Pulmonary oedema: pathophysiology and diagnosis. *The International Journal of Tuberculosis and Lung Disease*, 15(2): 155–60.

National Clinical Guideline Centre (2010) *Delirium: Diagnosis, Prevention and Management*. London: National Clinical Guideline Centre for Acute and Chronic Conditions.

National Kidney Foundation (2006) *Updates: Clinical Practice Guidelines and Recommendations*. New York: NKF.

NCEPOD (2009) *Adding Insult to Injury: A Review of the Care of Patients Who Died in Hospital with a Primary Diagnosis of Acute Kidney Injury*. Accessed at: www.ncepod.org.uk/2009report1/Downloads/AKI_report. pdf)

NCEPOD (2010) *National Confidential Enquiry into Patient Outcome and Death*. Accessed at: www.ncepod.org. uk/index.htm

NICE (National Institute for Health and Care Excellence) (2007) *Acutely Ill Patients in Hospital: Recognition of and Response to Acute Illness in Adults in Hospital, NICE Clinical Guideline 50*. London: NICE.

NICE (2008) *Lipid Modification, NICE Clinical Guideline 67*. London: NICE.

NICE (2010a) *Delirium: Diagnosis, Prevention and Management, NICE Clinical Guideline 103*. London: NICE.

NICE (2010b) *Quick Reference Guide to Delirium: Diagnosis, Prevention and Management, NICE Clinical Guideline 103*. London: NICE.

NICE (2010c) *Chronic Obstructive Pulmonary Disease, NICE Clinical Guideline 101*. London: NICE.

NICE (2010d) *A Review of Acutely Ill Patients in Hospital: Recognition of and Response to Acute Illness in Adults in Hospital, NICE Clinical Guideline 50*. London: NICE.

NICE (2011) *NICE Pathways*. Accessed at: www.pathways.nice.org.uk

NICE (2012) *The Epilepsies: The Diagnosis and Management of the Epilepsies in Adults and Children in Primary and Secondary Care, NICE Clinical Guideline 137*. London: NICE.

NICE (2013) *Prevention, Detection and Management of Acute Kidney Injury up to the Point of Renal Replacement Therapy, NICE Clinical Guideline 169*. London: NICE.

NICE (2014a) *Pneumonia: Diagnosis and Management of Community- and Hospital-Acquired Pneumonia in Adults, NICE Clinical Guideline 191*. London: NICE.

NICE (2014b) *Head Injury: Triage, Assessment, Investigation and Early Management of Head Injury in Infants, Children, Young People and Adults*. London: NICE.

NICE (2015) *Acute Coronary Syndrome Pathways*. London: NICE.

Nightingale, F (1860) *Notes on Nursing: What It Is What It Is Not*. New York: Appleton and Company. Accessed at: www.digital.library.upenn.edu/women/nightingale/nursing/nursing.html#XIII

NMC (Nursing and Midwifery Council) (2010) *Standards for Pre-registration Nursing Education*. London: NMC.

NMC (2015) *The Code: Professional Standards of Practice and Behaviour for Nurses and Midwives*. London: NMC.

NPSA (National Patient Safety Agency) (2007a) *Recognising and Responding Appropriately to Early Signs of Deterioration in Hospitalised Patients*. London: NPSA.

NPSA (2007b) *Safer Care for the Acutely Ill Patient: Learning from Serious Incidents*. London: NPSA.

O'Connor, M, Bucknall, T and Manias, E (2010) International variations in outcomes from sedation protocol research: where are we at and where do we go from here? *Intensive and Critical Care Nursing*, 26(4): 189–95.

O'Driscoll, BR, Howard, LS and Davison, AG (2008) *Guidelines for Emergency Oxygen Use in Adult Patients: Executive Summary*. London: British Thoracic Society; also in Thorax, 63 (Supplement VI): vi1–vi68.

Page, V (2008) *ICU Delirium: Why It Matters*. Accessed at: www.icudelirium.co.uk/why-it-matters

Patrozou, E and Opal, S (2010) What is inflammation? What is sepsis? What is MODS? in Deutschman, C and Neligan, P (eds) *Evidence-Based Practice in Critical Care*. Philadelphia, PA: Saunders.

Patschan, D and Muller, G (2015) Acute kidney injury. *Journal of Injury and Violence Research*, 7(1): 19–26.

Patschan, D, Patschan, S and Muller, G (2012) Inflammation and microvasculopathy in renal ischaemia reperfusion injury. *Journal of Transplantation*, 764154: 1–7.

Polosa, R and Thomson, NC (2013) Smoking and asthma: dangerous liaisons. *European Respiratory Journal*, 41: 716–26.

Prescott, A, Lewington, A and O' Donoghue, D (2012) Acute kidney injury: top ten tips. *Clinical Medicine*, 12(4): 328–32.

Public Health England (2014) *Urinary Tract Infection: Diagnosis Guide for Primary Care*. Accessed at: www.gov. uk/government/publications/urinary-tract-infection-diagnosis

Quirke, S, Coombs, M and McEldowney, R (2011) Suboptimal care of the acutely unwell ward patient: a concept analysis. *Journal of Advanced Nursing*, 67(8): 1834–45.

Ramsay, M, Savego, T, Simpson, B and Goodwin, R (1974) Controlled sedation with alphaxolone-alphadolone. *British Medical Journal*, 2(920): 656–9.

Rang, H, Dale, D, Ritter, J, Flower, R and Henderson, G (2012) *Rang and Dale's Pharmacology*. Edinburgh: Elsevier/Churchill Livingstone.

RCP (Royal College of Physicians) (2012) *Policy Responses and Statements: NHS Early Warning Score* (NEWS). Accessed at: www.rcpe. ac.uk/policy/2011/nhs-early-warning-score.php

RCP (Royal College of Physicians), BTS (British Thoracic Society) and ICS (Intensive Care Society) (2008) *The Use of Non-Invasive Ventilation in the Management of Patients with Chronic Obstructive Pulmonary Disease Admitted to Hospital with Acute Type II Respiratory Failure*. London: Royal College of Physicians.

Redden, M and Wotton, K (2002a) Third space shift in elderly patients undergoing gastrointestinal surgery: part 1 – pathophysiological mechanisms. *Contemporary Nurse*, 12(3): 275–83.

Redden, M and Wotton, K (2002b) Third space shift in elderly patients undergoing gastrointestinal surgery: part 2 – nursing assessment. *Contemporary Nurse*, 13(1): 50–60.

Renal Association (2013) *Chronic Kidney Disease Stages*. Accessed at: www.renal.org/information-resources/ the-uk-eckd-guide/ckd-stages#sthash.PsjK16Qq.dpbs

Resuscitation Council (UK) (2011) *Advanced Life Support*. Sixth edition. London: Resuscitation Council (UK).

Resuscitation Council (UK) (2015) *Guidelines and Guidance: A Systematic Approach to the Acutely Ill Patient (ABCDE Approach)*. Accessed at www.resus.org.uk/resuscitation-guidelines/a-systematic-approach-to-the-acutely-ill-patient-abcde

References

Richardson, A and Whatmore, J (2014) Nursing essential principles: continuous renal replacement therapy. *Nursing in Critical Care*, 20(1): 8–15.

Riker, R, Fraser, G, Simmons, L and Wilkins, M (2001) Validating the sedation agitation scale with the bispectral index and visual analogue scale in adult ICU patients after cardiac surgery. *Intensive Care Medicine*, 27(5): 853–8.

Rivara, FP, Mackenzie, EJ, Jurkovich, GJ, Nathens, AB, Wang, J and Scharfstein, DO (2008) Prevalence of pain in patients 1 year after major trauma. *Archives of Surgery*, 143(3): 282–7.

Rivers, E, Nguyen, B, Havstad, S et al. (2001) Early goal directed therapy in the treatment of severe sepsis and septic shock. *New England Journal of Medicine*, 344: 699–709.

Royal College of Nursing (2003) *Defining Nursing*. London: RCN.

Samuelson, K (2011) Unpleasant and pleasant memories of intensive care in adult mechanically ventilated patients: findings from 250 interviews. *Intensive and Critical Care Nursing*, 27: 76–84.

Scott, C (2003) *Setting safe nurse staffing levels: RCN research report*. London: Royal College of Nursing.

Sepsis Alliance (2014) *Sepsis: Understanding the Risk*. Accessed at: www.sepsisalliance.org/downloads/sepsis-risk.pdf

Sepsis Alliance (2015) *Life After Sepsis*. Accessed at: www.sepsisalliance.org/life_after_sepsis

Skaer, TL (1998) Cancer pain management. *American Journal of Pharmaceutical Education*, 62: 182–9.

Smith, G, Prytherch, D, Meredith, P, Schmidt, P and Featherstone, P (2013) The ability of the National Early Warning Score (NEWS) to discriminate patients at risk of early cardiac arrest, unanticipated intensive care unit admission and death. *Resuscitation*, 84: 465–70.

Smith, J (2009) How to keep score of acuity and dependency. *Nursing Management*, 16(8): 14–19.

Sneyers, B, Laterre, P, Bricq, E, Perreault, M, Wouters, D and Spinewine, A (2014) What stops us from following sedation recommendations in intensive care units? A multi-centric qualitative study. *Journal of Critical Care*, 29: 291–7.

Sung, J (2014) Acute gastrointestinal bleeding, in Bersten, A and Soni, N (eds) *Oh's Intensive Care Manual*. Seventh edition. Oxford: Butterworth Heinemann Elsevier.

Surviving Sepsis Campaign (SSC) (2015) *History*. Accessed at: www.survivingsepsis.org/About-SSC/Pages/History.aspx

Tait, D (2009) *A Gadamerian Hermeneutic Study of Nurses' Experiences of Recognising and Managing Patients with Clinical Deterioration and Critical Illness in a NHS Trust in Wales*. Unpublished doctoral thesis: University of Wales, Swansea.

Teasdale, G (2014) Forty years on: updating the Glasgow Coma Scale. *Nursing Times*, 110(42): 12–16.

Thomas, D, Cote, T and Lawhorne, L (2008) Understanding clinical dehydration and its treatment. *Journal of the American Medical Directors Association*, 9: 292–301.

Thompson, C and Dowding, D (2002) *Clinical Decision Making and Judgement in Nursing*. Edinburgh: Churchill Livingstone.

Tortora, G and Derrickson, B (2014) *Principles of Anatomy and Physiology*. Fourteenth edition. New York: John Wiley.

UK Sepsis Trust (2014) *Introducing Red Flag Sepsis, UK Sepsis Trust Clinical Toolkits 2014.* London: UK Sepsis Trust.

Umpierrez, GE, Isaacs, SD, Bazargan, N, You, X, Thaler, LM and Kitabchi, AE (2002) Hyperglycemia: an independent marker of in-hospital mortality in patients with undiagnosed diabetes. *The Journal of Clinical Endocrinology & Metabolism,* 87(3): 978–82.

Vasilevskis, E, Han, J, Hughes, C and Ely, E (2012) Epidemiology and risk factors for delirium across hospital settings. *Best Practice and Research Clinical Anaesthesiology,* 26: 277–87.

Vivek, M, Raiz, AM, Sujoy, G et al. (2011) Myxoedema coma: a new look into an old crisis. *Journal of Thyroid Research* 493462.

Walker, R, Gebregziabher, M, Martin-Harris, B and Egede, L (2015) Understanding the influence of psychological and socioeconomic factors on diabetes self-care using structured equation modelling. *Patient Education and Counselling,* 98: 34–40.

Wheeldon, A (2013) The respiratory system and associated disorders, in Muralitharan, N and Peate, I (eds) *Fundamentals of Applied Pathophysiology: An Essential Guide for Nursing and Healthcare Students.* Chichester: Wiley-Blackwell.

White, K and Arlt, W (2010) Adrenal crisis in treated Addison's disease: a predictable but undermanaged event. *European Society of Endocrinology,* 162: 115–20.

Whitehouse, T, Snelson, C and Grounds, M (2014) *Intensive Care Society Review of Best Practice for Analgesia and Sedation in Critical Care.* London: Intensive Care Society.

Whitlock, J, Rowland, S, Ellis, G and Evans, A (2011) Using the SKIN bundle to prevent pressure ulcers. *Nursing Times,* 107(35): 20–3.

Williams, T, Martin, S, Thomas, L et al. (2008) Duration of mechanical ventilation in an adult intensive care unit after introduction of sedation and pain scales. *American Journal of Critical Care,* 17(4): 349–56.

Wilson, B (2007) Nurses' knowledge of pain. *Journal of Clinical Nursing,* 16(6): 1012–20.

Winters, B, Eberlein, M, Leung, J, Needham, D, Pronovost, P and Sevransky, J (2010) Long-term mortality and quality of life in sepsis: a systematic review. *Critical Care Medicine,* 38(5): 1276–83.

Woodrow, P (2012) *Intensive Care Nursing: A Framework for Practice.* Third edition. London: Routledge.

Woodward, S and Waterhouse, C (2009) *Oxford Handbook of Neuroscience Nursing.* Oxford: Oxford University Press.

World Health Organization (2006) *Cancer Pain Relief.* Second edition. Geneva: WHO.

Zwarenstein, M, Goldman, J and Reeves, S (2009) *Interprofessional Collaboration: Effects of Practice-Based Interventions on Professional Practice and Healthcare Outcomes (Review).* Accessed at: www.onlinelibrary.wiley.com/doi/10.1002/14651858.CD000072.pub2/pdf/standard

Index